SEX AND SECLUSION, CLASS AND CUSTODY

PERSPECTIVES ON GENDER AND CLASS IN THE HISTORY OF BRITISH AND IRISH PSYCHIATRY

Steven Sturdy

Science Studies Unit
University of Edinburgh
July '05.

THE WELLCOME SERIES IN THE HISTORY OF MEDICINE

Forthcoming Titles:

The Cape Doctor in the Nineteenth Century:
A Social History
Edited by Harriet Deacon, Howard Phillips
and Elizabeth Van Heyningen

War, Medicine and Britain, 1600-1815
Edited by Geoff Hudson and Roy Porter

The *Clio Medica* series editors are
V. Nutton, C. J. Lawrence and M. Neve.
Please send all queries regarding the series to Michael Laycock,
The Wellcome Trust Centre for the History of Medicine at UCL,
24 Eversholt Street, London NW1 1AD, UK.

SEX AND SECLUSION, CLASS AND CUSTODY

PERSPECTIVES ON GENDER AND CLASS IN THE HISTORY OF BRITISH AND IRISH PSYCHIATRY

Edited by Jonathan Andrews and Anne Digby

Amsterdam – New York, NY 2004

First published in 2004
by Editions Rodopi B. V., Amsterdam – New York, NY 2004.

Jonathan Andrews and Anne Digby © 2004

Design and Typesetting by Michael Laycock,
The Wellcome Trust Centre for the History of Medicine at UCL.
Printed and bound in The Netherlands by Editions Rodopi B. V.,
Amsterdam – New York, NY 2004.

Index by Indexing Specialists (UK) Ltd.

British Library Cataloguing in Publication Data
A catalogue record for this book is available from the
British Library
ISBN 90-420-1176-9 (Paper)
ISBN 90-420-1186-6 (Bound)

'Sex and Seclusion, Class and Custody
Perspectives on Gender and Class in the History of
British and Irish Psychiatry' –
Amsterdam – New York, NY:
Rodopi. – ill.
(Clio Medica 73 / ISSN 0045-7183;
The Wellcome Series in the History of Medicine)

Front cover:
Front cover: Somerset County Asylum (England); mentally ill patients
dancing at a ball. Lithograph by K. Drake.
Image courtesy *Wellcome Library,* London.

© Editions Rodopi B. V., Amsterdam – New York, NY 2004
Printed in The Netherlands

All titles in the Clio Medica series (from 1999 onwards) are available to
download from the CatchWord website: http://www.ingenta.com

Contents

Acknowledgements

We are very grateful to the Wellcome Trust for providing the funding for the initial seminar series at Oxford Brookes University from which the seeds of this book germinated. We are also grateful to the anonymous readers who gave feedback on this volume *in utero*. Thanks to the various contributors for keeping faith with the book in its long period of generation. Thanks too to Michael Laycock for an excellent job with copy-editing and proof stages, and to Marieke Schilling at Rodopi for her calm support and patience.

Notes on Contributors

Jonathan Andrews is a Senior Lecturer in History, specialising in the History of Medicine, at Oxford Brookes. He has published widely in the history of psychiatry, including (jointly authored) *A History of Bethlem* (Routledge, 1997), *They're in the Trade of Lunacy* (Wellcome Institute, 1998), (with Andrew Scull), *Undertaker of the Mind* (University of California Press, 2001) and *Customers and Patrons of the Mad Trade* (University of California Press, 2003). He is currently working on criminal insanity in Britain during ca. 1860-1913.

Joan Busfield is a Professor in the Department of Sociology at the University of Essex and currently Dean of the University's Graduate School. She trained initially as a clinical psychologist at the Tavistock Clinic and then moved into sociology. She has published several books including *Managing Madness: Changing Ideas and Practice* (Hutchinson, 1986), *Men, Women and Madness: Understanding Gender and Mental Disorder* (Macmillan, 1996) and *Health and Health Care in Modern Britain* (Oxford University Press, 2000). She also edited a recent collection, *Rethinking the Sociology of Mental Health* (Blackwell, 2001) which was previously published as a special issue of *Sociology of Health and Illness* in September 2000.

Anne Digby is Research Professor in History at Oxford Brookes University. She has published widely in the social history of medicine including *Madness, Morality and Medicine* (Cambridge University Press, 1985), *Making a Medical Living* (Cambridge University Press, 1994) and *The Evolution of British General Practice, 1850-1948* (Oxford University Press, 1999). More recently, she has worked with Helen Sweet on a project examining different forms of medicine in South Africa. Currently, she is completing a book on this subject entitled 'Medicine, Culture and Society'.

3

Rab Houston is Professor of Early Modern History at St Andrews University. He has published extensively in the social history of early modern Britain and Europe, including the fields of literacy and education, urbanisation, historical demography, and social relationships. His most recent work has been on the history of mental disability, including *Madness and Society in Eighteenth-century Scotland* (Clarendon Press, 2000) and *Autism in History: The Case of Hugh Blair* (Blackwell Publishers, 2000). He also edited *The New Penguin History of Scotland* (Allen Lane, The Penguin Press in association with the National Museums of Scotland, 2001).

Mark Jackson is a Professor in the History of Medicine in the Department of History at the University of Exeter. After qualifying in medicine in 1985, he pursued doctoral research in the social history of infanticide. He has also researched the history of feeble-mindedness in Britain and is currently writing a book on the history of allergic diseases, such as asthma and hay fever, in the modern world. His publications include *New-born Child Murder* (Manchester University Press, 1996), *The Borderland of Imbecility* (Manchester University Press, 2000), and (ed.) *Infanticide* (Ashgate, 2002), as well as several edited volumes and numerous articles. He was Reviews Editor for *Social History of Medicine* between 1997 and 2001.

Marjorie Levine-Clark is an Assistant Professor of History at the University of Colorado at Denver. Her book *Beyond the Reproductive Body: The Politics of Women's Health and Work in Early Victorian England* is forthcoming from Ohio State University Press. She has published articles on women's health, female insanity, and gender and the Poor Law. Her current research focuses on gender, family, and welfare in the Black Country in the late-nineteenth and early-twentieth centuries.

Joseph Melling is Reader in the History of Industrial Health and Welfare and also Director of the Centre for Medical History at the University of Exeter. He has published widely in peer reviewed journals on the history of asylums and psychiatry, and jointly edited (with Bill Forsythe) *Insanity, Institutions and Society* (Routledge, 1999). His research is concerned with occupational health and labour relations as well as the history of insanity. He is presently working with Mark Bufton on the history of silicosis in British industry during the twentieth century and with Janet Greenlees on ill health in cotton textiles. He is also completing a book with Forsythe on the history of insanity in England.

Pamela Michael is a Lecturer in Health Studies and Social Policy in the School of Social Sciences, University of Wales, Bangor and is course director of a new degree in Health and Social Care. She also contributes to teaching on an M.A. in Women's Studies in the School of Lifelong Learning at Bangor. Pamela was formerly employed on a Wellcome Trust funded project on the history of the North Wales [psychiatric] Hospital, Denbigh and has published various articles and chapters on this subject and a full length monograph on *Care and Treatment of the Mentally Ill in North Wales, 1800-2000* (University of Wales Press, 2003).

Anne Shepherd is currently working at the Centre for Suicide Research, Department of Psychiatry, University of Oxford. Previously, she was Deputy Editor for *Reviews in History*, based at the Institute of Historical Research. She is currently finishing her PhD and (with David Wright) has recently published an article in *Medical History,* 46 (2002), 175–96, 'Madness, Suicide and the Victorian Asylum: Attempted Self-Murder in the Age of Non-Restraint'.

Lorraine Walsh is a Programme Director in Continuing Professional Development at the University of Dundee. Her current research interests include the philosophy of history; the use of C&IT within the tertiary level history curriculum; and continuing professional development for teachers in further and higher education. She has published a monograph and a range of articles and chapters on the history of insanity and the development of organised charity in the Scottish burgh, including *Patrons, Poverty and Profit* (Abertay, 2000).

Oonagh Walsh is a Lecturer in the School of History and History of Art at the University of Aberdeen. She is author of *Ireland's Independence, 1880-1923* (Routledge, 2002) and the forthcoming *To Forge or to Follow: Women of the Church of Ireland in Dublin, 1910-1926* (University College, Dublin Press, 2003). She has published a number of chapters and articles on the history of Irish psychiatry. Her edited works include *An Englishwoman in Belfast: Rosamond Stephen's Record of the Great*

War (Cork University Press, 2000) and the jointly edited *Gendering Scottish History: An International Approach* (Cruithne Press, 1999). She is currently completing an edited collection of writings on women's experiences of the Irish revolutions for Thommes Press.

David Wright holds the Hannah Chair in the History of Medicine, McMaster University, Hamilton, Canada. He has published widely on the history of developmental disability and the history of the confinement of the insane. His major publications include: *Mental Disability in Victorian England: The Earlswood Asylum, 1847-1901* (Oxford University Press, 2001) and three edited volumes: (with Anne Digby) *From Idiocy to Mental Deficiency: Historical Perspectives on People with Learning Disabilities* (Routledge, 1996); (with Peter Bartlett), *Outside the Walls of the Asylum: The History of Care in the Community, 1750-2000* (Athlone, 1999); and (with Roy Porter) *The Confinement of the Insane, International Perspectives: 1800-1965* (Cambridge, 2003). He is currently writing a book on the confinement of the insane in nineteenth-century England and conducting research on the historical epidemiology of mental disorders.

1

Introduction:
Gender and Class in the Historiography of British and Irish Psychiatry

Jonathan Andrews and Anne Digby

This volume had its origin in a stimulating seminar series devoted to historical perspectives on gender and class in the history of psychiatry. The papers presented outlined a number of important perspectives on the place of gender and class within the history of psychiatry and, more broadly, medicine and society. There were also considerable inter-relationships between the various thematic strands developed in the papers – so much so, that organisers, speakers and participants alike were keen to see a published outcome.

Although gender and class studies of medicine have attracted a wide range of scholarship in recent decades, and have selectively explored gendered and class aspects of mental illness and psychiatry, very few have addressed both themes in tandem. Widening provision at university level for the study of the history of medicine has not been adequately met by specific texts granting an easy, readable access to the types of questions being raised by historians concerned with how medicine or psychiatry has been mediated by, and has itself constructed, visions of gender and class. Not only students, but many scholars themselves have found it difficult to engage with the disparate literature on such themes. It is envisaged that this edited collection will bring together in one volume a group of inter-related perspectives to offer the reader an excellent overview of the essential constituents of gender and class-based approaches to the history of psychiatry.

Rather than adopting an exclusively class-oriented or gender-studies based approach to (psychiatric) history, most contributions have the distinctive strength of combining, comparing and contrasting these twin perspectives. Unlike some previously rather Anglo-centric and chronologically confined collections on British psychiatry, the book has the additional advantage of giving coverage to the (Dis)United Kingdom[1] as a whole, from the mid-eighteenth to the late-twentieth centuries. Indeed, to extend the thematic, chronological and geographical scope of the book, contributions from Houston, Melling and Michael in this volume were specially commissioned.

In the first part of this short introduction we will selectively draw out historiographical issues and themes which seem particularly relevant both for work in general in this field and for the essays collected here. We will also seek to suggest some key lines and directions for future research. We make no claim to offer a complete or entirely new schematic model for work in this field, but showcase a relatively representative sample. Finally, in the second part of the introduction we will provide the reader with a summary of the innovative and important elements in the collection's chapters, as well as draw out some of the significant links and differences in their themes.

Contexts

Gender perspectives on the history of British and Irish psychiatry and asylums were once dominated by a somewhat exclusive focus on women; on distorted, if not misogynistic, psychiatric constructions of femininity, and of specific, female-directed forms of treatment; on the creation of mental illness as a predominantly feminine disorder, and on male-orchestrated abuse of women and chauvinism within psychiatry and psychiatric institutions. Crudely conceived in some studies, psychiatry – analogously to the medical dismissal of witches as deluded crones, and the ousting of cunning women, female healers and midwives by male doctors, man-midwives and obstetricians[2] – was a tool in the subjugation of women and a denial of their avenues to knowledge or to the occupational roles held by men.[3] As Nancy Tomes pointed out in a recent historiographical survey, some of these early feminist histories were more manifesto than a measured historical evaluation of the gendered aspects of psychiatry. Yet they were nevertheless path-breaking in many ways, and not least because psychiatric history prior to the 1960s had been a virtually woman-free zone.[4]

More recent studies have to some degree built upon these earlier approaches. Their models whether of 'feminisation' of cultural representations,[5] or of the medicalisation of the female sex, are more thoroughly contextualised and better founded on empirical evidence. Yet, in a number of specific and more general contexts, recent surveys have queried the utility and relevance of gender and/or class as explanatory models for psychiatric history, some going to the extent of doubting that gender made much of a difference.[6] These historians have been quite critical of ideological feminist approaches, in particular their polemical employment for specific political purposes, and have gone about deconstructing and challenging their appeal.[7] Tomes and others have argued that the (re-)emergence of this critique amounts to a dangerous 'intellectual backlash' against feminism and feminist history, involving the marginalisation of 'feminist histories of psychiatry', and thus needs to be resisted. This is important because, as Tomes remarks, such histories have been vital in elucidating how medical and psychiatric theories were employed to devalue women's work and challenge their access to equal educational and employment opportunities, to curtail 'women's aspirations and to deride feminism [itself]'.[8] It is also significant because it impacts upon the balance of existing scholarship and on academic consensus regarding core directions for future research. Tomes' own survey, along with much of the recent historiography in the field, also suggests the need for more men to undertake research on gender and psychiatry, and for mainstream psychiatric historians to integrate more evenly insights derived from the approaches of feminist and women's history. Furthermore it calls for such research carefully to compare men and women, as well as, or rather than, women/men in isolation.

To exemplify how debates have gathered momentum and moved on in recent decades in one particular cluster of the historiography, one might emphasise how, previous (and some current) work on hysteria, neurasthenia and nervous ailments has tended to be preoccupied with the way illness was deployed to delimit female sex roles, to trap women within their gynaecology, as well as with the more extreme fictionalised representations of femininity.[9] This research has helped to provoke, while being complemented (or perhaps steadily superseded?) by, more recent studies which have paid more attention to hypochondriacal, hysterical, nervous and neurasthenic men.[10] These surveys have also illustrated the importance of both relating and distinguishing between sex and gender differences, of closely comparing women with men before arriving at confident findings as to gendered biases, and of not restricting gender analysis or even separate spheres models to women.[11] They have demonstrated the need for charting and explaining more carefully how both gendered and sex-specific models of mental illness might rise and decline only to re-emerge in vigorous new guises in later periods, as with ovarian explanations for hysteria. For example, Micale has shown how, subsequent to the anatomical discrediting of the 'wandering womb' in early modern times, sex differences and gynaecological theory became much less relevant to understandings of hysteria specifically, and mental and nervous illness more generally, only to be revived and reformulated from the end of the eighteenth into the nineteenth centuries via the findings of ovarian physiology. He has also demonstrated that sex-specific conceptualisations of hysteria were widened at the end of the nineteenth century to embrace males, as well as females.[12]

As a range of scholars from Porter and Rousseau[13] to Houston (in this volume) have pointed out, the nervous disorder known as 'vapours' was essentially conceptualised in both sex-specific and highly gendered terms in early modern medicine, and was also strongly class-bounded (tending to be reserved exclusively to genteel females). The historiography of suicide has also benefitted from recent approaches that have paid more attention to class and gender disparities, and to constructions of male as well as female behaviour. Indeed, suicide has been shown to be constructed by medical men as gendered in various significant ways across different historical time periods and national contexts, as well as being both committed/attempted and mediated divergently according to variant socio-cultural expectations of male and female conduct.[14] Similarly positive trends are observable in other allied spheres of study. For example, a concentration on the sexual surgeries visited upon women by psychiatrists in modern asylums and mental hospitals, has more recently been followed by more research on the analogous surgeries to treat masturbation, night-time emissions, phimosis, spermatorrhœa and the like in men, and their rationales in constructions of masculinity.[15] Historical examinations of war and psychiatry have only recently seen conceptions of masculinity as key to evaluations of and responses to shell-shock and mental illness in troops, and (as Busfield's chapter below reflects) have also begun to chart the impact of such particular typologies of psychiatric disorders on wider modern social and cultural notions of masculine identity. In recent times, researchers have branched out beyond previous preoccupations with shell-shock and the psycho-neuroses of war, to explore the gendered and class-centred aspects of stress and trauma more broadly.[16] Moreover, these studies have looked to a medley of other factors as well as gender, and often quite apart from gender, as having more substantially predicated the construction and treatment of prevailing diagnostic entities.

Path-breaking studies like those of Showalter and Small[17] of the cultural discourses surrounding madness in the eighteenth and nineteenth centuries have strongly emphasised their gendered content. Their work highlighted how madness was generally gendered terminologically and typologically – pointing to examples such as the predominant concern with male madness in literary and artistic productions prior to ca. 1700, and the increasing propensity thereafter to ascribe love's madness disproportionately to women. Similarly, these historians have argued, insanity derived from/excused by drunkenness tended more often to be posited as a male preserve, or else as confined in women to the degenerate, vicious and lower class. However, their studies were predominantly based on the constructions in elite artistic, literary and professional/medical source material. Recent research, which has relied on more documentary sources, has built on the earlier work of these scholars, but tackled these themes more circumspectly.

In the present collection, Houston finds a certain amount of documentary evidence in reports of what constituted insane conduct to support the presence of such gendered interpretations. On the other hand, Houston's work alerts us to the limits to gendered vocabularies of mental incapacity; and how domestically located were common-or-garden contemporary interpretations of abnormal, or 'mad' behaviour. Indeed, rather than imposed indiscriminately from above on those adjudged simply deviant or inferior because of sex or class differences, as Doerner and Foucault have asserted[18], 'social constructions of insanity were based on relatively conventional nuanced and contextualised ideas about appropriate behaviour for a certain social class and sex'. Houston's study argues that eighteenth-century madness was rarely conceived as sex specific, and that while 'understandings of mad behaviour were certainly gendered' this was 'not nearly as crudely as one might expect'. His study also emphasises the need for historians to test the assumptions of academic discourse about sex and class bias more carefully against what documentary sources reveal about common practices and commonsensical judgments of ordinary people. The frequent neglect of legal, familial and parochial records, especially those offering access to the testimonies of common folk, in mainstream histories of madness, in favour of the analysis of the discourses of medical, literary, artistic and philosophical writings, is something that existing and future generations of psychiatric historians continue to need to address and redress.

A good deal of the scholarship of past decades has continued to demonstrate the strong gender component in the definition and arbitration of new or expanded psychiatric categories (a good example being a recent study of kleptomania).[19] Some have gone so far as to argue that such expansions of the boundaries of what constituted insanity – especially when it came to milder, nervous illnesses – impacted more profoundly upon women, and that more women were being labelled as mentally incapacitated. Studies of twentieth-century psychiatry and psychiatric institutions continue to point out the inherent gendered prejudices in modern mental health systems, while the recent development of disability studies has seen the stigma and abuse often associated with mental illness and its treatment conceived as doubly and quintessentially a feminist and disability issue.[20] Since the 1970s, psychological and psychiatric studies have continued to devote a great deal of attention to sex differences in the origins and symptomatology of both major and minor mental problems and pathologies.[21]

However, other recent work which has adopted a gender focused perspective on the history of asylums and psychiatry, has also challenged the extent to which insanity was an especially 'Female Malady' – whether in Victorian times or any other historical period.[22] This research has counselled more caution and precision in defining those arenas, methods and technologies where gender constructions dominated.[23] Nevertheless, while chapters in this book question whether either nascent psychiatry or the asylum were predominantly instruments of class and/or gender oppression, most explore the significance of constructions of class and gender in biasing a range of lunacy/mental health arenas, from the representation and definition of insanity, and the admission and treatment of the insane in institutions,[24] to the policing of social norms outside the asylum. Many of the contributions in this volume also question the somewhat deterministic and ideologised formulations of previous scholarship.

There are clearly many areas of historical enquiry into psychiatry, however, where gender differences are pronounced and have not only merited, but demanded, historical explanation. For example, the oft alleged trans-historical tendency for depressive illness to be ascribed and/or reported more frequently in/by women has attracted a substantial degree of recent historical and sociological attention.[25] Similarly, historical research on the understandings of women as more strongly determined by their biological or gynaecological frailties, has illustrated how powerfully mental problems such as puerperal insanity, and infanticide, were gendered in medical and socio-cultural constructions.[26] Earlier research alerted historians to both the exaggerations – and the genuine grounds – for Georgian and Victorian concerns with wrongful confinement. But this too often left gender out, and a range of modern scholars have continued to find evidence that women were much more subject to false confinement, silencing and the settling of domestic conflicts in private madhouses. However, the evidence is often more debateable than might appear at first hand.[27]

A post-revisionist critique has influenced most of the chapters in this collection. This perspective has highlighted the overly ideologised and unconvincingly theorised approaches to issues of class and gender in asylum and psychiatric history. Most of this volume's chapters are therefore substantially based on empirical research in the archives, and quite a number represent detailed and highly nuanced case studies of one or two institutions. Previous revisionist studies have been censured for their lack of a firm or comprehensive grounding in a range of archival sources, and for their absence of historical specificity, and all the chapters here are careful to fully display their credentials in this respect.

However, a growing volley of criticism has emerged directed at this kind of 'new' or 'counter-revisionist' asylum historiography. While acknowledged as having added considerable depth and balance to our understanding of asylums, lunacy and various key historical agencies/actors, such research is often accused of being particularist, and too divorced from wider historical issues. Asylum studies have been criticised for becoming a narrow discipline, the asylum a subject (or 'island') in itself, by contrast with the place of the asylum in the writings of Foucault, Doerner, Rothman and Scull, where it tends to be approached as a means of comprehending the causes and processes of wider socio-cultural and economic change and development.[28] This new generation of psychiatric historiography is seen instead as being in danger of becoming rather myopically historicised, consciously anti-theory, and intellectually impoverished by comparison with the more ambitious, synthesising accounts of previous scholars, at the centre of whose agendas was the elaboration of more broadly applicable interpretive models. Andrew Scull in particular has provocatively upbraided historians for their lack of engagement with 'macro-social concerns', in favour of 'micro-researches', alleging that the 'new' histories of madness were inadequately framed against 'broader changes in English society's political, economic and social structures, and... the intellectual and cultural horizons of its people'.[29] Similarly, Anne Borsay has spoken of the 'resurgence of empiricism in [the] field', despite its self-confessed 'indebtedness to the sociological insights of [synthesisers such as]… Scull and Foucault'.[30]

Borsay has also criticised recent asylum studies for their lack of 'sustained discussion of how involvement in the care of the insane impacted upon class development', echoing a point made by Ingnatieff back in 1983 that the most 'essential question' for analysts of the asylum and '"total institution" is what part it plays in the reproduction of social order in the world beyond its walls'.[31] However, as Melling and Forsythe have observed, a strong class-informed analysis was somewhat lacking from Foucault's account of the rise of the asylum (despite its focus on idleness), as indeed was the significance of other factors such as kinship in influencing responses to insanity and life within psychiatric institutions.[32] Yet other historians have been held to err on the opposite extreme. For example, however 'pioneering' the work of Scull, according to Melling, his formulations tended towards reductivity, positing the asylum too much as 'an elaboration of class relations'. [33] This attempt to bridge the parallax by making class a key focus, and clarifying its role, without diminishing the complexities of agency and representation pertinent to the history of the asylum and psychiatry, echoes the perspectives and approaches to class and class-relations (in so far as they were reflected in the asylum) adopted in the present volume.

Historiographically, there have been many studies illustrating how divergences in the social origins and economic circumstances of the mentally disturbed and disabled met with significant and related (if not always clearly corresponding) differences in the treatment they were accorded.[34] Increasingly, historians have also shown the various ways in which a family's economic and demographic circumstances, including such issues as family/household structure, migration, employment and life-crisis cycles, affected a person's chances of being institutionalised – though clearly other factors such as geography were often just as important in terms of regional differences in experiences of institutionalisation.[35] On the other hand, rather fewer studies have compared in detail the fates of private, monied patients, with paupers and the poorer sort. Fewer still have fully explored the influence of diverse and divergent social circumstances on patients' release and the reuniting of families, and on the extent to which patients were genuinely, over long periods, reintegrated into communities. Such issues ought to be at the top of the agenda for future research in this field.

While some recent monographic studies of asylum and psychiatric history have devoted substantial sections to the factors of class and gender (and indeed race), or have employed gender and class-based analyses throughout, on the whole modern scholarship has tended to show marked disparities in the degree of engagement with such issues.[36] In large part, this is explicable by different approaches and preoccupations, but one might question how appropriate it is not only for synthetising studies of psychiatry, but even individual asylum histories, to reduce issues such as the class-dimension of contemporary debates about the disposal of the insane/defective, and the threat posed by the mentally ill/disabled to the moral or socio-economic order of British society to the sidelines. By making class a key focus, and clarifying its role – but without diminishing the complexities of agency and representation pertinent to the history of the asylum and psychiatry – the present volume aims to contribute to the further development of these fascinating but complex discussions. Keen to avoid previous methodological straightjackets, most of its chapters attempt to look well beyond asylum/psychiatric histories in framing their scrutiny of class and gender influences on psychiatry.

Far from eschewing completely the types of analyses of power relations and class that came to be understood (often and increasingly derogatively) under the convenient catch-all of 'social control', recent historians have tended to adopt both inspiration and points of departure from such approaches.[37] Long ago Jacques Donzelot elucidated how complicated forms of social control did not simply emanate from above, but were often asserted or heavily mediated by communities, households and families.[38] It has become customary in recent studies of the asylum, keen to avoid simplistic or sweeping conceptualisations of power, to trace with more precision the forms of social control that emanated from a range of actors/agencies, but also to stress the multiplicity of functions and interactions within the asylum and the variety of responses in the community to mental afflictions, apart from those that are comprehensible under the rubric of social control and class oppression.[39] This has meant looking from both above and below, and questioning to what extent such control was exercised and mediated by, or at the behest of, not only governmental, medical or legal authorities, but also the family, local magistrates and clergy, or parochial authorities. The over-arching and multiplying structures of the Poor Law (in particular) have now begun to be seen as perhaps more significant in determining the disposal of the insane in Victorian Britain, than the classificatory formulations of the practitioners of mental medicine.

While Scull in particular has emphasised the Victorian asylum as a dumping ground for a growing agglomeration of chronic pauper insane, contending that ties of kinship and traditional means of coping with mentally disordered family members were steadily eroded by the onward march of capitalism,[40] more recent surveys have paid more attention to the perdurability and adaptability of relational links and social ties, and the permeability of the asylum. These surveys have traced significant survival networks maintained by patients, both whilst inside the asylum with their households/kin and communities, and also later sustained outside the bounds of the asylum. They have suggested that there continued to be broader options and strategies available to families in dealing with mental problems besides the asylum. While even scholars like Walton doubted that large numbers of patients were successfully 'brought back' from the asylum, recent studies have stressed the frequency of discharge, but also the role of resistance and negotiation (as well as domination and denigration) for patients and their families during confinement in psychiatric institutions.[41] Melling has contended, that it is important for psychiatric historians to reveal the extent to which familial, class and other relational ties were positively renegotiated, and which therefore show 'the asylum as a terrain on which identities and interests remained contested rather than being merely contained or suffocated'.[42]

Far from being a mere agent of control, the asylum (like other contemporary social institutions) 'was itself part of a network of power in which there remained some scope for asymmetrical bargaining, resistance and collusion'.[43] As a number of recent Anglo and American studies have shown, in regions where (as the nineteenth century progressed) a close alliance was forged between the interest/concerns of the state and of medical, asylum and local authorities, there was a large scope via the asylum for central control of the insane's definition and treatment. Subsequent to committal, familial and community bargaining powers were often sharply curtailed. Even here, however, the role of families and communities in initiating and negotiating patients' committals, and in continuing to shape the asylum should not be underestimated. Indeed, James Moran contends that it is the responsibility of historians to recognise and explore 'the inequalities in the power and influence of each group [or agency]'.[44]

It has been some time since Laurence Ray, John Walton and others began to challenge the notion of the asylum either as an exclusive house of industry for the idle and work-shy, or as a 'museum' or 'warehouse' for an 'underclass' – the social (and biological) detritus, of the elderly, the vagrant/migrant, or the chronically unproductive.[45] Since then, historians have found a wealth of supporting evidence that patients were drawn from a wide range of socio-economic backgrounds. Only in the twentieth century did the asylum approximate to a psycho-geriatric home. As Bartlett has pointed out, asylums had both policing/quarantining and consciously reformative/reintegrative agendas, housing an antithetical mix of social undesirables on the one hand and respectable workers on the other. Others have begun to question the former orthodoxy that asylum attendants were uniformly drawn from the 'dregs of society'.[46] This interpretation seems to have derived from historians taking contemporary alienists and lunacy reformers somewhat uncritically at their word; as well as from a tendency to see asylum staff in isolation from analogous employment sectors; and to have been insufficiently based on detailed investigation of evolving working patterns in this employment sector.

Contributors to this volume engage with analogous issues largely through detailed case studies but have framed their chapters against the wider historiography of class and gender in British and Irish psychiatry/asylums. Yet the challenge remains for this and succeeding generations of asylum and psychiatric historians to build on the growing number of case studies in order to arrive at more general models of socio-economic change.

A further issue – only partially addressed by previous studies of class and psychiatry, and one which receives some coverage here – is the importance of class to the identity and status of asylum patients in particular, and to the mentally disordered more generally. An interesting but unresolved related issue is the degree to which we can refer to a class-consciousness amongst asylum patients, and to what extent this was divergently configured from class identities in other carceral institutions outside the bounds of the asylum. What was the impact of the asylum and its increasing accumulation of pauper lunatics in nineteenth-century Britain on class and class consciousness amongst inmates and their families, and what was its role in contemporary debates about these issues in wider society? Scholars have highlighted how the category of pauper lunatic was to some extent an artificial administrative construct/convenience.[47] On the one hand, the economic burden that lunacy brought with it was itself pauperising, and the label once applied had a habit of sticking. On the other hand, pauper status was more complicated than appears at first glance. Individuals designated as pauper insane might be supported in the asylum by a combination of parish rates, charitable support and family income, while the status of a pauper lunatic could be fluid and changeable. For, while chronic pauper populations were certainly accumulating in asylums, as work by Wright and others have shown, the majority of patients were discharged, many returning to employment and domestic duties within their communities.[48] Individuals and families who were confronted with the threat of being pauperised might refuse parochial aid or remove themselves from the rates. As Fennell's work has emphasised,[49] lunacy itself implied a distinct loss of status, in particular legal and consensual rights, which to some degree cut across class (and gender) boundaries.

There are a number of sites where we might find signs of a significant role for class identity/consciousness amongst the pauper/private insane. To some degree these are to be located within the strictly demarcated recreational and occupational activities of asylums, or within patient magazines and literary clubs often dominated by cliquish groups of genteel or literate middle-class patients.[50] Yet what evidence can we find of patients identifying and acting out common causes, and how far was what agitation there was mediated by class-based concerns? Early protest literature about lunacy certifications and asylums mostly emanated from private moneyed patients, whose narratives and court appeals were somewhat solitary voices (or 'cracks in the walls of silence'[51]). Indeed, outside of narrow bodies like The Alleged Lunatics Friends Society, there appear limited indications of patients forming common identities, especially pauper patients. Some pauper patients were clearly able to make sufficient common cause to pen protests, as did those in Barnhill Poorhouse, in Glasgow during the 1840s-60s.[52] Yet organised, collective agitation/complaints were rare in pauper asylums and lunatic wards, and seem only a very limited reflection of the forging of a common, let alone broadly class-centred, consciousness. Grievances focused on internal issues often narrowly and somewhat apolitically construed – such as food, heating and creature comforts and abuse/mistreatment – complaints common to most institutional populations. Furthermore, local parochial boards often responded dismissively to such complaints from the poor and insane, as when Barnhill's Governor Alexander Henderson testified before a 1909 Royal Commission blaming pauperism on the ignorance, lack of foresight, and wanton behaviour of the poor, rather than on prevailing economic or social factors such as unemployment or recession.[53] Furthermore, the ascription of lunacy was further apt to discredit or mitigate the seriousness of patient grievances in the eyes of authorities. Greater protection and responsiveness to patient complaints had been afforded through the ministrations of the central Lunacy Commission in England and Wales after 1845, and Scotland after 1857. In mixed and private asylums, private patients tended to be more worried about being lorded over by attendants not fit to be servants in their own households, than about wider issues as to basic human rights and privileges often denied them in the asylum. And vocal patient complaints about the monitoring, stopping and censoring of patient correspondence[54] were at least met to a degree in some asylums by the introduction of reforms such as patient letter boxes. Yet, much research still needs to be done on the way the ascription of lunacy and detention in an asylum impacted upon identity, and its class-based constituents.

Although an effort has been made to accord chronological breadth to this collection, most contributions concentrate on the Victorian and Edwardian period. To some extent this manifests a bias in current historical scholarship, in itself a reflection of the fact that it was this period which saw the most profound developments in institutional 'solutions' to insanity and the professionalisation of psychiatry. It is also a simple reflection of the substantial survival of large bodies of asylum and other psychiatric archival material not subject to the bars of confidentiality and closure restricting access to more modern health records. Since at least the 1980s, there has been a new sensitivity amongst a range of social, economic and political analysts to the importance of factors of ethnic and racial exclusions and social exclusion within the divided entity constituted by modern Britain. In Victorian times social exclusion and demarcation was no doubt more starkly reflected in segregative institutions like the asylum, and was often enshrined and bolstered by divisions within contemporary institutions.

Modern sociological, epidemiological and historical surveys, having previously placed a great deal of stress on social class and class conflicts/divisions in assessing the causation of mental illness and experiences within mental health services, have now begun to spend more time investigating other and related issues such as racial differences, social exclusion and social stress.[55] The chapters on twentieth-century developments in this volume (e.g. Busfield and Jackson) further highlight the historical propensity for the mentally ill and defective amongst the lower social classes to be more subject to institutionalisation, and the long historical denial amongst medical men and health administrators of such differential patterns, let alone the social roots and inequalities residing behind them. While engaging critically with some of the assumptions in the existing literature and the conceptual/social shifts it implies, these chapters further elucidate how the social loading of mental illness/defect was much more than simply the consequence of class relations, being closely linked to the processes of class formation.

Themes

As we have asserted in the contextual discussion, this collection is distinctive in a number of respects, and this section of our introduction examines this in greater detail. The collection provides a more nuanced interpretation of the hitherto rather crude equation of class and custodialism and, in its discussion of gender, it also gives greater visibility for men through a more symmetrical analysis of male as well as female experience. This collection employs both qualitative and quantitative approaches to examine the experiences of patients, and in this way offers both precision and depth to its analyses. And, by placing examination of both class and gender in the same volume, their complex intersections can be better appreciated together with the importance of context in framing them. The book's case histories span four countries and reveal how the psychiatric institution was an organisational prism that reflected broader trends in society. Discussion of the network of related establishments gives good insight into patient careers involving progression from prison or workhouse to asylum. Examination of the asylum admissions process poses interesting issues about the relationship of lay and medical knowledge, the creation of psychiatric knowledge, and the boundaries of professional power.

These historical and sociological analyses use varied and innovative sources. They highlight valuable issues concerning gendered or classist bias. For example, Rab Houston's analysis of madness and gender in eighteenth-century Scotland utilises an unusual source in the brieves or letters generated by eighteenth-century legal inquests concerning the alleged inability of people to manage their own affairs. These were designed to protect property and asked whether the subjects were furious (manic) or fatuous (idiotic or melancholy.) But this documentation reveals fascinating gender predispositions in that, when giving evidence in the courts, men commented on the public world but women on the private world of the household. That lay men and women provided information in the committal of the insane poses the question of whether these admissions certificates were commonsensical descriptions of individual behaviour or, as David Wright argues, more complex documents that reflected negotiations between families, doctors and poor law officers, thus suggesting a dynamic relationship between medical and lay knowledge. Within the asylum, case notes have proved to be a useful but not unproblematic source for the historian. They are predisposed towards the affluent and articulate patient, and so have an inbuilt social bias.[56]

In the first part of the introduction we have seen how earlier studies in psychiatric history viewed the asylum as a custodial – even 'total' – institution, emphasising the constituent processes of social control, by underlining relationships between social class and professional power. This class-based nature of the asylum system has also featured in more recent studies.[57] The collection of essays in this volume builds on this earlier work but modifies and extends it.

Using occupation as a proxy provides some information on the extent to which admissions reflected the class make-up of society. This is easier to discern with men than for women, since many females, more especially from the middle class, had no vocation recorded. In Holloway Sanatorium in Surrey, for example, eighty-five per cent of female patients in 1893 had no occupation assigned but were of 'good social standing' and, amongst the working-class clientele in Brookwood Asylum, nearly fifty per cent of women had no occupation. Among women in private establishments such as Wonford House in Devon, or Holloway the anachronistic label of 'gentlewoman' was much in evidence. For men the reflection of the occupational world in patient admission records was not exact. Pamela Michael suggests that amongst Victorian male inmates of the North Wales Lunatic Asylum at Denbigh transport workers, those in commercial occupations and also building labourers were over-represented. The dominance in occupational censuses of female domestic servants was replicated in this asylum, as was also the case in Brookwood. The presence of governesses and the wives of professional men in Brookwood hint at the social drift that was associated with asylum patients, where poverty might follow mental illness. Significantly, both governesses and domestic servants were peculiarly vulnerable in that, if they lost their job, their home also disappeared. In these circumstances the asylum might be a more respectable and discreet refuge for their poverty than the workhouse.

Notions of social hierarchy and class also influenced diagnoses. Mark Jackson examines the covert classist assumptions about uncontrolled criminality and sexuality in the lower classes, and argues that it was these preoccupations that drove the mental defective legislation of the Edwardian era. Another case study, this time by Joan Busfield, discusses the class-related types of war neurosis (or shell-shock) where hysteria was used as a label for ordinary ranks (whose bodily symptoms were highlighted), whereas the diagnosis for the officer class (whose psychological problems were emphasised), was neurasthenia

The institutional environment created for patients of different social classes was also very obviously differentiated, and mirrored that in the outside world. Those who could pay more received more. As Anne Shepherd's paired study of a private and a public asylum situated only ten miles from each other shows, the environment, the food, even the nature of the treatment showed dramatic contrasts. The Holloway Sanatorium at Virginia Water provided a luxurious, elegant and comfortable environment, with theatre, billiard room, and a winter garden, where the patient's psychiatric experience occurred in very different surroundings from that of the functional public institution at Brookwood. Occupational therapy was also class and gender specific. At Brookwood there was domestic work for women in kitchen, laundry, and sewing room, whereas at Holloway there was moral therapy. Here genteel occupations were assisted by companions possessing musical and artistic skills, and supplemented by carriage rides, walks, shopping, and excursions to places of interest. At Brookwood men did gardening and farm work whereas those at Holloway enjoyed seasonal sports including hunting. In the public asylum there was recourse to cheaper treatments (employment and exercise in the fresh air) together with chemotherapy for troublesome individuals, whereas the private establishment occupied their clientele with hydrotherapy or Swedish gymnastics.

During the 1890s social class was also articulated in the setting of the Dundee Royal Lunatic Asylum where Lorraine Walsh discusses the creation of Gray – later Gowrie – House as a separate facility for private patients. Her investigation indicates that equating private care with the middle-class was not necessarily straightforward, but that respectability and socially acceptable behaviour were also important determinants of patient selection. In an important reappraisal she demonstrates how private and pauper categories were not fixed and rigid, but rather were 'asylum constructions' that were not necessarily linked to the patient's social standing outside the institution's walls. Here the subsidy to private patients equalled half the monies the asylum gained from all boarding fees, and the fact that there was a very high ratio of subsidised to non-subsidised private patients 'demonstrates that the majority... did not match the accepted profile of the private patient.' She therefore challenges Andrew Scull's earlier interpretation that the pauper and private lunatic accurately reflected the class divisions of Victorian society.[58]

Ambiguities of class are also tellingly depicted in Joseph Melling's analysis of the public and private asylum in relation to the governess patient. This explores some of the elusiveness of class in that the governess was an individual drawn from the respectable middle-class, yet was someone who worked as an employee on the borderland between polite and servile society. Her admission to both private and public asylums exposed the tension between social aspiration (her concern to retain privacy and thus respectability within a private establishment), and economic ability (her incapacity to pay commercial fees after salaried employment where genteel conditions of work substituted for monetary reward), and thus her occasional reluctant recourse to a public institution.

That Victorian asylums were alleged to contain a larger proportion of their inmates from the ranks of governesses than any other occupation has provided a potent symbol of the supposedly insupportable tensions between femininity, work and domestic duty. As Joseph Melling suggests, this has contributed to the creation of a broader feminist interpretation of the asylum. This historiography included the argument by Chesler that the asylum was used to enforce social conformity on women,[59] and that by Showalter that 'madness is a female malady because it is experienced by more women than men'.[60] Critiques of these theses demonstrated that women were not in fact disproportionately represented in asylum populations, and helped to alert historians and sociologists to some of the contradictions inherent in overly social constructionist accounts of female insanity.[61] This volume extends revisionism by giving male and female patients equal coverage in discussion, and by exploring interactions of gender with class. Crucially, this provides a corrective to an earlier over-emphasis on middle- and upper- class women in discussions of female disorders related to insanity. Several case studies also investigate the relationship of cultural constructions of gender to the actual experiences of the patient population and their treatment regimes.

Men were almost as likely to be institutionalised as women, so that in the medium to long term numbers were virtually equivalent in the asylums analysed here, with the exception of case studies located in Wales and Ireland, where men predominated. The popular image of the victimised woman, still less the incarcerated wife, finds relatively little support in this volume. The unmarried – both men and women – were likely to be disproportionately well represented in Victorian public and private establishments for the mentally ill in Scotland, Wales and England. However, the Irish experience was slightly different, in that married women made up as many as half the females in the asylum. On the other hand there were rather shorter durations of stay for women in Irish asylums because they were admitted later in their illness and removed after a shorter period. Evidence suggests that in the Denbigh Asylum, and other asylums in late-Victorian Britain, women tended to stay slightly longer than men. By the mid-twentieth century, following the provisions of the British Mental Health Act of 1959, men generally predominated in legal sectioning.

The extent to which gender representations framed discussion on certification and admission was complicated. Houston concludes that there was little gendering of language in Scottish discussions of madness. Instead the vocabulary – of low spirits, fatuous, furious, daft, mad, silly, idiotic, deranged, troubled in mind, void of reason – suggested 'shared experiences'. However, a gendered understanding of behaviour and thus of madness was significant in eighteenth and early nineteenth-century Scotland, and nineteenth-century Wales. Deviance was interpreted less in terms of crossing the constructed boundaries of patriarchy, than in terms of defying the norms of behaviour of one's own sex.

Causes of insanity attributed to men and women showed strong similarities although with some significant variation in specifics. Both at the Connaught District Lunatic Asylum and the West Riding Lunatic Asylum stressful social predicaments were key factors for patients of each sex; disappointment or dispute were important at the former, and at each institution impoverishment was a very important precipitating cause. The emotional or moral causation of insanity was cited as very significant for both working-class and middle-class women in the Ballinasloe and Holloway establishments. Intemperance featured strongly as a causative agent amongst Irish and Scottish male patients, whereas equivalent middle-class cases in Holloway featured overwork and business worry. However, anxieties over respectability and work were features of both female and male cases in the West Riding Asylum.

The differential social presentations of men and women did not lead to a fundamental gendering of diagnosis, although some revealing divergences occurred. 'Mood' disorders were common in female admissions, whereas GPI, dementia, and idiocy featured amongst men. Interestingly, men and women shared common types of delusion but its content might be gendered, so that those of women were concerned with kin, family and household, whilst those of men were focussed on work, status and property. In Ireland Oonagh Walsh discovered that the delusions of married men in the asylum centred on the supposed infidelity of their wives. Social norms and expectations were therefore intriguingly reflected in gendered false beliefs.

Concepts of manhood feature in the essay by Joan Busfield, who argues that the diagnosis of shell-shock (later termed war neurosis and then post traumatic shock) initially posed a threat to society's concept of manliness. Later this came to be seen as a sacrifice that men made during the wars of the twentieth century. The social creation of normalities and pathologies, the constructions of sanity and mental incapacity, and the framing of disease thus revealed gendered dimensions. To a lesser extent this was also evident in therapeutics. Mid-twentieth century women were more subject than men to new physical treatments such as ECT, and were also prescribed new tranquillising drugs for diagnosed anxiety and depression. In seeking to explain their need for help women focussed on their interior world, thus obscuring their social circumstances, so that medication tended to serve as a palliative.

There were also certain gender differences with respect to outcomes. Female recovery rates were rather better than those of men, not least because women were often – though not invariably – admitted at an earlier stage of the disease. Paradoxically, however, a higher male death rate (particularly associated with cases of GPI or terminal syphilis), led to women predominating over men amongst chronic or long-stay patients. Women were not more liable to readmission than men, but the development of the option of voluntary boarding led to a greater take-up by discharged women. This indicates that a private institution such as Holloway was far from being perceived as a stereotypically oppressive institution.

The foregoing discussion already points to the fact that social class and gender permeated psychiatric ideas and practices and that, in analysing the complexity of patient experience, it is necessary to map the connections between them. This is even more clearly exemplified in selected aspects of case studies discussed below.

Marjorie Levine-Clark shows that the stereotype of only one sex, that of men, having their identity predicated on work status is misleading, because her sample of working-class women in the West

Riding Asylum felt pressures of unemployment and accompanying poverty very keenly. Indeed, they felt these endangered survival. 'Poverty and unemployment had as much of an impact on women's sense of identity as they did on men's' she argues, because work was central to their identities and well being. Her analysis of case notes suggests that poverty and female insanity were closely linked, with unemployment and other socio-economic factors being interpreted as causal influences in almost one in seven cases. Anxieties were not only directed to women's position in the labour market, and hence to calculations about their personal financial independence as workers, but also to their dependent status as wives – where fears of poverty were linked to the inability or refusal of husbands to provide for them.

A quite different subject provides material for an illuminating discussion of the intersection of class and gender. Mark Jackson dissects the intricate interplay of these concerns in framing Edwardian understanding of the feeble-minded in the landmark Mental Deficiency Act of 1913. Here 'the conflation of the feeble-minded with the supposedly promiscuous, criminal, and degenerate lower classes' contrasted with 'the moral superiority, professional expertise, and political authority of the middle classes'. Degenerationist fears about differential fertility between the working and middle classes were linked to concerns about women's sexuality and the spread of feeble-mindedness. Feeble-mindedness was seen as fundamentally a problem of class but was also interconnected with gendered anxieties about women. And, in what is in certain respects a complementary analysis, Joan Busfield looks at unacceptable conduct linked to criminal behaviour identified in men rather than women. This later diagnosis of psychopathic disorder (like that of feeble-mindedness) aligned perceived symptoms to an exaggeration of lower class behaviour or even of biological make-up.

Was it biological determinism or cultural conditioning that constituted predispositions towards so-called 'women's disorders' in insanity? In an analysis of over 1,700 admissions to the Buckinghamshire County Pauper Lunatic Asylum, David Wright finds no cases of ovarian madness or of climacteric insanity, fewer than one per cent of admissions suffering from hysteria or hysterical mania, and only two per cent of female admissions with puerperal insanity. The patient constituency of a county asylum like this one was overwhelmingly the lower stratum of society. Wright poses the strategic question of whether feminist concern over these kinds of disorders and related medical discourses about women's bodies has distorted the reality of women's past asylum experience. This is complemented by the discovery that anorexia was diagnosed more amongst the middle-class patients of Holloway Sanatorium than amongst the working class inmates of Brookwood. These illuminating findings indicate that too much has been made of the experiences of a small number of affluent patients, and thus that class as much as gender needs to be included in interpretations.

As well as class and gender, ethnicities are also highly relevant for a more inclusive analysis. This volume is distinctive in including case studies from Denbigh to Dundee and from Ballinasloe to Brookwood, thus embracing Scotland, and Ireland, as well as England and Wales. Asylums in different countries had distinct legal frameworks, and were embedded in particular social and ethnic contexts. This was also true of colonial milieus and, in the following chapters there are several brief cross-cultural references to colonial psychiatry. Mark Jackson refers to the belief that inbreeding contributed to feeble-mindedness, and remote areas facilitated this, whether in rural Britain or imperial Australia, New Zealand and Canada. In colonial asylums in South Africa the black patient's case records were often silent about the patient's history and hence about causes of illness, therefore providing a strong parallel with working-class patients in an English asylum such as Brookwood.[62] Much as in Ireland, the police or the prison were important intermediaries in the construction of a predominantly male population in the colonial asylum in Canada, Australia or South Africa.

British asylums were implanted in a complex of institutions within a public and private market, and referrals between them constituted a kind of rudimentary welfare network.[63] Patient careers – more particularly those of working-class inmates – frequently took them from the household through a variety of institutions including the workhouse and prison. In Ireland legislation criminalised the insane and labelled the majority of pauper insane as dangerous so that, for instance, seventy per cent of the women and almost eighty per cent of the men who entered the Connaught District Lunatic Asylum were admitted under the Dangerous Lunatics Act. By contrast, in England and Wales (as we have seen earlier in the first part of this introduction) the workhouse was the most important filter in identifying and creating the pauper lunatic. Amongst the patients in the Buckinghamshire Asylum David Wright finds that one quarter had been resident in the workhouse and another quarter had been held there for temporary security. In Brookwood one third of the single men came from London workhouses and these were individuals deemed difficult to control. Earlier work has demonstrated the close legal relationship between the poor law and asylum.[64] However, material conditions in the two establishments were dissimilar, since the superior eligibility of the asylum contrasted with the less eligibility of the workhouse. The rationale for the workhouse of the New Poor Law was predicated on the adult male inmate but, as we have seen in Marjorie Levine-Clark's case study, there were parallel expectations for women concerning work and dependency. And, women's fears of having to rely on a harsh system of poor relief that would strip them of their respectability itself contributed to female insanity and entry to the asylum.

The tight nineteenth-century regime of interlocking, interdependent institutions gave way to a more dispersed set of establishments in the twentieth century, when the asylum (now termed a mental or psychiatric hospital) was less central to social networks of care and custody. Joan Busfield emphasises that there was not a simple linear track of welfare regimes but suggests that development took place in four stages: from 1890 to 1929, custodialism was under attack with the development of voluntary admissions; between 1930 and 1953, the Mental Treatment Act of 1930 led to a more active therapeutic regime and assimilation of mental to physical illness; from 1954 to 1973, new chemically-synthesised psychotropic drugs kept florid symptoms under control and paved the way for community care of the mentally ill involving an expansion of the public sector; and finally, from 1974, an era of privatisation and commercialisation developed.

The mental institution responded flexibly to changing social requirements. The family could exploit the importance of kin in the normal committal process for its own special purposes, with ends that privileged the needs of relatives. Walton had earlier suggested that the working class used the asylum as a temporary refuge for their elderly relatives or a means for sick family members to regain their health.[65] Anne Shepherd states that Holloway was used by affluent English families for their social convenience as a respite or relief home, so that difficult members of the family were sent there when the rest of their relatives went on holiday. In addition, epileptic members of the family might be placed there when kith and kin thought that epileptic fits had reached a more than tolerable level. Links between affluence and the asylum were matched by those between impoverishment and insanity. In Ireland Oonagh Walsh suggests that the linked institutional network of poorhouse and madhouse was being deliberately used as 'a temporary means of respite' for women representing themselves as deserted wives with no means of support, when in fact their husbands were working as migrant labourers in England or Scotland. This is a similar finding to that on the English workhouse under the New Poor Law, where wives and mothers learned to exploit the mechanisms of poor relief to meet their need for material help through outdoor relief, whilst skilful manipulation avoided the more coercive and disciplinary option of indoor relief in the workhouse.[66]

Avoidance of the workhouse through recourse to the asylum was vital if reputation was an individual's main capital, as was the case with the mid-nineteenth century governess. Joseph Melling argues that she needed to avoid the public institution of county asylum or workhouse where news of her plight would adversely impinge on any future hopes of employment. Since the Devon governesses were unmarried and getting on in years, Melling surmises that the asylum was used as 'a refuge for the elderly exhausted governess with no other means of care'. In an interesting insight into the dynamics of occupational classes, governesses and specialist teachers were to be found mainly – although not exclusively – in the private asylum, whilst elementary teachers were located in the public one.

The Victorian social order impinged on the asylum in another important respect in that several cases studies show that its occupational therapy acted as a means of providing for socio-economic needs. Recovery was then effectively defined as having taken place when former patients could fend for themselves in the labour market. The asylum has been conceived as an instrument of a class society in which deviant members were disciplined.[67] Lorraine Walsh's study of the Dundee Royal Lunatic Asylum demonstrates that social class heavily influenced routes into and out of the asylum. And, as both Pamela Michael and Anne Shepherd show, the asylum also operated within a gendered society where women could be committed by their male relatives for so-called situational improprieties – cursing, noisy, erotic, or troublesome conduct. They were classified according to whether their behaviour fitted gendered norms, their therapy had a disciplinary edge, and they were seen to have 'recovered' when they were again quiet and obedient.

The asylum also offered a disciplinary model, not so much as an actual instrument of social control as an ever-present possibility as a coercive site, for those currently outside its walls. Pamela Michael outlines how, for an older generation, the threat of the asylum was a potent corrective tool; mothers used the asylum to threaten misbehaving children. More significantly for this analysis, the asylum was employed in North Wales to police the prescribed boundaries of class and gender, so that those with unrealistic hopes were brought back into line. Impossible expectations of a life beyond customary roles led to a warning that the individual would be cast out of society – dispossessed of even the harsh realities of the working-class household – through being exiled into the world of the mad. There impractical fantasies would blend in with the delusions of the certified mad.

The case studies presented in this volume thus provide complementary investigations that pose fresh questions, probe new issues and together create a powerful and cohesive synthesis. They suggest that within the asylum women occupied more complex roles than the earlier stereotype of powerless victims subdued by arbitrary diagnoses, whilst the working classes play more varied and interesting parts than that of disciplined deviants. The asylum itself appears as a multi-faceted establishment that operated within a changing network of social institutions. As a microcosm of society, the asylum was also found to throw light on ordinary values and standards of behaviour. The intersection of lay and professional worlds revealed in these analyses modifies an earlier view of a monopoly of professional power, but indicates instead the extent to which doctors responded to the class and gender divisions of society. These readings on the multiple functions of the asylum and the varied experiences of its patients provide new perspectives but also leave some questions for more detailed investigation. This future agenda could usefully pursue such issues as patient careers, the impact of voluntary admission on the character of the asylum, or the extent to which the asylum refashioned a custodial into a medical image.

If previous studies have remained rather locked-in the asylum, and fallen into the narrow trap of reproducing micro-historical case study after case study, this volume serves to further underline the importance of the wider context for the case study. There is plainly a growing recognition of the need for researchers to look well outside their more specific contexts (while not stretching the point or representativeness of their analyses), and to think more carefully about how their individual study adjusts/agrees with other studies from similar/divergent contexts. And there seems little doubt that thinking more fundamentally in terms of madness and society than madness and the asylum would help future researchers – as it has helped contributors to this present collection – to broaden the appeal and resonance of their work.

Notes

1. See e.g. C. Kinealy, *A Disunited Kingdom?: England, Ireland, Scotland and Wales, 1800-1949* (Cambridge: Cambridge University Press, 1999); R. Hudson and A. M. Williams, *Divided Britain* (London: Belhaven, 1989; 2nd edn, Chichester: John Wiley, 1995); L. McDowell, P. Sarre and C. Hamnett (eds), *Divided Nation: Social and Cultural Change in Britain: A Reader* (London: Hodder and Stoughton in association with the Open University, 1989).

2. See e.g. J. Donnison, *Midwives and Medical Men: A History of the Struggle for the Control of Childbirth* (2nd edn, London: Historical Publications, 1988), first published as *Midwives and Medical Men: A History of Inter-Professional Rivalries and Women's Rights* (London: Heinemann Educational, 1977); B. Ehrenreich and D. English, *Witches, Midwives, and Nurses: A History of Women Healers* (2nd edn, Old Westbury, N.Y.: The Feminist Press, 1973). For a more recent and nuanced edited collection on midwifery and reproduction over the past 300 years, see M.M. Lay et al. (ed.), *Body Talk: Rhetoric, Technology, Reproduction* (Madison, Wis.: University of Wisconsin Press, 2000). For an interesting recent historiographical survey of historical approaches to witchcraft, which analyses the divergent approaches of male and female historians, see E. Whitney, 'The Witch "she"/the Historian "he": Gender and the Historiography of the European Witch-Hunts', *Journal of Women's History*, 7 (1995), 77–101.

3. For examples, see e.g. P. Chesler, *Women and Madness* (New York: Avon Books, 1972). See also H. Allen, 'Psychiatry and the Construction of the Feminine', in P. Miller and N. Rose (eds), *The Power of Psychiatry* (Cambridge: Polity Press, 1986); R. Shafter, 'Women and Madness: A Social Historical Perspective', *Issues in Ego Psychology*, 12 (1989), 77-82. For more recent and rather unsophisticated ideologised feminist assaults on psychiatry and its history, see e.g. Jane Ussher, *Women's Madness. Misogyny or Mental Illness* (Hemel Hempstead: Harvester, 1991); M. Caminero-Santangelo, *The Madwoman Can't Speak, or, Why Insanity is not Subversive* (Ithaca; London: Cornell University Press, 1998); J. Evans, 'Well-Conducted, Rational and Industrious: Female Insanity and its Treatment at the North Riding Pauper Lunatic Asylum, 1865-83: Cure or Custody' (York: MA diss., 1996). There is of course a huge literature on individual cases of psychiatric abuse of women that we cannot attempt to summarise here, though one which was traditionally reserved primarily to famous women writers

31

and artists, from Mary Wollstonecraft's fictional Maria to the real lives of Margery Kempe, Charlotte Perkins Gilman, Virginia Woolf and Sylvia Plath. As an example of a rarer 'male-feminist' venture into this field of mad-doctor bashing, see S. Trombley, *All That Summer She Was Mad. Virginia Woolf: Female Victim of Male Medicine* (New York: The Continuum Publishing Company, 1982). This for long remained the only study to give sustained attention to the motives and opinions of Woolf's doctors. Approaches applying psycho-history, psychoanalysis and feminist approaches to similarly negative assessments of the role of her doctors, are found in, A.H. Bond, *Who Killed Virginia Woolf?: A Psychobiography* (New York, N.Y.: Human Sciences Press, c1989). See also R. Bowlby, *Still Crazy After all these Years: Women, Writing, and Psychoanalysis* (London; New York: Routledge, 1992). However, more balanced biographical surveys are provided in T.C. Caramagno, *The Flight of the Mind: Virginia Woolf's Art and Manic-Depressive Illness* (University of California Press, 1992); E. Abel, *Virginia Woolf and the Fictions of Psychoanalysis* (Chicago: University of Chicago Press, 1989).

4. N. Tomes, 'Feminist Histories of Psychiatry', in M. S. Micale and R. Porter (eds), *Discovering the History of Psychiatry* (New York; Oxford: OUP, 1994), 348-83. For a more recent gender studies survey of literature on women and madness, in particular that relating to narrative accounts, see also S. McKay and F. Bonner, 'Telling Stories – Women, Madness and English Culture 1830-1980', *Women's Studies International Forum*, 22 (1999), 563–71.

5. E.g. J.E. Kromm, 'The Feminisation of Madness in Visual Representation', *Feminist Studies*, 20, 3 (1994), 507-33; Kromm, 'Studies in the Iconography of Madness, 1600-1900' (PhD Thesis, Emory University, 1984).

6. E.g. J.P. Eigen, 'Criminal Lunacy in Early Modern England: Did Gender Make a Difference?', *International Journal of Law and Psychiatry*, 21 (1998), 409–19.

7. For another comprehensive survey of the historiography and an agenda setting, 'state of the nation' type, survey of work in the field, see e.g. N. Tomes, 'Historical Perspectives on Women and Mental Illness', in R. Apple (ed.), *Women, Health, and Medicine in America: A Historical Handbook* (New York: Garland, 1990), 143–71.

8. Tomes, *op. cit.* (note 4), 376.

9. E.g. E. Showalter, *Hystories: Hysterical Epidemics and Modern Culture* (London : Picador; New York: Columbia University Press, 1997); M.N. Evans, *Fits and Starts: A Genealogy of Hysteria in Modern France* (Ithaca: Cornell University Press, 1991); C. Smith-Rosenberg,

'The Hysterical Woman: Sex Roles and Role Conflict in Nineteenth-Century America', in *Health and Disease: A Reader* (Milton Keynes: 1984), 25–33, reprinted in C. Smith-Rosenberg, *Disorderly Conduct: Visions of Gender in Victorian America* (Oxford: Oxford University Press, 1985), 197–216. For a not dissimilar approach in a more recent study, see M.A. Simmons, 'Fictions of Femininity: Fin-de-siécle Representations of Hysteria' (Ph. D diss., City University of New York, 1996). See also S. L. Gilman, H. King, R. Porter, G.S. Rousseau and E. Showalter, *Hysteria Beyond Freud* (Berkeley & Los Angeles, California: University of California Press, 1993).

10. See e.g. J. Oppenheim, who pens extremely well-balanced chapters on nervous men and nervous women in her *'Shattered Nerves': Doctors, Patients, and Depression in Victorian England* (Oxford: Oxford University Press, 1991). See also the work of M.S. Micale on hysteria, e.g. *Approaching Hysteria. Disease and Its Interpretations* (Princeton, NJ: Princeton University Press, 1995). For excellent surveys of past historiography and future agendas for research in this area, see Micale, 'Hysteria and its Historiography: A Review of Past and Present Writings', *History of Science*, 27 (1989), 223–61 and 319–51; Micale, 'Hysteria and its Historiography: The Future Perspective', *History of Psychiatry*, 1 (1990), 33–124.

11. For a recent American survey which applies the separate spheres model to understanding psychiatric visions of masculinity, see J.S. Hughes, 'The Madness of Separate Spheres: Insanity and Masculinity in Victorian Alabama', in M.C. Carnes and C. Griffen (eds), *Meanings for Manhood: Constructions of Masculinity in Victorian America* (Chicago: University of Chicago Press, 1990), 53–66.

12. M.S. Micale, refs in note 10; Micale, 'Hysteria Male/Hysteria Female: Reflections on Comparative Gender Constructions in Nineteenth-Century France and Britain', in M. Benjamin (ed), *Science and Sensibility: Gender and Scientific Enquiry, 1780-1945* (Cambridge: Basil Blackwell, 1991), 200–39; Micale, 'Charcot and the Idea of Hysteria in the Male: Gender, Mental Science, and Medical Diagnosis in Late Nineteenth-Century France', *Medical History*, 34 (1990), 363–411. Micale's forthcoming *Hysterical Males: Medicine and Masculine Nervous Illness from the Renaissance to Freud* (Yale University Press), will undoubtedly comprise a useful *longue durée* synthesis of the intersection of hysteria and masculinity. See, also, J. Goldstein, 'The Uses of Male Hysteria: Medical and Literary Discourse in Nineteenth-Century France', in *French Medical Culture in the Nineteenth Century* (*Clio Medica*, 25; Amsterdam,

Netherlands: Rodopi, 1994) and in *Representations*, 34 (1991),
134–65; R.J. Gilmour, 'Strong Men, Soldiers and Homosexuals:
Gender, Hysteria and the Social Construction of Mental Health'
(unpublished paper, University of York, 1992), see
http://www.yorku.ca/history/rgilmour/ithink/academic/papers/strong
men.htm; and Chapter 2 by R.A. Houston in this volume.

13. R. Porter, *Mind-Forg'd Manacles: A History of Madness in England
from the Restoration to the Regency* (London: The Athlone Press,
1987); G. S. Rousseau, 'Depression's forgotten genealogy', *History of
Psychiatry*, 11, 1, 41 (2000), 71–106; G.J. Barker-Benfield, *The
Culture of Sensibility: Sex and Society in Eighteenth-Century Britain*
(Chicago: University of Chicago Press, 1992). See, also, G.S.
Rousseau, '"A Strange Pathology": Hysteria in the Early Modern
World, 1500-1800', in S.L. Gilman *et al.*, *Hysteria Beyond Freud*,
91–224; and E. Showalter, 'Hysteria, feminism and gender', in *ibid.*,
286–344.

14. See e.g. H.I. Kushner, 'Suicide, Gender, and the Fear of Modernity
in Nineteenth-Century Medical and Social Thought', *Journal of
Social History*, 26, 3 (1993), 461–90; Kushner, 'Gender and the
Irrelevance of Medical Innovation: The Social Construction of
Suicide as a Male Behaviour in Nineteenth Century Psychiatry', in
*Medicine and Change: Historical and Sociological Studies of Medical
Innovation'* (L'innovation en médecine: études historiques et
sociologiques; Montrouge, France: John Libbey Eurotext, c1993;
Colloques de l'Institut national de la santé et de la recherche
médicale, vol. 220), 421–45. For a magisterial study of English
suicide, which pays close heed to gender and class factors, see M.
MacDonald and T.R. Murphy, *Sleepless Souls: Suicide in Early
Modern England* (Oxford; New York: Clarendon/Oxford University
Press, 1990). See, also, G. Minois, *History of Suicide: Voluntary Death
in Western Culture*, trans. Lydia G. Cochrane (Baltimore; London:
Johns Hopkins University Press, 1999). For the modern period, see
especially M.J. Clarke, 'The History of Suicide in England and
Wales 1850-1961, with Special Reference to Suicide by Poisoning'
(University of Oxford, PhD thesis, 1993), 2 vols. For a rather dryer
history, see Olive Anderson, *Suicide in Victorian and Edwardian
England* (Clarendon Press: Oxford, 1987).

15. See e.g. L.A. Hall, *Hidden Anxieties: Male Sexuality, 1900-1950*
(Cambridge: Polity Press, 1991); Hall, 'Forbidden by God, Despised
by Man: Masturbation, Medical Warnings, Moral Panic and
Manhood in Great Britain, 1850-1950', *Journal of the History of
Sexuality*, 2 (1991-92), 365–87. See also the discussion of

masturbation in T. C. Parker, *Sexing the Text: The Rhetoric of Sexual Difference in British Literature, 1700-1750* (Albany: State University of New York Press, 2000). For a more clinical viewpoint, see E.H. Hare, *On the History of Lunacy: The Nineteenth Century and After* (London: Gabbay, 1998). For the place of medical conceptualisations of masculinity/femininity in the formation of sexology, see e.g. L. Bland and L. Doan (eds), *Sexology in Culture: Labelling Bodies and Desires* (Cambridge: Polity Press, 1998). For an American perspective on medicine, psychiatry and male sexual function/dysfunction, see e.g. F. Hodges, 'A History of Spermatorrhœa: The Evolution and Legacy of Medical Conceptualisations of a Venereal Disease and Male Debility in Nineteenth-Century America' (Oxford D.Phil, 2000).

16. E.g. J. Bourke, *Dismembering the Male: Men's Bodies, Britain and the Great War* (London: Reaktion, 1996); Bourke, 'Disciplining the Emotions: Fear, Psychiatry and the Second World War', in R. Cooter, M. Harrison and S. Sturdy (eds), *War, Medicine and Modernity* (Stroud: Sutton, 1998), 225–38; M. Thomson, 'Status, Manpower and Mental Fitness: Mental Deficiency in the First World War', in Cooter, Harrison and Sturdy, *idem*, 149–66; J. Winter (ed.), *Journal of Contemporary History*, Shell-Shock Issue, 35 (2000); B. Shephard, *A War of Nerves: Soldiers and Psychiatrists 1914-1994* (London: Jonathan Cape, 2000). For previous (and some recent) studies where gender is relatively peripheral to the analysis, see e.g. T. Bogacz, 'War Neurosis and Cultural Change in England, 1914-22: The Work of the War Office Committee of Enquiry into "Shell-Shock" ', *Journal of Contemporary History*, 24 (1989), 227–56; H. Merskey, 'Shell-Shock', in G. Berrios and H. Freeman (eds), *150 Years of British Psychiatry, 1841-1991* (London: Gaskell, 1991), 245–67; A. Babington, *Shell-Shock: A History of the Changing Attitudes to War Neurosis* (London: Leo Cooper, 1997). For a political and class-centred analysis, see e.g. J. Crouthamel, 'War Neurosis Versus Savings Psychosis: Working-Class Politics and Psychological Trauma in Weimar Germany', *Journal of Contemporary History*, 37 (2002), 163-82. For trauma and combat stress, see e.g. P. Lerner and M. S. Micale (eds), *Traumatic Pasts: History, Psychiatry, and Trauma in the Modern Age* (Cambridge: Cambridge Studies in the History of Medicine, 2001); H. Binneveld, *From Shell Shock to Combat Stress: A Comparative History of Military Psychiatry* (Amsterdam: Amsterdam University Press, 1997).

17. E. Showalter, *The Female Malady. Women, Madness and English Culture 1830-1980* (London: Virago Press, 1987; 1st edn, New York:

Pantheon Books, 1985). In this book and other writings, Showalter did much to elucidate the prevalence of Ophelia-like constructions of female melancholia in eighteenth and nineteenth-century writings and artistic productions on insanity. See also Showalter, 'Representing Ophelia: Women, Madness and the Responsibilities of Feminist Criticism', in P. Parker and G. Hartman (eds), *Shakespeare and the Question of Theory* (London; New York: Methuen.1985), 77–94; H. Small, *Love's Madness: Medicine, the Novel, and Female Insanity, 1800-1865* (Oxford: Clarendon Press; New York: Oxford University Press, 1996); B.G. Lyons, 'The Iconography of Ophelia', *English Literary History* 44 (1977), 60–74.

18. K. Dörner, *Madmen and the Bourgeoisie: A Social History of Insanity and Psychiatry*, trans. J. Neugroschel and J. Steinberg (Oxford, Basil Blackwell, 1981), first pub. as *Bürger und Ire* (1969); Dörner, 'The Role of Psychiatry in Solving the Social Question, 1790-1990', in L. De Goei and J. Vijselaar (eds), *Proceedings of the 1st European Congress on the History of Psychiatry and Mental Health Care* (Rotterdam: Erasmus Publishing, 1993), 331–7; M. Foucault, *Madness and Civilisation: A History of Insanity in the Age of Reason* (New York, Random House, 1965), trans. and abridged by Richard Howard from *Folie et Déraison: Histoire de la Folie à L'Age Classique* (Paris: Librairie Plon, 1961).

19. T. Whitlock, 'Gender, Medicine, and Consumer Culture in Victorian England: Creating the Kleptomaniac', *Albion*, 31 (1999), 413–37.

20. E.g. J. McNamara, 'Out of Order: Madness is a Feminist and a Disability Issue', in J. Morris (ed.), *Encounters With Strangers: Feminism and Disability* (London: The Women's Press, 1996), 194–205.

21. For example, E. S. Gomberg and V. Franks (eds), *Gender and Disordered Behavior: Sex Differences in Psychopathology* (New York: Brunner/Mazel, 1979); M. Briscoe, *Sex Differences in Psychological Well-Being* (Cambridge; New York: Cambridge University Press, 1982; *Psychological Medicine*, Monograph Supplement, 1); R. Jenkins, *Sex Differences in Minor Psychiatric Morbidity* (Cambridge: Cambridge University Press, 1985)

22. Showalter, *op. cit.* (note 17). Many of the essential ingredients of her arguments that there were (disproportionately) more women in Victorian asylums (especially pauper asylums) are first encountered in her article 'Victorian Women and Insanity', *Victorian Studies*, 23 (1979-80), 157–81, subsequently reprinted in Andrew Scull (ed.), *Madhouses, Mad-doctors, and Madmen: The Social History of*

Psychiatry in the Victorian Era (London: Athlone Press, 1981), 313–36.

23. See e.g. J. Busfield, 'The Female Malady? Men, Women, and Madness in Nineteenth Century Britain', *Sociology*, 28 (1994), 259–77. For Busfield's account of gender issues in twentieth-century mental health, see her *Men, Women and Madness: Understanding Gender and Mental Disorder* (London: Macmillan, 1996).

24. For a recent antipodean study which takes a gender-based approach to asylum committals, see B. Labrum, 'Looking Beyond the Asylum: Gender and the Process of Committal to Auckland, 1870-1910', *New Zealand Journal of History*, 26 (1992), 125–44.

25. On nineteenth-century 'depression', see e.g. Oppenheim, *op. cit.* (note 10). Interestingly the word 'depression', though in the book's sub-title, is not in the index, Oppenheim preferring more common contemporary terms such as 'nervous exhaustion/breakdown'. For more sustained linkage between Victorian and ensuing modern constructions and patterns of depressive illness, see e.g. M.J. van Lieburg, *Woman and Depression: Impressions from the History of a Connection* (Rotterdam: Erasmus, 1992); M. Steen, 'Historical Perspectives on Women and Mental Illness and Prevention of Depression in Women, Using a Feminist Framework', *Issues in Mental Health Nursing*, 12 (October–December 1991), 359-74. See also N. Tomes, 'Devils in the Heart: A Nineteenth-Century Perspective on Women and Depression', *Transactions and Studies of the College of Physicians of Philadelphia.*, 5 ser., 13 (1991), 363–86; Tomes, 'Women and Depression: A Historical Perspective', in *History of Psychiatric Diagnoses: Proceedings of the 16th International Symposium on the Comparative History of Medicine – East and West: September 1-8, 1991, Susono-shi, Shizuoka* (Japan, Tokyo: 1997), 55–83.

26. See e.g. H. Marland, '"Destined to a Perfect Recovery": The Confinement of Puerperal Insanity in the Nineteenth Century', in J. Melling and W. Forsythe (eds), *Insanity, Institutions and Society, 1800-1914: A Social History of Madness in Comparative Perspective* (London; New York: Routledge, 1999), 137–56; Marland, 'At Home with Puerperal Mania: The Domestic Treatment of the Insanity of Childbirth in the Nineteenth Century', in D. Wright and P. Bartlett (eds), *Outside the Walls of the Asylum: The History of Care in the Community* (London: Athlone Press, 1999), 45–65; M. Jackson (ed.), *Infanticide: Historical Perspectives on Child Murder and Concealment, 1550-2000* (Aldershot: Ashgate, 2002). For an excellent American study, see N. Theriot, 'Diagnosing Unnatural

Motherhood: Nineteenth-Century Physicians and "Puerperal
Insanity"', *American Studies*, 26 (1990), 69–88, reprinted in
J.W. Leavitt (ed.), *Women and Health in America* (2nd edn,
Madison: University of Wisconsin Press, 1999), 405–21. For more
general background on scientific and medical constructions of the
female mind/body and its illnesses, see e.g. L. Jordanova, *Sexual
Visions: Images of Gender in Science and Medicine Between the
Eighteenth and Twentieth Centuries* (Brighton: Harvester, 1989);
L. Schiebinger, *The Mind Has No Sex: Women in the Origins of
Modern Science* (Cambridge, Mass.: Harvard University Press, 1991,
orig. 1989); T. Laqueur, *Making Sex: Body and Gender from the
Greeks to Freud* (Cambridge, Mass.: Harvard University Press, 1990);
L.S. Dixon, *Perilous Chastity: Women and Illness in Pre-Enlightenment
Art and Medicine* (Ithaca: Cornell University Press, 1995).

27. For a degree of scepticism about the extent of false confinement in
Victorian Britain, but also for a good early analysis of the genuine
grounds for suspicions, see P. McCandless, 'Liberty and Lunacy: The
Victorians and Wrongful Confinement', in Scull, *op. cit.* (note 22),
339–62 and in *Journal of Social History*, 11 (1977-78), 366–86.
McCandless strikingly rather ignored questions about gendered bias
in such confinements. W.L. Parry-Jones, *The Trade in Lunacy. A
Study of Private Madhouses in England in the Eighteenth and
Nineteenth Centuries* (London: Routledge and Kegan Paul/Toronto:
University of Toronto Press, 1972) was also relatively dismissive,
asking few questions about gender-bias, and tending to address male
and female patients/proprietors alike. For thoroughly gendered
recent accounts, see e.g. E. Foyster, 'At the Limits of Liberty:
Married Women and Confinement in Eighteenth-Century England',
Continuity and Change, 17 (2002), 39–62; M.J. Kurata, 'Wrongful
Confinement: The Betrayal of Women by Men, Medicine and Law',
in K.O. Garrigan (ed.), *Victorian Scandals: Representations of Gender
and Class* (Athens : Univ. Ohio Pr., 1992), 43–68. Others make a
rather more 'ambiguous' case for gender bias in committals; e.g. J.J.
Schwieso, '"Religious Fanaticism" and Wrongful Confinement in
Victorian England: The Affair of Louisa Nottidge', *Social History of
Medicine*, 9 (1996), 159–174.

28. See e.g. T. E. Brown, 'Dance of the Dialectic? Some Reflections
(Polemic and Otherwise) on the Present State of Nineteenth-
Century Asylum Studies', *Canadian Bulletin of Medical History*, 11
(1994), 267-95; http://home.cc.umanitoba.ca/~sprague/brown.htm.

29. A. Scull, 'Rethinking the History of Asylumdom', in Melling and
Forsythe (eds), *op. cit.* (note 26), 295–315: 297–9.

30. Anne Borsay, review of Melling and Forsythe (eds), *op. cit.* (note 26), in *Reviews in History*, 83 (1999).
31. M. Ignatief, 'State, Civil Society, and Total Institutions: A Critique of Recent Social Histories of Punishment', in N. Morris and M. Tonry (eds), *Crime and Justice: An Annual Review of Research* (Chicago: University of Chicago Press, 1981), 13; reprinted in S. Cohen and A. Scull (eds), *Social Control and the State* (Oxford: Basil Blackwell, 1983), 75–117. See, also, Brown, *op. cit.* (note 28), 270, who cites this viewpoint of Ignatief.
32. Melling and Forsythe (eds), *op. cit.* (note 26), 2–3: Foucault is accused of offering a 'limited analysis of class politics' and 'marginalizing the agency of social classes, kinship networks and political movements'.
33. Melling, author's response, *Reviews in History* (1999).
34. For individual institutional studies which elucidate such differences, see e.g. A. Digby, *Madness, Morality and Medicine: A Study of the York Retreat, 1796-1914* (Cambridge, Cambridge University Press, 1985); C. Mackenzie, 'Social Factors in the Admission, Discharge, and Continuing stay of Patients at Ticehurst Asylum, 1845-1917', in Bynum, Porter and Shepherd (eds), *Anatomy of Madness*, ii, 147–76; Mackenzie, *Psychiatry for the Rich. A History of Ticehurst Private Asylum, 1792-1917* (London and New York: Routledge, 1992). For some superb North American examples, see e.g. E. Dwyer, *Homes for the Mad: Life Inside Two Nineteenth-Century Asylums* (New Brunswick, N.J.: Rutgers University Press, 1987), which nicely contrasts male:female and pauper:private patients; and R.W. Fox, *So Far Disordered in Mind: Insanity in California, 1870-1930* (Berkeley: University of California Press, 1978). For some other rare comparative studies of pauper and private patients, see Shepherd and Walsh in this volume.
35. See e.g. J. Melling, 'The Road to the Asylum: Institutions, Distance and the Administration of Pauper Lunacy in Devon, 1845-1914', *Journal of Historical Geography*, 25 (1999), 298–332; B. Forsythe, J. Melling and R. Adair, 'The New Poor Law and the County Lunatic Asylum – the Devon Experience', *Social History of Medicine*, 9 (1996), 335–56; R. Adair, B. Forsythe and J. Melling, 'Migration, Family Structure and Pauper Lunacy in Victorian England: Admissions to the Devon County Pauper Lunatic Asylum, 1845-1900', *Continuity and Change*, 12 (1997), 373–401; Adair, Forsythe and Melling, 'A Danger to the Public?: Disposing of Pauper Lunatics in late-Victorian and Edwardian England: Plympton St. Mary Union and the Devon County Asylum, 1867-1914', *Medical History*, 42

(1998), 1–25; D. Wright, 'Getting Out of the Asylum: Understanding the Confinement of the Insane in the Nineteenth Century', *Social History of Medicine*, 10 (April 1997), 137-55; Wright, *Mental Disability in Victorian England: The Earlswood Asylum, 1847-1901* (Oxford: Clarendon Press, 2001).

36. For example, Mark Jackson's *The Borderland of Imbecility: Medicine, Society, and the Fabrication of the Feeble Mind in late Victorian and Edwardian England* (Manchester; New York: Manchester University Press, 2000) explores class and gender factors in great depth and regularly emphasises their importance in discourse about the social threat posed by the defective, and cross-relates gender and class constructions in his text. By contrast, David Wright, whose methodological orientations are rather different, makes little mention of these factors in his *Mental Disability in Victorian England, op. cit.* (note 35), (gender being allocated just two pages in his index under the heading 'patients', while class receives no special entry). Of course, it might be argued that individual scholars should not necessarily feel it incumbent upon themselves to foreground class and gender (despite the frequent appeals of some critics and conference goers for them to do so), while class and gender-based analysis of psychiatry and mental disorder have themselves been subject to criticism for a tendency to ignore or downplay other significant factors. Those historians who have preferred to concentrate on demographic and socio-economic factors, and on mechanisms and influences affecting networks of support in households and communities, have often provided equally (if not more) telling models for understanding the history of mental disability, as those provided by class and gender analyses. For a recent European study where class and gender figure strongly in accounting historically for the making of madness, see e.g. A. Goldberg, *Sex, Religion, and the Making of Modern Madness. The Eberbach Asylum and German Society 1815-1849* (Oxford: Oxford University Press, 1999). For other Anglo and North American studies which have paid substantial attention to the importance of class (and, perhaps to a lesser extent, gender) in mediating psychiatry and asylum management, in particular in the prevalent biases within hereditarian, degenerationist and eugenic theories of mental illness, see e.g. I. Dowbiggin, *Keeping America Sane: Psychiatry and Eugenics in the United States and Canada* (Cornell University Press, 1997); G.V. O'Brien, 'Protecting the Social Body: Use of the Organism Metaphor in Fighting the "Menace of the Feebleminded"', *Mental Retardation*, 37 (1999), 188–200; D. Pick, *Faces of Degeneration: A*

European Disorder, c. 1848-c.1918 (Cambridge: Cambridge University Press, 1989); D.J. Childs, *Modernism and Eugenics: Woolf, Eliot, Yeats, and the Culture of Degeneration* (Cambridge: Cambridge University Press, 2001); M. Jackson, 'Images of Deviance: Visual Representations of Mental Defectives in Early Twentieth-Century Medical Texts', *British Journal for the History of Science*, 28 (1995), 319–37; M. Thomson, *The Problem of Mental Deficiency: Eugenics, Democracy, and Social Policy in Britain c.1870-1959* (Oxford: Clarendon Press, 1998). See also G.E. Allen, 'Genetics, Eugenics and Class Struggle', *Genetics*, 79 (1975), 29–45; S. F. Weiss, 'Race and Class in Fritz Lenz's Eugenics', *Medizinhistorisches Journal*, 27 (1992), 5–25.

37. For qualified critiques, see e.g. D.J. Rothman, 'Social Control: The Uses and Abuses of the Concept in the History of Incarceration', *Rice University Studies*, 67 (1981), 9–20; A. Scull, 'Madness and Segregative Control: The Rise of the Insane Asylum', *Social Problems*, 24 (1977), 337–51; Scull, *The Most Solitary of Afflictions. Madness and Society in Britain, 1700-1900* (New Haven & London: Yale UP, 1993), esp. 77–8, 391–2. For more emphatic statements of departure, see e.g. C.M. McGovern, 'The Myths of Social Control and Custodial Oppression', *Journal of Social History*, 20 (1986), 3–23, reprinted as 'The Myths of Social Control and Custodial Oppression: Patterns of Psychiatric Medicine in Late Nineteenth-Century Institutions', in P.N. Stearns (ed.), *Expanding the Past: A Reader in Social History* (New York: New York University Press, 1988), 193–213; L. Cordon, 'Conclusion: Social Control and the "Powers of the Weak"', in Cordon, *Heroes of Their Own Lives: The Politics and History of Family Violence* (New York: Penguin Books, 1989; orig. New York: Viking, 1988), 289–99; D.E. Chunn and S.A.M. Gavigan, 'Social Control: Analytic Tool or Analytic Quagmire', *Contemporary Crises*, 12 (1988), 107–24.

38. J. Donzelot, *The Policing of Families* (trans. from the French by R. Hurley; London: Hutchinson, 1980).

39. E.g. C.M. McGovern, 'The Community, the Hospital and the Working Class Patient: The Multiple Uses of the Asylum in Nineteenth-Century America', *Pennsylvania History*, 54 (1987), 17–33; B. Luckin, 'Towards a Social History of Institutionalisation', *Social History*, 8 (1983), 87–94.

40. For a classic article which effectively distils such a viewpoint, see A. Scull, 'A Convenient Place to Get Rid of Inconvenient People: The Victorian Lunatic Asylum', in A.D. King (ed.), *Buildings and Society* (London: Routledge and Kegan Paul, 1980), 37–60.

41. E.g. J.K. Walton, 'Casting out and Bringing Back in Victorian England: Pauper Lunatics, 1840-70', in W. Bynum, R. Porter and M. Shepherd (eds), *The Anatomy of Madness: Essays in the History of Psychiatry* (London and New York: Tavistock, 1985- 88), 3 vols, ii, 132–46; D. Wright and P. Bartlett (eds), *op. cit.* (note 26); Wright, 'Getting Out of the Asylum', *op. cit.* (note 35), 137–55.

42. Melling, author's response, *Reviews in History*, 83 (1999).

43. *Ibid.*

44. J.E. Moran, *Committed to the State Asylum. Insanity and Society in Nineteenth-Century Quebec and Ontario* (Montreal & Kingston; London; Ithaca, McGill-Queen's University Press, 2000), 170, 172.

45. L.J. Ray, 'Models of Madness in Victorian Asylum Practice', *Archives of European Sociology*, xxii (1981), 229–64; Walton, 'Casting Out', *op. cit.* (note 40).

46. P. Bartlett, *The Poor Law of Lunacy: The Administration of Pauper Lunatics in Mid-Nineteenth Century England* (London: Leicester University Press, 1999); Bartlett, 'The Asylum, the Workhouse and the Voice of the Insane Poor in Nineteenth Century England', *International Journal of Law and Psychiatry*, 21 (1998), 421–32; D. Wright, 'The Dregs of Society?': Occupational Patterns of Male Asylum Attendants in Victorian England', *International History of Nursing Journal*, 1, 4 (Summer 1996), 5–19; L.D. Smith, 'Behind Closed Doors: Lunatic Asylum Keepers, 1800-1860', *Social History of Medicine*, 1 (1988), 301–27. For a North American perspective on the roles and social backgrounds of asylum keepers, see e.g. J. Moran, 'The Keepers of the Insane: The Role of Attendants at the Toronto Provincial Asylum, 1875-1905', *Histoire Sociale/Social History*, 28 (1995), 51–75.

47. E.g. Bartlett, *op. cit.* (note 46); Bartlett, 'The Asylum, the Workhouse and the Voice of the Insane Poor in Nineteenth Century England', *International Journal of Law and Psychiatry*, 21 (1998), 421–32; Forsythe, Melling and Adair, *op. cit.* (note 35).

48. D. Wright, 'The Discharge of Pauper Lunatics from County Asylums in mid-Victorian England: The Case of Buckinghamshire, 1853-72' in Melling and Forsythe, *op. cit.* (note 26), 93–112; Wright, 'Getting Out of the Asylum', *op. cit.* (note 35).

49. P. Fennell, *Treatment Without Consent: Law, Psychiatry and the Treatment of Mentally Disordered People Since 1845* (London; New York: Routledge, 1996).

50. See e.g. M. Barfoot and A.W. Beveridge, '"Our Most Notable Inmate": John Willis Mason at the Royal Edinburgh Asylum, 1864-1901', *History of Psychiatry*, 4 (1993), 159–208; A. Beveridge and

M. Williams, 'Inside "The Lunatic Manufacturing Company": The Persecuted World of John Gilmour', *History of Psychiatry*, 13 (2002), 19–50: 31–3; M. Williams, *History of Crichton Royal Hospital, 1839-1989* (Dumfries: Dumfries and Galloway Health Board, 1989); J. Andrews, 'The Patient Population', in J. Andrews and I. Smith (eds), *"Let there be light again": A History of Gartnavel Royal Hospital* (Glasgow: Gartnavel Royal Hospital, 1993), 103–17.

51. See A. Ingram, *The Madhouse of Language. Writing and Reading Madness in the Eighteenth Century* (London & New York: Routledge, 1991).

52. Like many Scottish poorhouses, Barnhill Poorhouse (Barony Parish Poorhouse) had lunatic wards from early on in the nineteenth century. Repeated complaints about the house governor and local parochial board's management of the institution, emanating from patients as well as medical men, during the 1840s and 50s, made regular appearances in the *Glasgow Sentinel*, a local newspaper. See records of the poorhouse at Strathclyde Regional Archives, Mitchell Library, Glasgow, LR22D.130 1860; LR24D.55 1861; D-HEW 2/7/1 Minutes of Barnhill Poorhouse Committee; E. Milner, `Retrospect of the Doings of Barony Parochial Board', C103564 and C166825; J. McKenzie, 'Barnhill A Scottish Poorhouse' (Glasgow: STRO, 1989), unpublished typescript. While there are signs of ordinary paupers and tradesmen getting together to protest or assert rights, as in 1857 (D-HEW 2/7/1 22/6/1857) when the weavers complained to the Board of Supervision about the inadequacies of their diet, calling themselves 'members of the working classes', there are much fewer instances of such collaboration from the lunatic wards.

53. See McKenzie, *op. cit.* (note 52).

54. See e.g. A. Beveridge, 'Life in the Asylum: Patients' Letters from Morningside, 1873-1908', *History of Psychiatry*, 9 (1998), 431–69; A.W. Beveridge and M. Barfoot, 'Madness at the Crossroads: John Home's Letters from the Royal Edinburgh Asylum, 1886-7', in *Psychological Medicine*, 20 (1990), 263–84; J. Andrews, '"They're in the Trade of Lunacy... They "cannot interfere" – they say': The Scottish Lunacy Commissioners and Lunacy Reform in Nineteenth-century Scotland* (London: Wellcome Institute for the History of Medicine, Occasional Publication No. 8, 1998), 55–8; J. Andrews and I. Smith, *op. cit.* (note 50), 108–9.

55. G. Parry, 'Paid Employment, Social Stress and Mental Health in Working Class Women with Young Children' (Ph.D. thesis, University of Sheffield, Dept. of Psychology, MRC Social and

Applied Psychology Unit, 1987); M. C. Angermeyer (ed.), *From Social Class to Social Stress: New Developments in Psychiatric Epidemiology* (Berlin; New York: Springer-Verlag, c1987).

56. For example, J. Andrews, 'Glasgow Royal Asylum's Case Notes: What they do and don't Convey about the Experience of Insanity in the Nineteenth Century', *Social History of Medicine*, 11 (1998), 255–81.

57. For example, A. Scull, *Most Solitary of Afflictions, op. cit.* (note 37), 354–5: J. Andrews, 'Raising the Tone of Asylumdom. Maintaining and Expelling Pauper Lunatics at the Glasgow Royal Asylum in the Nineteenth Century', in Melling and Forsythe (eds), Melling and Forsythe, *op. cit.* (note 26), 200–22; Andrews, 'A Failure to Flourish? David Yellowlees and the Glasgow School of Psychiatry: Part 2', *History of Psychiatry*, 8 (1997), 333–60: 347.

58. Scull, *ibid.*, 354–5.

59. E.g. P. Chesler, *op. cit.* (note 3).

60. Showalter, *op. cit.* (note 17), 3.

61. N. Tomes, *op. cit.* (note 4); J. Busfield, 'Sexism and Psychiatry', *Sociology*, 23 (1989), 34364; Busfield, 'Mental Illness as Social Product or Social Construct: A Contradiction in Feminists' Arguments?', *Sociology of Health and Illness*, 10 (1988), 521–42; Showalter, *op. cit.* (note 17); Busfield, *op. cit.* (note 23).

62. S. Swartz, 'The Black Insane at the Cape', *Journal of African Studies*, 21 (1955), 399-415; Swartz, 'Colonialism and the Production of Psychiatric Knowledge in the Cape, 1891-1920' (unpublished PhD thesis, UCT, 1996), 121.

63. See, for example, R. Adair *et al.*, 'A Danger to the Public?', *op. cit.* (note 34), 3.

64. P. Bartlett, *op. cit.* (note 46).

65. J. Walton, 'Lunacy in the Industrial Revolution: A Study of Admissions in Lancashire, 1848-1850', *Journal of Social History*, 13 (1979), 1–22; Walton, 'Casting Out', *op. cit.* (note 40).

66. See, for example, A. Digby, 'Poverty, Health, and the Politics of Gender in Britain 1870-1948', in A. Digby and J. Stewart (eds), *Gender, Health and Welfare* (London; New York: Routledge, 1996; reissued, 1998), 67–90.

67. S. Cohen and A. Scull (eds), *Social Control and the State: Historical and Comparative Essays* (Oxford: 1983).

2

Class, Gender and Madness in Eighteenth-Century Scotland[1]

Robert Allan Houston

This chapter uses a wide range of qualitative and quantitative sources from eighteenth-century Scotland to ask whether identifying someone as mad was an arbitrary means of exerting power over them. Separate sections analyse the effect of gender and class on the constructions of mental disability. The conclusion is that rather than providing evidence of a crude bourgeois and/or male conspiracy, understandings of mental incapacity reveal in a subtle and nuanced way the nature and extent of distinctions between people based on their social status, age, occupation and sex.

I

This chapter seeks to test some enduring and strongly held beliefs about what it meant to call someone mad, and about how the mentally incapable were identified in the past. Most of these assumptions come out of the so-called 'anti-psychiatry' movement of the 1960s, and are manifested more in 'historically informed' literary and sociological studies rather than in the discipline of history itself.[2] They include the idea that what is called insanity is just a cultural artefact rather than at least partly a physical syndrome. Thus, being classed as insane was an arbitrary act perpetrated on men and women who simply failed to conform. Women in particular were the victims of repressive doctors and asylums; the way men and women alike were defined as mentally disabled imposed the standards of one sex and/or class on another; and living in an unequal society placed a unique strain upon the lives of those in subordinate positions.[3]

Other chapters in the book will address these issues in whole or in part. The aim of this one is to ask in what sense, if any, was madness 'a female malady' and to what extent was its definition a 'bourgeois' or 'élite' one? Most of the analysis is qualitative, including an assessment of the language used to describe mental incapacity. It is clear that, by almost all quantitative measures, males were more likely than females to be classified as mentally disabled and to be institutionalised on that account.[4] Unfortunately, there is no unbiased eighteenth-century evidence that would allow quantification of the chances of different social groups experiencing mental problems.[5] Yet there is now abundant evidence that the institutionalised insane were treated differently according to their wealth and social origins.[6] And a family's economic and demographic circumstances affected a person's chances of being institutionalised. Historians are therefore justified in asking whether similar gender- and class-related influences operated in identifying mental problems.

II

Conventional histories of psychiatry have relied largely or entirely on institutional sources: asylum admission records (specifically completed questionnaires), case books and annual reports.[7] While this chapter deploys such material, it focuses more on identifications of madness outside the asylum. Public asylums contained a majority of paupers, but most licensed private asylums were for the better-off middling and upper ranks whose families also resorted to the second source used here. That is civil court inquests known as 'cognitions', which resembled proceedings before Chancery in eighteenth-century England. If people were allegedly unable to manage their own affairs, their relatives could ask for a formal legal procedure to test whether they were 'fatuous' (idiotic or melancholic) or 'furious' (manic).[8] Relatives purchased a 'brieve' or writ from Chancery ordering a judge to hold inquest by a jury of fifteen laymen into the questions raised in it, and to return or 'retour' the answers. Proof depended on witness statements, and (normally) a personal interrogation of the subject of the inquest by the jury.[9] A curator or tutor, usually an adult male relative, was nominated to watch over the idiot or lunatic – the equivalent of an English 'committee of the person/estate'.[10]

Between 1701 and 1818 a total of 164 individuals (thirty-three of them women) became the subject of tutories and curatories on the grounds of idiocy or furiosity, producing 500 often lengthy depositions. Those described as 'of' a place (indicating they owned land there), or who had a title, comprised forty-seven per cent of subjects (men and women together). The next largest category comprised merchants and craftsmen (twenty-seven per cent), followed by sixteen per cent who were professionals (including army and navy officers); the remaining ten per cent were made up of tenant farmers and 'residenters'. However, the social composition of witnesses was much more representative of the population, with one in four being merchants or artisans, one in five tenant farmers and one in ten servants. Cognitions and asylum documents are supplemented by insanity defences in criminal cases, family papers, further civil court documents about marriage, contracts and disputed inheritance, newspaper reports, medical texts, literary fiction, and certain prescriptive writings about how sane people should behave.

III

Understandings of mental incapacity show clear if subtle evidence of gendering in eighteenth-century Scottish society. Inquests were concerned with the ability of a man or woman to look after their own affairs and particularly to spend money consciously and wisely. Significantly, the opinions of women were rarely reported when it came to the affairs of men. Sisters very occasionally pronounced on money matters in the courts, but other women generally did not. It is most unusual for women's views about the capacities of a man to be recorded, but conventional for men to expound on female ability, even if they had only known the subject briefly, as was often the case with doctors who gave evidence.

Whether that is because women were not asked or because their reply was not thought worthy of inclusion in the written record, the end is the same. In a rare instance where a female relative gave evidence in a case, Alexander Goldie's younger sister Mary offered the court her thoughts on the rate at which he spent money. Questioned by Goldie himself, she said 'that she kept house for him for seven years. She thinks that his family expenses have been much higher for some years past than they were while the deponent [witness] kept house for him'. Shocked at the expenditure of 'a brother she loves', she told him that it was a mistake to keep a house in Edinburgh and one in the country, both staffed by servants.[11] She made some general remarks to the effect that her brother was not a drinker, but that on a recent occasion he seemed 'to be in a very great passion and carried off... not quite composed in his judgement'. What is telling is that her commentary on his affairs (as opposed to fears for his sanity) is exclusively concerned with how Goldie ran his household(s).

In reality, his household expenses were small beer when compared with his other prodigal acts. From other sources such as deeds (contracts) and from the depositions given by men it is clear that he had systematically anticipated revenues from his tenants in

Dumfriesshire and was involved in some highly speculative business enterprises in England. Mary was silent about these, either through ignorance or because it was not her place to pass remark on what was not within her sphere. According to the physician Alexander Monro, in an advice manual written for his daughter's benefit: 'The household economy is certainly the wife's province'.[12] Whether women like Mary Goldie had internalised this view of their role because she did not want to encroach on – or had simply been excluded from mentioning – a male preserve, the division of perceived or experienced roles between domains or spheres is clear.[13] Gendering in the discussion of business affairs shows that this sphere was, in a sense, 'private' to men whereas the household (which also had a public face) was particular to women.[14] This is a surprising finding in view of the overwhelming evidence that early-modern women were actively involved in economic affairs either as workers or, for the better off, as 'interventionist house-managers' or as the keepers and recorders of household and business accounts.[15]

This argument can be extended into a related area. Witnesses only thought fit to comment about capacity to 'work' (as opposed to 'manage affairs') when talking about females. Two women, one young and one old, looked after Barbara Hill. Both thought her 'in a state of idiocy, unable to utter a word of sense or to do any kind of work not even to put off and on her own clothes'.[16] To be sure, idleness was frowned upon in both sexes, but the social construction of profitable pastimes varied between men and women. While the word was the same, men's 'work' was different from women's. The Royal Lunatic Asylum, Montrose (chartered in 1810), drew two-thirds of its patients from the ranks of paupers. Males who chose to work were sent to the garden in summer while females: 'are much employed in spinning flax, and those who can enjoy such amusement, are allowed to read, draw, or play at draughts or cards, but never for money'.[17] One woman brought a brieve against herself in the 1720s in order to prove her mental capacity. She was described by a man who had known her since her infancy: 'He has heard her read distinctly, seen her work stockings and go about her other affairs as an ordinary woman uses to do, discourse and give pertinent answers'.[18] Prescriptive writings again reinforce this picture. In his advice to his daughter, Alexander Monro set out a section headed 'Women's Work'. 'Sowing, spinning, knotting, stockins, knitting, washing and dressing linens, platting caps, shaping frocks, gowns etc, pastry cookery and all the other parts of what is called Women's work are so evidently necessary to be known by every woman and so useful in all the different stations of life.'[19] There is, of course, a social class dimension here (and in many other aspects of identifying mental problems), but the gendered application of the word 'work' is telling.

Understandings of mad behaviour were certainly gendered, but not nearly as crudely as one might expect. As part of the evidence he gave to justify his conclusion that Cecilia Stevenson was 'silly or fatuous in mind', Mr John Aitken, physician in Edinburgh, 'presented a doll to her which she took in her hand, seemed very fond of it and betrayed her fondness in childish gesticulations'.[20] Before concluding that he was imposing a gendered criterion, it should be noted that six of the other eight witnesses were women. They were unanimous that, in their words, Cecilia was childish and silly. A widow who knew her opined: 'at no time did she behave herself in the manner as girls of her age did'. This statement is also a reminder that definitions of incapacity accommodated behaviour that changed with age as well as differed between classes and sexes. Some might torture the evidence and posit that the female witnesses were only imposing a male view of what women should be. Such an argument depends on unsubstantiated notions of false consciousness. Women were judged mentally incapable not by the standards of men, but of other women. Females were classed as insane not because they crossed patriarchally imposed boundaries, but because they transcended the norms of their own sex.

Male and female interpretation of women's economic incapacity was domestically located. The origin of their illness was held by those around them to lie with events in the same domain. Three of the twenty-eight women admitted to Dundee Asylum in the year beginning 1 April 1820 were said to have been made mad by 'domestic affliction', but no males were so labelled.[21] The same gendered pattern is visible at Glasgow where women like Esther McCallum were thought to have been turned mad because of unhappy marriages: she 'seems dissatisfied with her marriage and generally dwells on that subject'.[22] Marital break-up or abuse is mentioned in four other female cases admitted to Glasgow Asylum in its first year, but not at all for men. In a domestic context men handed out abuse rather than took it. In the month before he was admitted to Glasgow Asylum in October 1816 William Fife tried to cut his sister-in-law's throat and to strangle his own children.[23]

It is noticeable that emotional causes of insanity, notably bereavement, were more likely to be cited as an explanation of a female's descent into madness.[24] James Maxtone of Cultoquhey had grown up with Christian Graeme and both were over sixty years of age at the time she was 'cognosced' [literally 'recognised', but here 'certified']. After the death of her brother, Alexander Graeme, merchant in Glasgow, about thirty years before, Maxtone recalled: 'she fell into low spirits and shut herself up from society and in a short time thereafter she became totally deranged in her mind and insane... totally incapable of managing any matter of the smallest importance'.[25] In this context, Dr William Buchan's gendered outline of environmental aetiology (specifically grief-inspired madness) is telling.

> Nervous disorders often proceed from affections of the mind, as grief, disappointments, anxiety, intense study etc.... I have known more hysteric and hypochondriac patients, who dated the commencement of their disorders from the loss of a husband, a favourite child, or from some disappointment in life, than from any other cause... whatever weakens the body, or depresses the spirits, may occasion nervous disorders.[26]

Buchan's book, *Domestic medicine; or, the Family Physician...*, first published in 1769, was a best seller, running to twenty-one editions between then and 1813.

One emotion affecting both sexes was unrequited love, presented in the sources as a cause and symptom of derangement or melancholy for both men and women. A third of Robert Burton's 1621 *Anatomy of Melancholy* was devoted to 'love melancholy', though he conceived this as a masculine condition.[27] Burton reflected that love madness was 'Full of fear, anxiety, doubt, care, peevishness, suspicion, it turns a man into a woman.'[28] Men were more compromised than women were because, by losing their rationality, they became more feminine.[29] An emotion long viewed with a measure of suspicion, love became more respectable and more openly discussed during the second half of the eighteenth century. The man of sensibility could demonstrate sensitivity by loving, as for example in Henry Mackenzie's *The Man of Feeling* (1771), written and set in London by a Scots-born and Scots-educated author. The ninth edition of Buchan's *Domestic Medicine* (1786) has a passage 'of love' in the section 'of the passions'. The first edition has no such passage.[30]

Novels were being borrowed from Scottish university libraries (which were male space) from the 1750s, yet that literary form was seen as principally female. In works such as *Julia de Roubingé* (1771), Henry Mackenzie focused primarily on a female audience, though he was also trying to reach out to men. In *The Man of Feeling*, Harley is persuaded against his better feelings to visit London's Bethlem.[31] There he encounters a woman made mad by a parental veto on her marrying her lover, followed by his death of a fever soon after going to the West Indies to make his fortune. In the mid-eighteenth century and beyond, love was an open topic for discussion. At the end of the eighteenth century and the beginning of the nineteenth, stories about women who turned insane after losing their lovers became popular. James Hogg's *Three Perils of Woman* (Edinburgh, 1823) is an example,[32] while Dr Alexander Morison's *Outlines of Lectures on Mental Diseases* (Edinburgh, 1825) explored the connection between love and insanity at a scholarly medical level.[33] According to Helen Small, the woman who lost her mind became the most common representative figure of the insane in late-Georgian literature.[34] Until the late-eighteenth or early-nineteenth century, the dominant literary and artistic construction of madness had been male.[35]

In the documentary sources consulted for this study, being in love was never suggested as a cause of madness in itself, but it was thought that the frustration of thwarted emotions could result in odd behaviour. The few examples of 'love madness' in the court cases and asylum documents show that this particular emotion was attributed to both men and women. Among twenty-eight female and twenty-two male entrants to Dundee Asylum in its first year 'disappointment in love' was said to be the cause of the lunacy of one young person of each sex.[36] For both sexes, love could also be a symptom. The perception of love-madness in literature may have been increasingly gendered, but in the sources used here it was not.[37]

If emotional causation is more commonly attributed to women, it was only of men that over-indulgence in drink was cited as a proximate cause. Civil court witnesses only ever mention drink as an explanation or exculpation of erratic or exuberant behaviour among men. Among the causes of the largely manic behaviour displayed by the first entrants to Dundee Asylum 'intemperance' was attributed to eight of twenty-two men compared with just one woman out of twenty-eight – and even here it was coupled with 'hereditary predisposition'.[38] Not surprisingly, some historians have taken such attributions literally as evidence of the gendered nature of behaviour. 'Escaping through alcohol was a male behaviour pattern.'[39] The problem here is that the clinical validity of these explanations cannot be verified. Instead they are useful as social indicators. More accurately, drinking was conventionally thought to be a male preserve or only felt to be appropriate to use as an excuse for male mania.

Dissipation had a certain cachet for men, which it certainly did not for women. As Alexander Monro wrote to his daughter, discreet tippling was not unknown among the fairer sex. Monro nevertheless counselled: 'downright drunkenness… is so monstrous in women that few of these of condition [breeding] are guilty of it'.[40]

Scotland was not short of male or female drinkers. In the fourth volume of Paisley Town's Hospital Minutes there are two cases where men petitioned to be allowed to place their wives in the cells in order to keep them off strong drink – neither was said to be mad.[41] For example, John Smith alleged 'that his wife has fallen into the practice of immoderate drinking so as to become outrageous and violent on both her husband and children and petitioned that she be admitted for a time into the hospital in order that she may be kept from spirituous liquors'. Smith promised to pay for her keep and affirmed 'that he has the concurrence of his wife's relations and the sanction of the magistrates'.[42] Most Scots drank and excessive consumption took place among men and women.

Other pathologies affected both sexes. Men and women might both commit suicide, and a desire to end one's existence was seen as a strong indicator of derangement. Yet the civil court witnesses only attributed suicidal tendencies to men. It cannot be that women as a whole had internalised the convention that they should not contemplate self-violence, because some plainly did.[43] Among thirty-five women entrants recorded in Glasgow Asylum admission papers in 1815 one had tried to 'harm' herself and three had talked about it. Harming oneself can, of course, mean mutilation short of a full attempt at suicide ('parasuicide'), but it is clear from the context that the question was designed to elicit a reply about self-destructive tendencies.[44] Jane Ewing 'frequently wishes to be killed but does not attempt any violence on herself or others' while Mrs Allan from Airth 'mentioned that something advises her to go drown herself'.[45] Nevertheless, there remains a gendered element to the observations made. Men, who were perhaps unaware of a woman's desire for death or reluctant to make that attribution in writing, wrote most of the replies to the twelve questions posed about potential entrants. For there is a marked contrast between the sexes, a desire for suicide or an actual attempt being mentioned for one male in four of the fifty-two entrants over twelve months 1816-17.[46] As with drinking, there may have been more suicide among men than women, but the differences in the distribution of the underlying phenomenon cannot have been a great as the construction suggests.[47]

Newspaper evidence helps to refine understanding of the social constructions placed on suicide. Female suicide was apparently more newsworthy than male. An impressionistic sampling of turn-of-the-century newspapers shows many more reported suicides by women than men.[48] Perhaps this is a reflection of the 'real' suicide rate;[49] perhaps it was less shaming or financially damaging to a family if a woman was judged to have killed herself; perhaps it was reported because female suicide was thought particularly shocking. The last possibility is the most likely. The disparity between the attribution of suicidal leanings, and the reality of reported (or likely) suicide patterns suggests that it was thought inappropriate to attribute a desire to kill oneself to women. On the contrary, sisters like Mary Goldie could reinforce their nurturative image by warning about the possibility of suicide.[50] She spoke of her 'fears and apprehensions that Mr Goldie might make some attempt upon his life while under low spirits'.

'Low spirits' was one euphemism for depression in the rich and varied vocabulary of mental incapacity. People employed adjectives or nouns such as 'fatuous' or 'furious' or 'insane', which had specific legal meanings. There were also other more colloquial words such as 'daft', 'mad', 'idiotic', 'deranged', 'silly'; or phrases such as 'troubled in mind', 'void of reason', 'out of his senses', 'not right'. In addition there were terms that could be deployed of behaviour which was unusual without necessarily being psycho-pathological. Examples include 'raised', 'distempered', 'outrageous', 'crazed' (literally, broken), 'distracted', or 'wild'.[51]

The most striking thing about vocabulary is how little gendering there was. In medical theory there were psychosomatic conditions like hysteria that had once been thought specific to females.[52] However, the growing stress on hysteria as a nervous rather than a uterine complaint meant it was no longer regarded as sex-specific in the eighteenth century.[53] Similarly, the word 'mad' was not sex-specific, but it was certainly gendered. Used sparingly in any context, it was applied to women twice as often as to men. The only word that is sex-specific is 'vapour' or its derivatives. When asked to comment on the capacities of Margaret Crawford, Andrew Sproul, writer in Edinburgh, said he 'observed her to be constantly vapourish and imagining things that never happened'.[54] In Cheyne's opinion: 'when the symptoms are many, various, changeable, shifting from one place to another, and imitating the symptoms of almost every other distemper described, if they are attended with no other apparent, real determined original distemper... then they may properly be called *Vapours*'.[55] Cheyne wrote just prior to the Margaret Crawford case and at a time when others were commenting that vapours were becoming fashionable. To be 'vapourish' could indicate breeding.[56]

IV

Assumptions about social class are no less apparent in eighteenth-century identifications of mental incapacity. Women were not simply judged by the standards of other women. Their behaviour was also contrasted with females of comparable age and social status. The same is true of men and it is hard to maintain that a definition of abnormality belonging to one social class predominated over others. In civil court cognitions, a bourgeois or élite definition of incapacity predominated, but only in so far as it applied to the bourgeoisie or members of the professional and landed élite who formed the bulk of subjects. There was a dominant definition of mental incapacity, but it was not the only one because perceptions of inability were socially related.

These generalisations hold true for all walks of eighteenth-century life. William Adam, portioner of Slachristock, owned part of a small estate in Stirlingshire. Witnesses produced to prove his mental capacity (against his family's efforts to show he was simple and weak-minded) focused on his elementary business ability. John Brown told how he 'has sometime sold nails to William Adam the alleged idiot and that he [William] made the bargain and paid for them as other country men did and that he counted the money right enough'.[57] Another man observed that William sold butter and cheese at market, bought meal from him 'and paid for it as other country men did'. William Adam was judged as a countryman because that was his social position. He was a minor landowner who bought and sold produce and livestock, and collected rent. He could do that perfectly well, but his mind was too weak to resist impositions from his brother-in-law and he was cognosced to protect his property. Emphasising the socially relative nature of judgements of incapacity, and showing a measure of circumspection, a recently arrived neighbour said of William: 'he has known wiser men and greater fools than he'. Other farmers were similarly judged. Joseph Howie was a minor landowner with a farm near Glasgow whose behaviour was intermittently erratic. Witnesses in the case generally thought he ran his affairs rather well. His daughter Christian was no clearer about Joseph's circumstances than any other female talking about men's affairs, only offering that he 'was in use to have as good crops as others'.[58]

Notions of thrift and profligacy were similarly tied to occupation and social status. Criteria of ability to manage one's affairs depended on one's station of life, meaning that the allegedly incapable were judged according to their social position. In the case of William Adam, a land-owning farmer required basic numeracy and an ability to judge crops and livestock. To take other examples, a merchant had to be able to do advantageous deals, a surgeon-apothecary to weigh and dispense drugs in an appropriate and timely fashion. Robert Russell, merchant in Edinburgh, gave evidence in a Court of Session case to 'reduce' (reverse) some inappropriate and damaging contracts entered into by John Blair, son to the deceased John Blair, surgeon in Edinburgh. Russell told the court he 'thinks him a foolish man; that from his actions he judges him a silly weak man; that he has dealt with Mr Blair and found him not to prig [haggle] down the prices he asked, and took little notice of the quality of the things'.[59] Blair tried his hand as a merchant, apothecary and surgeon, showing little aptitude for any of these occupations because he was 'a weak scatter brained lad'. His time as a surgeon's apprentice was short. His master bought him a set of weights to weigh drugs, 'yet he made no use of the weights, but mixed the drugs at random; and that when the doctor had ordered him to carry medicine to a patient at night, he would delay sometimes going with it till next morning; and that the doctor said... [that] he would never do any good'.[60]

The more lowly were judged on their ability to labour and to serve. Peter Gilchrist laboured on the roads with Alexander Steill and averred that he: 'has always worked diligently at these roads and still continues to do so, and is peaceable and as able to do the business of the roads as any other person employed at them'.[61] Steill received the same wages as others and if, according to another witness, he had been able to work less hard than others it was because his brother kept him under-nourished. Alexander only did hard manual labour – breaking, loading, and unloading stones – but he did it competently. He was 'a good workman'.

Attempts to impose criteria of capacity appropriate to workmen on those of higher status were no more successful than trying to foist upper-class standards on the lowly. Take the case of Hugh Blair, the son and heir of a landowner from Kirkcudbrightshire in south west Scotland, whose arranged marriage was annulled in 1747 on the grounds that he lacked the wit to give that informed consent necessary to a valid union.[62] Mr Robert Monteith, minister at Longformacus, had seen him bringing stone from a quarry to build walls that did not enclose anything and thus served no purpose. A weaver, Andrew Taggart, did not question the purpose of the wall. Instead he confined himself to a consideration of whether it was 'ill or well built'. It is possible that Hugh really was competent at building dry-stone dykes, but, without guidance, his erections had no function. One of the Blair tenants thought Hugh a good worker in the fields: 'in time of harvest the said Hugh helps to stack the corn when the deponent who was stacking could not over take it and that any stacks he put up appeared to the deponent at a distance to be as well set as his own'.

In the end, it did not really matter whether Hugh was good with his hands. His labours outside the home generally seemed to have no purpose, to be based on imitation rather than understanding, and to have been compulsive rather than discriminating. Almost every witness picked out some apparently trivial or pointless act: he 'frequently brought in ash wands to use as flails on the corn sheaves but they were quite unfit for that purpose. Sometimes he used scrap cloth and wood to make windmills such as bairns [children] ordinarily divert themselves with or are stuck up in corn fields to frighten away the birds... sometimes [he] tried to mend wheelbarrows with these scrap materials.' Those who opined that Hugh could fix the latch of the kitchen door 'as sufficient as any tradesman would have done', build stacks of cut corn, erect dry-stone walls as well as anyone, or carry stones to fill a hole in the road, ignored the fact that such manual tasks were inappropriate for a landowner's eldest son. There were many other examples of activities unsuited to a landowner. On a visit to Kirkcudbright town, a witness saw him sitting upon a stair foot beside an 'apple wife' who was selling her fruit, and remarked that this was 'a very odd place for a gentleman to sit'. There were other indicators that Hugh did not know how to behave correctly for a man in his social position. Poor people might gather dried dung for their fires, but those of Blair's standing bought peat, wood, or coal for heating. Had they required such fuel, they would not have gone looking for it themselves as Hugh often did.

An example from the top of the social hierarchy reinforces the class-related definition of incapacity. Dr Charles Stuart, an elderly Edinburgh physician, opined that Francis Stuart, Lord Doune, 'would be very liable to imposition; that any person might be disposed to practice upon him', and that he was 'incapable of judging between what might be for his benefit and what would prove injurious to him'. Stuart was cognosced just before his twenty-first birthday when he was legally still a minor, but he had title and lands in his own right and required a curator to sanction his actions.

Towards the end of his evidence, Dr Stuart told how well educated his namesake was. He could translate English into Latin and French into English 'but in the transactions of life the deponent should consider Lord Doune as incapable of management even if he stood in a much lower rank of society'.

Social constructions of insanity were based on nuanced and contextualised ideas about appropriate behaviour for a certain social class and sex. To this can be added a person's age. To use a case cited above, Cecilia Stevenson did not behave like other young women of twenty years old who came from a professional background. In another inquest Dr Alexander Monro told how he called to see David Balfour Hay at his mother's house in 1801. Hay had been wounded in Holland. Monro found: 'he complained much and seemed much alarmed about himself, more than is usual with young men, particularly those of the army and he seemed rather to be confused in his ideas'.[63] Fine gradations can also be found in the trials of criminal lunatics. As evidence of Robert Thomson's unusual mental state the teenager Elizabeth Dickson opined that he: 'used for the most part to be very sorrowful and not merry as other young men of his age were'.[64]

Medical writers reinforced such conventional judgements. An anonymous physician, writing in the second half of the eighteenth century, believed that in the young 'we may suppose the motion of the spirits brisk and free, the temper of mind is suitable; cheerful, merry, frolicsome, kind, generous, prodigal, full of hope, daring, bold and heedless', but in old age 'grave, serious, froward, selfish, unfeeling, full of doubt, distrust and caution'.[65] Eighteenth-century physicians were well aware of age-related patterns of mental problems. George Cheyne believed that those who passed the 'meridian of life' (thirty-five or thirty-six) without any 'mortal distemper' would probably not develop one.[66] Robert Whytt opined that 'old people, in whom the nerves have become less sensible, are little afflicted with those disorders', citing Cheyne in his support.[67] Andrew Duncan's lectures also covered the characteristics of the melancholic temperament and the stages of life at which it commonly occurred.[68] Yet, if certain disorders appeared to spare the elderly, old age could have other deleterious effects. William Cullen classified: '*amentia senilis* [as] from decay of perception and memory, in old age'.[69] However there were otherwise no disorders where age was a formally defining characteristic. Dr Peter Wright, physician in Glasgow, was rare in offering both a diagnosis and a cause that specifically mentioned old age: 'he observed that the said Rebecca

Glen was altogether or in a great measure in a state of childhood and deprived of her memory and judgement... [and that] her fatuity foresaid proceeds from a failing in nature'.[70] His comment reflects the conventional assumption that somatic factors influenced psychology: in the Glen case it was evident physical degeneration in a woman aged seventy-two years.

V

Klaus Dörner has claimed that contemporaries called people mad when they really meant something else.

> The Age of Reason... put all forms of unreason, which in the Middle Ages had been part of a divine world and in the Renaissance a secularising world... beyond the pale of the rational world – under lock and key. Beggars and vagabonds, those without property, jobs or trades, criminals, political gadflies and heretics, prostitutes, libertines, syphilitics, alcoholics, lunatics, idiots, and eccentrics, but also deflowered daughters, and spendthrift sons were thus rendered harmless and virtually invisible.[71]

This chapter offers no support to such an argument. Far from being 'an arbitrary matter',[72] or 'imprecise and... freely adaptable',[73] the definition of lunacy or idiocy was rather precise. Not every 'idle or eccentric person [was called] either a madman or a fool',[74] but nor was the choice contemporaries made based on an accidental or random attribution of those labels to anyone of whom they did not approve. Instead they applied them to those who displayed certain rather specific patterns of speech and action, which betrayed an underlying lack of rationality. While most or even all eighteenth-century Scots had the potential to be thought insane, not all were. Witnesses and jurors, comprising friends, neighbours, acquaintances and strangers, reaffirmed their own normality by pronouncing on the madness of some and the sanity of others, rather than indiscriminately defining all who came before them as mad or stupid. Scottish society had many simple means, formal and informal, of disciplining anomalous behaviour. If an accusation of madness is seen as a way of disciplining deviants, then it becomes necessary to explain why this was used in preference to some other weapon. An accusation of mental incapacity is best seen as a direct result of the accuser perceiving the accused to have mental problems, rather than an indirect result of some other factor such as the accused's wealth, sex, or religious beliefs.[75]

Social class and sex were, nevertheless, relevant to both identifying madness and attributing a cause to it. The propensity to define someone as insane might be a reflection of the threat their behaviour poses to certain power structures, but that is only one understanding of the relationship between sufferers and those who identify them. Indeed, the cornerstone of definition for eighteenth-century people was that insane behaviour was beyond the control of the sufferer.[76] The insane or mentally disabled were not simply unusual in belief and behaviour, but suffered from a defect of judgement which made the basis of their speech and action irrational. Thus, madness can only ever have been an implicit social protest.

The social constructions which sane people placed on the behaviour of the insane are better seen as indications of their expectations about normality based on a condition they regard as 'real', but pathological and worthy of care and treatment.[77] In this sense, identifying madness was not an oppressive act, but one that can nevertheless tell the historian about social values. Rather than providing evidence of a crude bourgeois and/or male conspiracy, understandings of mental incapacity in eighteenth-century Scotland reveal in a subtle and nuanced way the nature and extent of distinctions between people based on their social status, occupation and sex. The process of identifying mental incapacity tells the historian much about the perceptions of the sane, but the way they rationalised the judgement of incapacity was crucially determined by the class and sex of the person so defined. Just as the mad were treated according to their wealth and status when in asylums, so did their social position determine the process of formally identifying their mental disability.[78]

Notes

1. The research on which this chapter is based was made possible by funds provided by the Trustees of the Leverhulme Foundation. I am grateful to David Adamson, Jonathan Andrews, Elizabeth Foyster, Mark Jackson, Marjorie Levine-Clark, Sarah Pearsall, Alexandra Shepard, Lorraine Walsh, Oonagh Walsh, David Wright and Keith Wrightson for comments on earlier drafts and to the seminar audiences in the universities of Adelaide, Cork, Liverpool, and Manchester Metropolitan where much earlier versions were delivered as papers. A complementary article to this chapter has appeared. R. A. Houston, 'Madness and Gender in the Long Eighteenth Century', *Social History*, 27 (2002), 309–26.

2. T.S. Szasz, *The Myth of Mental Illness: Foundations of a Theory of Personal Conduct* (New York: Harper & Row, 1961); Szasz, *The Manufacture Of Madness. A Comparative Study of the Inquisition and the Mental Health Movement* (London: Routledge and Kegan Paul, 1971); R.E. Vatz and L.S. Weinberg, 'The Rhetorical Paradigm in Psychiatric History: Thomas Szasz and the Myth of Mental Illness', in M. S. Micale and R. Porter (eds), *Discovering the History of Psychiatry* (Oxford: Oxford University Press, 1994), 311–30; K. Dörner, *Madmen and the Bourgeoisie. A Social History of Insanity and Psychiatry* translated by J. Neugroschel and J. Steinberg (Oxford: Oxford University Press, 1981. First published 1969); P. Chesler, *Women and Madness* (New York: Avon Books, 1972); E. Showalter, *The Female Malady: Women, Madness, and English Culture, 1830-1980* (London: Virago, 1987).

3. For critical overviews see N. Tomes, 'Feminist Histories of Psychiatry', in M.S. Micale and R. Porter (eds), *Discovering the History of Psychiatry* (Oxford: Oxford University Press, 1994), 348–83. See also M.S. Micale, 'Hysteria and its Historiography: a Review of Past and Present Writings (II)', *History of Science,* 27 (1989), 319–51; M. MacDonald, 'Women and Madness in Tudor and Stuart England', *Social Research,* 53, 2 (1986), 261–81; A. Laurence, 'Women's Psychological Disorders in Seventeenth-Century Britain', in A. Angerman *et al.* (eds), *Current Issues in Women's History* (London: Routledge: 1989), 203–19; C. Vanja, 'Gender and Mental Diseases in Early Modern Society: the Hessian Hospitals', in L. de Goei and J. Vijselaar (eds), *Proceedings of the 1st European Congress on the History of Psychiatry and Mental Health Care* (Rotterdam: Erasmus Publishing, 1993), 71–5; J. Busfield, *Men, Women and Madness: Understanding Gender and Mental Disorder* (London: Macmillan, 1996). See also J. Busfield, 'The Female Malady? Men, Women, and Madness in Nineteenth Century Britain', *Sociology,* 28 (1994), 259–77.

4. Houston, *op. cit.* (note 1), 313–17.

5. Busfield, *Men, Women and Madness, op. cit.* (note 3), 25–7 and elsewhere, deals with social class and the distribution of mental disorder in more modern times. Her analysis, while excellent, approaches this subject from quite a different angle to that of this chapter.

6. R.A. Houston, '"Not Simple boarding": Care of the Mentally Incapacitated in Scotland During the Long Eighteenth Century', in P. Bartlett and D. Wright (eds) *Outside the Walls of the Asylum: the History of Care in the Community, 1750-2000* (London: Athlone,

1999), 19–44; Houston, 'Institutional Care for the Insane and Idiots in Scotland before 1820', *History of Psychiatry*, 12 (2001), 3–31, 177–97. There is an interesting new slant on this topic in an article on Germany, A. Goldberg, 'Conventions of Madness: *Bürgerlichkeit* and the Asylum in the Vormärz', *Central European History*, 33, 2 (2000), 173–93.

7. All source types are discussed in detail in R.A. Houston, *Madness and Society in Eighteenth-Century Scotland* (Oxford: Oxford University Press, 2000), chapter 2.

8. *An Introduction to Scottish Legal History* Stair Society vol. 20 (Edinburgh: Stair Society, 1958), 170–3. P. Gouldesbrough, *Formulary of Old Scots Legal Documents* Stair Society 36 (Edinburgh: Stair Society, 1985), 74. W. Bell, *Dictionary and Digest of the Law of Scotland* (4th edition, Edinburgh: Bell & Bradfute, 1838), 112–13. D.M. Walker (ed), *The Institutions of the Law of Scotland... by James, Viscount of Stair... 1693* (Edinburgh: Stair Society, 1981), 702-11.

9. For a full discussion of the procedure see R.A. Houston, 'Professions and the Identification of Mental Incapacity in Eighteenth-Century Scotland', *Journal of Historical Sociology*, 14 (2002), 441–66.

10. T.G. Davies, 'Judging the Sanity of an Individual: Some South Wales Civil Legal Actions of Psychiatric Interest', *National Library of Wales Journal*, 29 (1996), 455.

11. National Archives of Scotland (NAS) SC39/47/2, Alexander Goldie (1765).

12. P.A.G. Monro (ed), 'The Professor's Daughter. An Essay on Female Conduct by Alexander Monro (*primus*)', *Proceedings of the Royal College of Physicians of Edinburgh*, 26, 1 (1996, supplement 2), 104.

13. M.B. Norton, 'Eighteenth-century American Women in Peace and War: the Case of the Loyalists', *William and Mary Quarterly*, 33 (1976), 386–409, offers a similar finding, albeit based on claims from loyalist American exiles in England, 1774–89. She observes: 'what the women displayed were relative degrees of ignorance... [of] the broader aspects of their families' financial affairs' (397). She concludes (408–9) that 'late-eighteenth-century women had internalised the roles laid out for them in polite literature of the day. Their experience was largely confined to their households, either because they chose that course or because they were forced into it'.

14. MacDonald, *op. cit.* (note 3), 273, writes of early-modern England that people tended 'to see normal sex roles manifested in abnormal behavior'. R.A. Houston, 'Women in the Economy and Society of Scotland, 1500-1800', in R.A. Houston and I.D. Whyte (eds), *Scottish Society, 1500-1800* (Cambridge: Cambridge University Press,

1989), 118-47; R. Marshall, *Virgins and Viragos. A History of Women in Scotland from 1080 to 1980* (London: Collins, 1983). See also S. Hindle, 'The Shaming of Margaret Knowsley: Gossip, Gender and the Experience of Authority in Early Modern England', *Continuity and Change*, 9 (1994), 391–419, esp. 392, 408–9.

15. A. Vickery, 'Golden Age to Separate Spheres? A Review of the Categories and Chronology of English Women's History', *Historical Journal*, 36 (1993), 383–414, offers a lucid discussion of this issue. Pages 409-12 are particularly relevant to the origins and nature of the 'separation of the public sphere of male power and the private sphere of female influence'. L.E. Klein, 'Gender and the Public/Private Distinction in the Eighteenth Century: Some Questions about Evidence and Procedure', *Eighteenth-Century Studies*, 29 (1995), 97–109, warns of the perils of dichotomisation.

16. NAS SC49/57/4, Barbara Hill (1776). L.K. Kerber, 'Separate Spheres, Female Worlds, Woman's Place: The Rhetoric of Women's History', *The Journal of American History*, 75 (1988), 9–39.

17 *PP* 1816, VI, 376. See L.D. Smith, *'Cure, Comfort and Safe Custody': Public Lunatic Asylums in Early Nineteenth Century England* (London: Leicester University Press, 1999), 227–46, on the provision of 'useful occupations' in early-nineteenth-century English public asylums.

18 Edinburgh City Archives, Merchant Company no. 264. NAS SC39/36/1, Bessie Watson (1723).

19. Monro, *op. cit.* (note 12), 12.

20. NAS SC39/37/9, Cecilia Stevenson (1783).

21. *First Report… Dundee Asylum… 1820-1*, 5.

22. Greater Glasgow Health Board (GGHB) HB13/7/183.

23. GGHB HB13/7/184. Frances, Countess of Mar, was declared a lunatic in March 1730, having married John Erskine in 1714. According to her brother-in-law, she declared: 'in the beginning of her illness, loudly and oftner than once, that her husband's bad usage had turned her mad'. Quoted in *The Complete Peerage*, 8 (London, 1932), 428. Showalter, *op. cit.* (note 2), 3, takes such causal attributions literally, rather than treating them as socially constructed understandings.

24. E. Malcolm, 'Women and Madness in Ireland, 1600-1850', in M. MacCurtain and M. O'Dowd (eds), *Women in Early Modern Ireland* (Edinburgh: Edinburgh University Press, 1991), 324, finds a similar emphasis among the writings of William Hallaran about Cork Asylum. Smith, *Public Lunatic Asylums*, 105–7, 110–1, also notes the emphasis on emotional causes for English females in the early-

nineteenth century, though the analysis lacks statistical support.

25. NAS SC49/57/5, Christian Graeme (1787).

26. William Buchan, *Domestic Medicine; or, the Family Physician...* (Edinburgh: Balfour, Auld and Smellie, 1769), 509.

27. See L. Gowing, *Domestic Dangers: Women, Words and Sex in Early Modern London* (Oxford: Oxford University Press, 1996), 176–7, for examples of gendering within love madness in seventeenth-century England. Malcolm, *op. cit.* (note 24), 318–21, chooses to stress sexual lust rather than love as an ultimate cause in Irish women. This may be because female sexuality was perceived as more aggressive by males in the seventeenth century than it was to be in the eighteenth century. Vanja, *op. cit.* (note 3), 74, stresses female chastity (or its absence) as a prime indicator of madness in early-modern Hesse, along with violations of norms about dress and discrete behaviour.

28. Quoted in E.A. Foyster, *Manhood in Early Modern England: Honour, Sex and Marriage* (London: Longman, 1999), 56.

29. G. Rousseau, 'Depression's Forgotten Genealogy: Notes towards a History of Depression', *History of Psychiatry*, 9 (2000), 71–106, uses literary sources to argue that melancholy was conceived in female terms in the sixteenth and seventeenth centuries and only became integrated with male madness in the eighteenth century.

30. The addition was made to the second edition. C. J. Lawrence, 'William Buchan: Medicine Laid Open', *Medical History*, 19, 1 (1975), 22.

31. H. Mackenzie, *The Man of Feeling* (1771) (ed.) B. Vickers (Oxford: Oxford University Press, 1967), 29–35.

32. J. Hogg, *The Three Perils of Woman, or Love, Leasing, and Jealousy* (1823) (ed.), D. Groves, A. Hasler, and D. S. Mack (Edinburgh: Edinburgh University Press, 1995). See especially circles 7 and 8 of 'Peril First: Love'.

33. See H. Small, *Love's Madness. Medicine, the Novel, and Female Insanity, 1800-1865* (Oxford: Oxford University Press, 1996), 33–71. For further discussion, see R. Porter, 'Love, Sex, and Madness in Eighteenth-Century England', *Social Research*, 53 (1986), 211–42. Porter notes that sex was almost never an attributed cause of madness in England until the nineteenth century, a finding which would seem also to apply to Scotland. Showalter sees the repression of female sexuality as a core goal of Victorian psychiatry. Showalter, *op. cit.* (note 2), 75–6 and *passim*.

34. Small, *ibid.*, 33–71.

35. J.E. Kromm, 'The Feminization of Madness in Visual Representation', *Feminist Studies* 20, 3 (1994), 507-35. Showalter,

op. cit. (note 2), 8; C.T. Neely, '"Documents in Madness": Reading Madness and Gender in Shakespeare's Tragedies and Early Modern Culture', *Shakespeare Quarterly*, 42 (1991), 315-38. According to MacDonald, sixteenth- and seventeenth-century English madness 'wore a masculine visage'. MacDonald, *op. cit.* (note 3), 262.

36. *First Report… Dundee Asylum… 1820-1*, 5. Alexander Crichton, *An Inquiry into the Nature and Origin of Mental Derangement*, 2 vols. (London: T. Cadell & W. Davies, 1798), vol. 2, 319–20, cautioned that disappointed or unsuccessful love caused madness much less frequently than was commonly supposed, because grief was a temporary phenomenon.

37. See M. MacDonald, 'Ophelia's Maimèd Rites', *Shakespeare Quarterly*, 37 (1986), 309-17, on the misuse of historical context by literary scholars.

38. *First Report… Dundee Asylum… 1820-1*, 5. See A. Digby, 'Quantitative and Qualitative Perspectives on the Asylum', in R. Porter and A. Wear (eds), *Problems and Methods in the History of Medicine* (London: Croom Helm, 1987), 165–7, on the problems of interpreting asylum records about causation. Malcolm, *op. cit.* (note 24), 324, finds a less gendered attribution of causes at Cork Asylum, 1798-1818, at least regarding alcohol abuse. However, admissions to St Patrick's Hospital Dublin, 1841-50 more closely resemble the sex-related causes found for Scotland. *Ibid.*, 326-8.

39. Y. Ripa, *Women and Madness. The Incarceration of Women in Nineteenth-Century France* (Cambridge: Polity Press, 1990 translation), 78.

40. Monro, *op. cit.* (note 12), 56.

41. Paisley Main Library, Town Hospital Minute Books, 1801-19, 4 May 1807, 7 January 1817.

42. *Ibid.*, 7 January 1817. For another example see 4 May 1807. There are also examples of wives asking for their alcoholic husbands to be detoxified.

43. Ripa, *op. cit.* (note 39), 77-8.

44. Modern suicidologists have another category – 'subintentioned death' – which includes, for example, alcoholics who are aware that they are damaging their health, but refuse to desist or seek help. G. C. Davison and J.M. Neale, *Abnormal Psychology* (1974. 6th edn, New York: Wiley, 1994), 250–1.

45. GGHB HB13/7/183.

46. GGHB HB13/7/1. HB13/7/184.

47. Modern American studies show that between three and four times as many men as women kill themselves, but three times as many

women as men attempt suicide without dying. Davison and Neale, *op. cit.* (note 44), 249. Of seventeenth-century England, Laurence, 'Women's Psychological Disorders', 214, notes that 'Suicidal feelings... are more often mentioned in women's diaries and testimonies than men's'.

48. The subject was much discussed around this time, with the publication of Charles Moore's substantial work and a host of lesser contributions, including 'Historical Remarks on Suicide', *The Edinburgh Magazine*, 14 (December 1799), 446–9.

49. While there is no research on this topic for eighteenth-century Scotland, it seems likely that more males than females took their own lives. Estimates of the extent of the sex imbalance vary. M. MacDonald and T.R. Murphy, *Sleepless Souls. Suicide in Early Modern England* (Oxford: Oxford University Press, 1990), 247, suggest a ratio of approximately two males to every female for England. P.E.H. Hair, 'Deaths from Violence in Britain: a Tentative Secular Survey', *Population Studies* 1 (1971), 15–16, offers historical estimates for England ranging from parity to 4:1. In the third quarter of the nineteenth century males in England and Wales were three or four times as likely to commit suicide as females. However the rate of female suicide was higher in Scotland and among the highest in Europe. S.A.K. Strahan, *Suicide and Insanity* (London: 1894), 177–8. Vanja, *op. cit.* (note 3), 73, says that in her study 'all the melancholic men and women tried to commit suicide', but gives no further information.

50. On the neglected role of females as carers for the mentally disabled see Houston, *op. cit.* (note 6), 41–3. It is suggested that the quasi-professional standing of female madhouse keepers gave them an authority that transcended the normal limitations of their sex in a profoundly gendered society.

51. For a brief general discussion of terms see A. Leff, 'Clean Around the Bend: the Etymology of Jargon and Slang Terms for Madness', *History of Psychiatry*, 11 (2000), 155–62.

52. G. B. Risse, 'Hysteria at the Edinburgh Infirmary: the Construction and Treatment of a Disease, 1770-1800', *Medical History*, 32 (1988), 1-22. K.E. Williams, 'Hysteria in Seventeenth-Century Case Records and Unpublished Manuscripts', *History of Psychiatry*, 1 (1990), 383–401, shows for England that this idea had its roots in the seventeenth century. Some doctors thought men could be sufferers while medical representations of the condition being confined to women who were not sexually active was not replicated among recorded cases. See also R. Whytt, *Observations on the Nature,*

Causes, and Cures of the Disorders which have been Commonly called Nervous, Hypochondriac, or Hysteric (Edinburgh: J. Balfour, 1765); R.A. Houston, 'Therapies for Mental Ailments in Eighteenth-Century Scotland', *Proceedings of the Royal College of Physicians of Edinburgh,* 28 (1998), 555–68.

53. This point is driven home for the nineteenth century by M.S. Micale, 'Hysteria Male/Hysteria Female: Reflections on Comparative Gender Constructions in Nineteenth-Century France and Britain', in M. Benjamin (ed), *Science and Sensibility: Gender and Scientific Enquiry, 1780-1945* (Cambridge: Basil Blackwell, 1991), 200-39. See also J. Oppenheim, *'Shattered Nerves': Doctors, Patients, and Depression in Victorian England* (Oxford: Oxford University Press, 1991).

54. NAS SC39/36/2, Margaret Crawford (1737).

55. G. Cheyne, *The English Malady: or a Treatise of Nervous Diseases of all Kinds, as Spleen, Vapours, Lowness of Spirits, Hypochondriacal, and Hysterical Distempers etc.* (London: G. Strahan, 1733), 192–204: 'Of the spleen, vapours, lowness or spirits, hysterical, or hypochondriacal disorders'. Quotation at 195–6. Symptoms included restlessness and dispiritedness as well as physical signs. *Ibid.,* 205–17.

56. R. Porter, *Mind-Forg'd Manacles. A History of Madness in England from the Restoration to the Regency* (Harmondsworth: Penguin, 1987), 86. See also 50–1, 105–6, and V. Skultans, *English Madness. Ideas on Insanity, 1580-1890* (London: Routledge and Kegan Paul, 1979), 28-9.

57. NAS SC67/42/1, William Adam (1723).

58. NAS SC36/74/1, Joseph Howie (1764).

59. Signet Library SP22/18, 'Answers for John Blair… 5 March 1756', 5.

60. Signet Library SP56/50, 'State of the process of reduction…', 36–7.

61 NAS SC39/47/6, Alexander Steill (1804).

62. R.A. Houston and U. Frith, *Autism in History. The Case of Hugh Blair* (Oxford: Blackwell, 2000).

63. NAS SC39/47/7, David Balfour Hay (1807).

64. NAS JC3/3, 18 June 1739.

65. Royal College of Physicians of Edinburgh, Anonyma 16, 22. See also W. Cullen, *First Lines of the Practice of Physic,* 4 vols (1778-84. 4th edition, Edinburgh: C. Elliot, 1784), vol. 3, 255. 'In youth, the mind is cheerful, active, rash, and moveable; but as life advances, the mind by degrees becomes more serious, slow, cautious, and steady; till at length, in old age, the gloomy, timid, distrustful, and obstinate state of melancholic temperament is more exquisitely formed.'

66. Cheyne, *op. cit.* (note 55), 22.
67. Whytt, *op. cit.* (note 52), 118.
68. A. Duncan, *Heads of Lectures on the Theory and Practice of Medicine* (4th edition: Edinburgh: Watson, Elder and Company, 1790), 180–1.
69. W. Cullen, *Nosology: or a Systematic Arrangement of Diseases… Translated from the Latin…* (Edinburgh: William Creech, 1800), 130-1. NAS SC39/47/4 and SC39/36/12, Frances Deans (1792).
70. NAS SC36/74/2, Rebecca Glen (1773). For another example of age-related mental failings see SC49/57/4, Barbara Hill (1776).
71. Doerner, *op. cit.* (note 2), 14–15.
72. *Ibid.*, 16. See also A.T. Scull, *The Most Solitary of Afflictions. Madness and Society in Britain, 1700-1900* (London: Yale University Press, 1993), 345-50. These findings do not support Digby's argument: 'Until the late nineteenth century there existed at best only a blunted perception of difference between the imbecilic and the harmless or chronic lunatic, or between the congenitally handicapped and the senile demented'; Digby, 'Contexts and Perspectives', 7. This study tends more towards Andrews, who argues for a more precise definition in the same volume; Andrews, 'Identifying and Providing for the Mentally Disabled', 65–87.
73. Szasz, *Manufacture of Madness, op. cit. (note 2),* xix.
74. Doerner, *op. cit.* (note 2), 16. Szasz, *ibid.,* 14–15. See also M. Ingram, '"Scolding Women Cucked or Washed": A Crisis in Gender Relations in Early Modern England?', in J. Kermode and G. Walker (eds), *Women, Crime and the Courts in Early Modern England* (London: University of North Carolina Press, 1994), 48–80. Ingram argues that accusations of scolding were directed specifically at 'disruptive behaviour well beyond the normal range', rather than broadly deployed: 'as an attempt to impose tight controls on women's speech'; *ibid.,* 67. Ingram makes clear the distinction between conscious abuse and insane actions, for which the accused could not be held responsible; *ibid.,* 71.
75. Similar points are made by S. Clark, *Thinking with Demons. The Idea of Witchcraft in Early Modern Europe* (Oxford: Oxford University Press, 1997), 108-11. The connection between madness and religion is discussed in Houston, *op. cit.* (note 7), ch. 7.
76. Busfield, 'The Female Malady?', *op. cit.* (note 3), 261. That madness and a lack of intent are linked is clearly shown by J.P. Eigen, 'Intentionality and Insanity: What the Eighteenth-Century Jury Heard', in W.F. Bynum, R. Porter and M. Shepherd (eds), *The Anatomy of Madness. Essays in the History of Psychiatry, Volume II:*

Institutions and Society (London: Tavistock, 1985), 34–49. Similarly the fact that apparently possessed young people demonstrated behaviour which implicitly inverted social conventions about their status does not necessarily mean that this was their intention. J. A. Sharpe, 'Disruption in the Well-Ordered Household: Age, Authority, and Possessed Young People', in P. Griffiths, A. Fox and S. Hindle (eds), *The Experience of Authority in Early Modern England* (London: Macmillan, 1996), 187–212. While allowing the possibility of 'genuine symptoms' Sharpe seems to assume that in most cases the possession could not be real and therefore all manifestations must either be affected or, if believed, learned 'along the culturally known and approved lines'. *Ibid.*, 204. Since Sharpe himself calls for psychiatric insights, it would seem that his argument does not allow the possibility of involuntary and genuine belief, albeit with culturally coloured manifestations.

77. A culturally focused approach is neatly justified by Hodgkin, who uses the term madness 'to invoke a constellation of ideas around mental disorder which have a degree of historical continuity, over and above the various diagnostic categories around which such disorder is constituted'. K. Hodgkin, 'The Labyrinth and the Pit', *History Workshop Journal* 51 (2001), 37–63: 57.

78. See Houston, '"Not simple boarding"', *op. cit.* (note 6), and Houston, 'Institutional Care', *passim.*

3

Gender and Insanity in Nineteenth-Century Ireland

Oonagh Walsh

The nineteenth century was a period of considerable social, political, and economic change in Ireland, change that was demonstrated with particular force in relation to the care of the insane. This chapter seeks to examine some of the means through which the insane were re-figured in nineteenth-century Irish society, and looks in particular at popular conceptions of danger, the gender specificity or otherwise of insanity, and the question of celibacy as a precipitating factor in mental illness. The chapter seeks to engage with the ongoing debate in the history of psychiatry over the relative importance of gender as a factor in the admission, treatment, and discharge of the insane.

Introduction

The nineteenth century saw dramatic changes within Irish society. From 1800 the new constitutional relationship established by the Act of Union altered English administrative attitudes towards Ireland, which had far-reaching economic, legal and social consequences. The early years saw the establishment of a Poor Law system,[1] the development of a national system of education,[2] and the consolidation of a medical service in the form of a dispensary system throughout the country.[3] Mid-century saw over five years of horrifying famine, accompanied by widespread starvation, disease and emigration, which altered irrevocably traditional Irish patterns of marriage, inheritance and social custom.[4] However, one of the most dramatic developments, as far as the history of medicine in Ireland is concerned, was the expansion of the pauper lunatic system. Twenty-two new institutions for the care of the pauper insane were constructed, the majority in the decades between 1820 and 1860, with a continual enlargement of individual asylums continuing throughout the century. In 1830 there were beds for 791 pauper lunatics in Ireland: by 1896 this had increased to 13,620.[5] There were also a small number of private asylums throughout the country, offering accommodation for a very limited number of private, paying patients. In 1853 these amounted to only 123 individuals,[6] with a further 300 paying patients housed in Swift's Hospital[7] and the Retreat.[8] Thus the bulk of Ireland's mentally ill were catered for in large, pauper institutions, which although they demonstrated certain regional differences,[9] operated under identical regulations and decrees, laid down by the office of the Lord Lieutenant.

This chapter seeks to examine certain gendered dimensions of the asylum system in nineteenth-century Ireland, both public and private. After setting the historical context, and in particular emphasising those aspects of change which directly impacted upon the respective status of men and women in Irish society, I will turn to a discussion of gender bias within the asylum system. My main concern is with the question of whether the process of institutionalisation favoured males or females, in terms of admission, treatment, recovery and release. I then want to discuss the concept of 'danger' and the insane, with particular reference to the gendered interpretation of the Dangerous Lunatics Act of 1838. This will be followed by an examination of certain gender-specific manifestations of insanity, especially those which were associated with marital status. The chapter relates principally to the 1850s and the 1870s, and draws upon the Asylum Inspectors' Reports, and the records of the Connaught District Lunatic Asylum in Ballinasloe, Co. Galway, as well as reports from the Central Criminal Lunatic Asylum in Dundrum, Dublin. A word about sources: While admission figures provide a useful guide to relative rates of mental illness for men and women, they are not infallible. A key complaint of the asylum inspectors was the lack of institutional accommodation available throughout the country. There were always more applicants than there were beds, so that the less serious cases were simply not admitted. The admission records which survive therefore provide a picture of the 'successful' cases, not necessarily one of actual need.[10] Admissions to Irish district asylums occurred in two main ways. The first, which accounted for a minority of cases, was through a process of application by a relative or friend of the patient to the asylum manager. The person seeking admission had to attest to the patient's inability to pay for their support, and agree that they, or another, would assume responsibility for the patient on release. The form had to be accompanied by a medical certificate indicating the patient's state of mind, and the manager (through the physician and the asylum board) had the right to refuse admission.[11] The second means was under the Dangerous Lunatics Act (DLA) of 1838, under which the majority of pauper patients were admitted, and over which the asylum authorities had little or no control, since they could not refuse to admit a dangerous lunatic. The DLA led therefore to a huge rise in admissions, many of whom were clearly not 'dangerous'.[12] This piece of legislation was to have the greatest impact upon the asylum system, and mark Ireland as distinct from the remainder of the United Kingdom. Here, lunatics admitted under the DLA were criminalised in addition to being tagged as insane, as they were admitted to prison before being transferred to the asylum.

I

In the aftermath of the Famine, Irish farmers and labourers began to adjust to changed circumstances. Not the least of these was an alteration in the system of property inheritance, which created after 1850 a large number of young men who had little prospect of ever becoming landowners or even tenants in their own right. Thanks to the abundant and easily-grown potato,[13] the subdivision of land in the early nineteenth century had been common, allowing for early marriage amongst the landless cottier class. In an industrially undeveloped country such as Ireland, there was a strong sense of obligation on the part of a father to divide his property amongst his children, a tendency which was noted by contemporary observers as fraught with potential dangers:

> One great obstacle to improvement... and which is too general in Ireland, is their notion of the *equal and unalienable right of all their children to the inheritance of their father's property, whether land or goods.*[14] This opinion, so just and reasonable in theory but so ruinous and absurd in practice, is interwoven in such a manner in the constitution of their minds, that it is next to impossible to eradicate it. In spite of every argument, the smaller Irish occupiers continue to divide their farms among their children, and these divide on, till division is no longer practicable; and in the course of two or three generations, the most thriving family must necessarily go to ruin.[15]

After the famine, however, the system of land inheritance altered, with a much more widespread adoption of the system of impartible inheritance. Broadly speaking, this resulted in large numbers of children facing two unpalatable options: emigration, or the prospect of remaining as a landless labourer either on the family farm, or as an employee on another holding. In theory, these changes in land inheritance should have had the most negative effect upon women, since after 1850 their chances of inheritance were greatly reduced. It has been argued that Irishwomen's standing deteriorated as land ownership became the 'distinguishing criterion for status': '...on general principle... as property, lineage and inheritance become more important concerns for the family, the position of women deteriorates and the authority of fathers and the position of sons within the family grows stronger'.[16] However, although women may have been largely excluded from the process of inheritance,[17] they appear to have adapted to, and indeed exploited, the options open to them in a more vigorous manner than their brothers. The most dramatic of these was, of course, emigration.[18] In fact, young single women formed the majority of emigrants from Ireland in the later nineteenth century, with a particularly heavy loss from the west of the country.[19] They prepared themselves from an early age for work abroad, taking full advantage of educational opportunities which would equip them for life in Britain, America and Australia.[20] Part of their willingness to leave the country entirely may stem from not merely an acceptance that they were unlikely to inherit property, but from the obvious fact that they would leave the family home in any case upon marriage. Women traditionally shared their in-laws' home, assuming responsibility for their husband's parents, and were therefore psychologically prepared for change.[21] Indeed it has even been suggested that Irishwomen had less close links with their mothers than Irishmen as a result of this expectation.[22] Whatever the truth, preparation for a life of relative mobility may be said to have made young Irishwomen, despite their limited economic opportunities, psychologically more resilient than men.

This would certainly appear to be supported on the evidence of admission figures to the Ballinasloe asylum. Although early work on the history of psychiatry suggests that women were the principal subjects of asylums, with Elaine Showalter in particular emphasising the apparent bias in female admissions over male,[23] it was in fact men who formed the majority of admissions throughout the nineteenth century. Between 1850 and 1880 for example, male admissions consistently outnumbered female, in certain years forming over sixty per cent of admissions, but never achieving parity.[24] Furthermore, it was young single men, those who under more prosperous economic circumstances would have been marrying and raising families, who filled the asylum at Ballinasloe.[25] In certain years, the unmarried made up almost eighty per cent of male admissions, suggesting that the stress of circumstances, and the frustration of expectations, may have influenced movement into the asylum.[26] These factors did not however appear to have the same impact upon both sexes, with women apparently coping rather better with post-famine changes than men.

Changes in land inheritance, it has been alleged, resulted in a greater degree of intermarriage in Ireland after the famine, as families attempted to keep property within a narrowly defined unit.[27] If a sustained pattern of intermarriage did indeed take place, one would expect an increase of hereditary insanity, the diagnoses feared most by the asylum authorities. The lunacy inspectors themselves noted a particular propensity towards insanity in families with a history of intermarriage:

> Having investigated into the history of lunacy as regards certain families, from our personal knowledge of the members affected by it in asylums, we would refer to continued intermarriages and direct hereditary predisposition, no inconsiderable amount of the cases that have come under our observation, the malady frequently developing itself in the third and fourth generation, and, what may appear extraordinary, leaving the second unaffected.[28]

In the nineteenth century, insanity was believed to be passed in the female line, although it could effect children of either sex equally. The forms of admission used to process patients thus paid particular attention to the question of a family history of insanity, and whether female patients had already had children. But did this fear of lunatics literally reproducing themselves have any basis in fact? The records at Ballinasloe suggest not. In the 1870s and 1880s, decades in which one might expect to see an increase in the number of patients suffering from hereditary insanity[29] the actual numbers thus diagnosed were few. They formed just eight per cent of the total admissions, and, most interestingly, males and females manifested hereditary insanity in exactly equal numbers.[30]

It was not just pauper institutions such as Ballinasloe which saw large imbalances in male and female patient numbers. As early as the 1850s, the Asylum Inspectors remarked frequently upon the great disparity in admissions to private asylums in Ireland, with men outnumbering women at proportions of three to one, and even four to one in some cases. Male predominance in private asylums may reflect their greater economic importance, and a greater willingness on the part of families to pay for their treatment. This would certainly appear to be borne out by the professions of individuals admitted to private institutions. In 1853, of 245 male patients throughout the country, the majority were in relatively high-earning occupations, had private incomes, or were in positions of considerable responsibility and authority.[31] However, it may also indicate that women could be more easily treated at home than men. This was clearly the case in pauper asylums, where one finds that men were more likely to be admitted for their first violent attack, and women both admitted at a later stage in their illness, and more likely to be removed from the institution frequently, than men.[32]

The inspectors made efforts to explain differences in admission rates in several ways. Many believed that men were simply more prone to violence and excess, but others offered alternative interpretations. One suggested for example that greater male numbers was a direct consequence of the freedom they enjoyed to indulge their vices: given the same opportunity, he implied, female numbers would correspondingly rise:

> This [excess of males], we think, may in some measure be accounted for by the fact, that in the more affluent grades of society, men, having greater opportunities and being under less personal control than females, indulge more frequently in a course of life which occasionally leads to that perversity of action and idea recognised under the term of moral insanity.[33]

However, the inspectors noted that although women were admitted to private asylums in fewer numbers, they tended to benefit disproportionately from conditions there:

> ...there exists a greater recuperative power among females admitted into private asylums than among males... Our experience would refer the explanation of this discrepancy to the fact that, while moral causes, such as grief, love, anxiety, disappointment, etc., etc., more largely predispose females of the better classes – from their superior education and more refined sensibilities – to mental disease, provided there is no fixed hereditary tendency to insanity, time, quietude, and, above all, absence from the immediate exciting causes, gradually effect a cure.[34]

In Ballinasloe, across the nineteenth century, women were released more frequently than men, and spent shorter periods of time in the asylum. On average, women spent between three and eight months there, and were more frequently released on the request of relatives than men. These figures pertain only to short-term patients. There is no gender difference as far as long stay inmates were concerned. For both men and women, residence within the asylum for longer than five years almost invariably meant that they would remain there until their deaths.

Although men and women displayed differing patterns of admission and release, what is clear from the evidence at Ballinasloe is that their illnesses were, in the majority of cases, prompted by the stress of immediate circumstances. In 1872, only eight out of a total of nineteen alleged causes of insanity had a physiological basis; the remainder were prompted by highly individual circumstances.[35] In other words, biology was less significant in terms of admission than factors such as economic position, family disputes, or what the forms of admission termed 'disappointments' of various kinds. However, men and women did appear to respond differently to certain shared circumstances.

In an impoverished country such as Ireland, with little industrial development and few large urban centres in comparison with England, poverty and its associated stresses were often suggested as possible causes of insanity. However, the impact of poverty was believed by inspectors to be far greater upon women than men. The forms of admission to Ballinasloe reflect this, with 'poverty' used in explanation for the admission of women much more than men. But a simple alteration of material circumstances did not eradicate the problem, for example, even when the immediate threat of starvation or destitution was removed – through the unpleasant expedient of admission to a poorhouse – women continued to suffer psychological stress linked to poverty:

> Of those classified as lunatics in poorhouses, nearly two-thirds are of the female sex. Generally speaking, they are harmless, decrepit, and chronic cases; occasionally, however, their malady assumes an active character, when the usual course is taken for their transmission to the district asylum to which they belong.[36]

It is difficult to draw an explicit link between impoverishment and insanity, particularly since many of the women designated insane in poorhouses were long-term residents who, towards the end of their lives, became senile or depressed. Entry to the workhouse was not therefore in the first instance a result of insanity, but of poverty. Women were indeed believed to be more vulnerable to the effects of abandonment and desertion than men, although there is in fact little evidence to suggest that the loss of a husband contributed significantly to mental illness amongst Irishwomen. Moreover, some historians have suggested that many of those women described as deserted, and admitted to institutions such as workhouses on the grounds that they had no other means of support, were in fact deliberately using the poorhouse system as a temporary means of respite in times of economic difficulty. This strategy was supported by their husbands, many of whom were working in England and Scotland.[37]

Despite this frequent uncertainty regarding diagnoses, a definite pattern of difference between male and female designation is clear. The most obvious is the division between patients described as suffering from insanity relating to moral causes, and those whose illness had a physical basis. Women formed on average almost seventy per cent of the former category throughout the country, while men accounted for almost sixty per cent of the latter. Moral causes included poverty related stress, grief, bereavement and so on, while physical causes ranged from injury to the head, sunstroke, over-exertion, and alcohol abuse. Indeed, this final category, intemperance, accounted for as many as half of the male admissions to Ballinasloe throughout the century, and the figures were even higher at other periods in various asylums throughout the country.[38] Given the concern prevalent amongst asylum authorities to pin-point the cause of insanity, they seized upon an apparently clear reason for female illness:

> Love, from misguided affections and disappointed hopes, is a much
> more fertile source of the disease, particularly among the female sex,
> who, from their habits and sensibilities, are more susceptible than
> men of those influences recognised under the designation of moral.[39]

But was this actually true? The presumption that women would be more likely to suffer from these types of moral pressures accorded with general nineteenth-century expectations of feminine behaviour.[40] In this way, social and cultural factors may have been more important in determining illness than biological predisposition. If the category of intemperance, which related almost exclusively to men, is removed, then one finds that men and women were diagnosed in almost equal numbers in the moral and physical categories.[41] There was a great deal of stigma associated with alcohol as far as nineteenth-century Irishwomen were concerned.[42] Women rarely frequented public houses,[43] and those who did were associated well into the twentieth century with prostitution. Thus their absence from the 'physical' category, and their over-representation in the 'moral', may be more accurately assigned to public hostility towards women and drink (and an allied acceptance of male abuse), than an actual accordance with typically Victorian expectations of behaviour.

II

If popular concepts of appropriate behaviour conditioned both asylum authorities and the general public to expect male and female illness to take distinct forms, then nowhere should this be more clear than in the application of the Dangerous Lunatics Act (DLA). I now want to turn to the issue of how lunatics, male and female, were represented, through the distorting prism of the DLA. The insane have been construed in the past as inherently dangerous, as indeed they often remain in the public imagination today.[44] But this was made explicit in nineteenth-century Ireland, where lunacy legislation automatically criminalised the insane, and labelled the majority of pauper inmates 'dangerous'. The Dangerous Lunatics Act allowed for the arrest of any individual 'discovered and apprehended... under circumstances denoting a derangement of mind, and a purpose of committing an indictable crime'. The subject was brought before two justices of the peace, and if they agreed that the 'accused' was indeed dangerous, they could have them admitted to Gaol and thence to the nearest district asylum.[45] There was no need to secure a medical opinion, and the gaol and asylum had no right to refuse admission to such a patient. This ease of committal rapidly ensured that it became the most common means of admission to Irish asylums, but its real danger lay in the power it placed in the hands of individuals to commit others. It also irrevocably designated these asylum admissions as 'dangerous', regardless of whether or not the individual had committed or even attempted a dangerous act. In fact, many patients admitted to institutions showed no evidence of violent or dangerous behaviour following admission,[46] and indeed were acknowledged by asylum staff to be entirely pacific. The question I now want to address is whether there was any discernible difference in perceptions of the danger posed by male and female lunatics, or if the simple act of charging an individual under the DLA overrode conventional gender expectations.

If we look at admissions to the Ballinasloe asylum in the 1870s, the picture is not immediately clear. The proportion of males and females admitted under the DLA varied from year to year, with for example thirty-one women and twenty-seven men designated 'dangerous' in 1872, and twenty-two women and forty-five men thus described the following year. However throughout the decade on average seventy per cent of women and almost eighty per cent of men were admitted to Ballinasloe under the DLA. Their reasons for admission varied considerably. The problem in determining degrees of danger is that the key evidence was provided principally by the person seeking the committal, who frequently made allegations which could not be independently checked. In fact, this accounted for the majority of cases admitted to Ballinasloe. Both the asylum inspectors and the representatives of law and order in Connaught[47] frequently stressed the need to remove dangerous lunatics from the community at large.[48] However, an examination of the admission warrants indicates that the threat represented by lunatics, both male and female, towards strangers, was actually very low. In 1872-3 there were eight attacks in total upon strangers, six of which were committed by men, and two by a woman. In one of the latter cases, a woman attacked an infant in the workhouse where she was an inmate, and the assault appears to have stemmed from the loss of her own child shortly before. Violence appears therefore to have been largely contained within the family, the main exception being those individuals who assaulted fellow inmates of workhouses (twenty out of 170). Within the family, sisters appear to have been least likely to be the target (in only six cases), and brothers the most (in twenty-two cases, with two additional instances of attacks on brother-in-laws). However, this may merely reflect the more active role taken by men in subduing patients. Parents of both sexes were equally likely to be attacked, although daughters appear less prone to commit parental assault. The increasing number of unmarried men and women in Irish society is also reflected in this pattern: in other countries, assaults by the insane appear to be against spouses to a much greater extent.[49] Thus individuals in a state of excitement, for whatever reason, appear to have attacked those nearest to them – their immediate family – and not strangers.

However, the most striking difference in gender terms with regard to the perceived and actual danger offered by lunatics occurs with regard to self-harm. There were twenty exclusively suicidal cases in the two years (1872-3), all admitted under the DLA, and eighteen of whom were women.[50] In addition, ten further women were noted as 'dangerous to self and others'; a designation applied to only four men. Thus in terms of the security of the public at large, women represented a relatively minor threat. Furthermore, much of the violence they offered was potential rather than actual, in that they far more frequently made verbal threats against family members than they attempted to carry out. One 19-year-old woman, for example, 'put [her mother] in fear and terror', according to the admission warrant, but the only evidence of insanity offered was that she 'is in the habit of going away and remaining away for some days'.[51] In a number of cases where an actual assault took place, it stemmed from attempts by others to prevent suicide, rather than as a premeditated attack on the part of the patient. A woman who 'did violently attack and bite, and otherwise assault [her husband]' on May 26, 1872, did so because he was 'endeavouring to prevent her from going to drown herself, which she is constantly threatening to do'.[52] Similarly a 16-year-old girl 'assaulted [her father] and others in a most violent manner', because they stopped her from burning herself and 'grasping a knife to cut her heart out'.[53] I do not wish to suggest that these instances of violent behaviour are somehow less significant than others, simply because they were self-directed, but I do want to stress that the type of violence offered by male and female patients could differ to a great extent.

III

Perhaps the clearest instance of gendered difference in relation to danger may be seen in the case of the Criminal Lunatic Asylum in Dundrum, Dublin. Opened in 1850 'for [the treatment of] insane persons charged with offences in Ireland',[54] the construction of the institution was prompted by a belief that criminal lunatics required particular supervision which was not available in the district asylums. However the Criminal Asylum was deliberately designed to encourage cure and rehabilitation, not merely to serve as a quasi-prison, and to this end it was less fortified than many of the district asylums.[55] As a consequence there were far more staff per patient than in the district institutions, and a greatly increased expenditure per patient as a result.[56] The inspectors urged that only the genuinely criminally insane be admitted – from the year it opened, some criminals attempted to use it as a means of avoiding imprisonment,[57] believing that they would be released without charge once they 'recovered'.[58] In fact, it was extremely difficult to secure release from the Criminal Asylum. The inspectors had to recommend each case to the Lord Lieutenant after the patient had been sane for a period of at least four years, and even then very few were liberated. Curiously, one of the keenest arguments in favour of the release of such inmates was a firm undertaking to emigrate.[59] This was inclined to result in the release of men rather than women, as most of those thus pardoned were men of considerable means, who could afford to go abroad to begin new lives for themselves.[60] For example, in 1892 a physician charged with the murder of his wife used his influential contacts to secure his release only six years after the murder, because he was able to show that he would emigrate to South Africa.[61]

Within the Criminal Asylum, male patients far outnumbered female. The institution was supposed to be reserved for 'cases of a grave character', and theoretically all lunatics convicted of a criminal offence could have been transferred there. However, the workings of the Dangerous Lunatics Act would have made the majority of asylum inmates eligible for admission to the Criminal Asylum, so the practical decisions regarding suitability were left to the discretion of the Lord Lieutenant. On a crude level, it is clear that one of the principal tests applied with regard to admission was the successful attempt to take life. The majority of patients admitted to the district asylums were accused of representing a threat to the lives of others, but these individuals either failed to carry out their threat, or were arrested before they could do so. Those convicted of murder but found insane on remand or at trial were sent to the Criminal Asylum. There was however a striking difference between the types of crimes committed by male and female inmates at the Criminal Asylum, which would seem to indicate a gendered division of insanity. What is particularly noteworthy is that contrary to the assertion that women were more prone to insanity as a result of physiology, they were in these cases judged to be acting under intolerable pressure which led to a temporary breakdown, from which they were likely to rapidly recover.[62] Men, on the other hand, were presented as labouring under more serious and less tractable types of illness, which had a higher relapse rate and were far more difficult to cure. Males were in the vast majority of cases convicted of crimes of violence, ranging from murder to assault. Women were convicted for crimes against property in the main, with the notable exception of those convicted of infanticide. More importantly, the women committed to Dundrum for the murder of their children were in almost all of the cases listed unmarried, and had concealed their pregnancies. The authorities were remarkably sympathetic towards these women, recognising the limits to which they had been pushed by the stigma of unmarried motherhood:

> Great commiseration is no doubt, due to many who come within this category; for we can fully imagine how shame and anguish must weigh on an unfortunate and betrayed female, with enfeebled system, what strong temptations induce her to evade the censure of the world in the

Table 3.1
Offences Committed by Patients in the Central Criminal Asylum,
1855 and 1857[63]

	Male	Female	Total
Homicide	60 (83%)	12 (17%)	72
Infanticide	0 (0%)	19 (100%)	19
Violent Assault	51 (81%)	12 (19%)	63
Burglary, Arson, etc.	57 (58%)	41 (42%)	98

destruction of the evidence of her guilt, by a crime that outrages her most powerful instinct, maternal love of her offspring.[64]

Even allowing for a high Victorian attitude to infanticide (the women are regarded more favourably because they clearly demonstrate signs of remorse and shame), there is nevertheless a clear recognition that stress led directly to the crime and, moreover, the insanity which accompanied it was short-lived and directed against a very specific target. This raised great difficulties with regard to the release of such women. Arguing that they deserved to be treated 'with the utmost leniency', the question remained: when could a person charged with such a serious crime safely be released? 'Is such a person – sane immediately after the act, sane at trial, and sane on admission – to remain for life – or, if not for life, for what period – the inmate of an asylum, and the associate of lunatics?'[65] It was the sheer unnaturalness of this act which convinced authorities that the woman posed no further threat.

The crimes committed by patients sent to the Criminal Asylum do suggest a gendered division of insanity, and a greater propensity towards violent crime on the part of men, as shown in Table 3.1. Male inmates of the Criminal Asylum were regarded as being far more dangerous than the female, and in fact several of the men had been convicted of multiple murders. By far the most common victim was the patient's wife – in 1855, eight out of nine men sent there for murder had killed their wives. Indeed, a plea of insanity was more likely to be accepted if the victim was a wife. Murder of strangers, or of non-family members, was likely to result in a straightforward murder conviction, with the individual sent either to prison or for execution.[66] However, the readiness to understand, if not excuse, infanticide in females points to a disturbing attitude towards the crime of murder. Infanticide was treated sympathetically because it

81

was so contrary to gendered expectations that it automatically implied an act of insanity. Wife-murder on the other hand was a more 'normal' crime, in that a man might commit it without being presumed insane. One last important point to be made regarding the gendered nature of insanity in Dundrum. The asylum inspectors presumed that men would be admitted to the institution in greater numbers than women, because of an alleged propensity towards violence. Thus more accommodation was set aside for male than female patients, with only one-third of beds reserved for women.[67] A gender bias was therefore, quite literally, built into the Dundrum asylum, a fact which raises questions regarding the importance of gender presumption on the part of officials when it came to evaluating the insane.

IV

It has been argued that 'marriage protected both men and women from asylum admission in nineteenth-century Ireland'.[68] Marital status was certainly an important factor in determining admissions and length of stay for each patient within the asylum. As mentioned above, regardless of sex, the unmarried were the most likely to be admitted to the asylum, and were most likely to remain there for the longest periods. However there is a striking difference between the experiences of married men and women, as far as permanent release from the institution was concerned. Married men were far more likely to be removed by their families, while married women stood a greatly increased chance of remaining there until their deaths. This would appear at first glance to run contrary to the popular perception of Irish motherhood in the nineteenth century, which placed a great deal of emphasis upon the sanctity of the home, and the crucial role played by the mother in maintaining the family unit. Between 1868 and 1881, 175 men and 147 women died in the asylum after stays of between three months and ten years. The marital status of these individuals is interesting. Of the men, almost seventy per cent were single. Of the women, however, just over fifty per cent were single. Married women were also admitted more frequently than married men. Throughout the nineteenth century, rates for the admission of married men rarely rose above thirty per cent of the male total. Married women on the other hand accounted on average for fifty per cent of female admissions. Thus marriage could be said to protect men from admission, but it clearly did not do the same for women. However, marriage did not make women any more vulnerable to admission than their single counterparts, and it did have the benefit of ensuring that they were removed more frequently from the institution. Even when families were grown, offspring were the most likely to seek the release of their mothers from the Ballinasloe asylum. The reasons for this greater willingness to remove mothers over fathers (aside from those cases of removal of husbands, as principal breadwinners) are unclear. It may be as simple as a greater sense of responsibility, or indeed affection, on the part of grown children, as in the case of a son, now resident in the United States, who sought the release of his mother some thirty years after her committal. She had actually been admitted for attempting to murder him as a baby, and by the time he reached adulthood, she no longer believed that she had any children. He was advised that to remove her would cause her great distress, so he left her in Ballinasloe, keeping contact with the staff there until her death.

Patients admitted to Ballinasloe suffered from a wide range of symptoms, and manifested their illnesses in all sorts of ways. However, marriage appeared to encourage certain, quite specific delusions, amongst particular patients. One interesting instance is the number of husbands who accused their wives, without foundation, of having affairs with other men, an accusation rarely made by wives against their husbands. For example, in a case admitted in June 1895, a man accused his wife both of attempting to poison him, and of having an affair with a local pensioner.[69] Another patient admitted the following month made a similar allegation, claiming in justification for stabbing his wife with a pitchfork that 'he saw a man in bed with his wife and would have stabbed him instead of his wife with the fork but that he [the other man] had a revolver with him and men at the windows watching to shoot him'.[70] The patient claimed that he had unimpeachable testimony as to his wife's infidelity: 'As well as he can understand his wife told the curate himself in his presence that she misconducted herself with a man; the priest can witness it; he [the patient] is overlooking it and also the people being behind the ditches to injure him'. Despite his claim the following year that 'he now professes himself ready to go back to live with his wife and mind his children "and will forgive all"', the physician judged that he had not recovered. In fact, his delusions[71] worsened, and he remained in the asylum until his death. Earlier in the year, another patient alleged that 'his wife was too great with several young men and that one of them was in bed with her one night and he watched till morning but could not catch him... He used [to] hear people saying things of her and heard his landlord was too free with his wife'.[72] The patient was suffering from religious delusions in addition to his suspicions regarding his wife. After six months in the asylum, the religious preoccupation diminished, 'but throughout a latent or repressed delusion against his wife persists'. He was nevertheless released, but was readmitted seven months later, after attempting to burn his wife and children alive in their home. Shortly after his readmission, his wife wrote a plaintive letter to the physician:

> Dear Sir, I beg pardon to trouble you again as I had a sade [sic] story every day since I brought home... my husband every day and night killing us. Me and my children should sleep in the out house and I trying to rare [rear] my family but I hope dear Doctor you will never let him out to punished [sic] me again... He burn [sic] the house over us.

In other cases, allegations that a wife had not given due deference to her husband were made in explanation for violent behaviour. One man who 'has recently taken to drink without any obvious reason and has been reduced to a state of purposeless indecision and restlessness by it' was admitted for attempting to stab his wife, himself and his daughter.[73] He was removed from the asylum by her on the first occasion, but he again attacked her with a pair of shears and was readmitted. The conflict between the spouses, which the patient alleged earlier was over 'monetary affairs', appears on closer examination to be perceived challenges to his paternal authority. In 1897 and 1898 he claimed to the physician that his wife had driven him to the asylum by her unreasonable behaviour. '[He] is distrustful of his wife and "doubts she might drink"... Says he "lost his spirit" when he went home and found how his wife squandered his money when he was away and sold a young horse he expected big money for and would give him no account of it: She would take other people's advice rather than his and go off drinking with women but not with men – he had nothing against her that way. He worked very hard all his life and "fortuned"[74] three sisters and got them married'. In 1909, a year before his death in the asylum, he still complained that 'his wife disobeyed his orders'. Thus the rebellious wife was the explanation for his illness, not any predisposing element in his own character.[75] There is of course another context for these anxieties regarding the trustworthiness of wives, and the dangers of assault from hidden watchers. From the late 1870s onwards, a campaign to further tenant rights emerged in Ireland. It depended upon agrarian outrages to a significant degree, and there were attacks upon crops

and livestock, as well as land agents and landlords.[76] The cases
described above may well reflect nothing more than male anxiety
regarding female sexuality, but the belief that men were hiding in
ditches, watching the house, and preparing to attack the patient, may
well be sparked by the very real danger which lay in wait for certain
individuals, especially in rural areas. It is noteworthy that women
were involved to a significant degree in Land League activities, often
playing a direct role in attacks.[77] The government were reluctant to
imprison women, fearing a backlash, with the result that female
activists met with less overt opposition to their activities.[78] This
greatly expanded role for women may have effected the manner in
which they were viewed by disturbed male relatives, leading to an
increased sense of threat.

Although marriage may have produced a particular set of
delusions, the unmarried faced their own particular problems. In the
nineteenth century many commentators believed that celibacy itself
was a possible cause of insanity. Noting that the single markedly
outnumbered the married in terms of admission to institutions, the
inspectors of asylums noted in 1853 that:

> ...independent of congenital mental disease, and that which
> supervenes before puberty, insanity may be regarded as an affection
> of the more early or marriageable rather than of the later stages of
> life; at the same time the unsettledness of a single state, particularly
> if attended with disappointments and the want of domestic
> occupations – may occasionally, at certain ages, and in certain
> constitutions, produce deleterious effects on the mind.[79]

However, there is little evidence to support this thesis when one
looks at the case of married women, who were, as noted above,
admitted to the asylum in almost equal numbers with single women.
It moreover presumes a typically Victorian attitude towards sexuality
– that men were adversely affected by a lack of sexual indulgence
(within the strict limits of marriage) while women were
comparatively unaffected.

The question of celibacy as a predisposing factor in insanity was
taken seriously by asylum inspectors, though. As the century
progressed, a curious feature of asylum admission began to come to
the attention of the authorities, which appeared to strengthen the
notion that an unmarried, celibate life, could be detrimental to
mental health. In 1853 it was noted that a significant minority of
patients in private asylums were clerics. Interestingly, it was not

asserted that religion itself was the exciting cause, rather the restricted lifestyle of the professed religious.

> ...we should say the proportion under the heading clerical or religious largely predominates, being possibly about the proportion of one lunatic to three hundred sane individuals in that immediate community; it would, however, be a mistake to assume that the delusions of the individuals in question turn on purely divine or metaphysical points, they almost invariably refer to much more sublunary objects. As an instance, indicative of the many, we might adduce the case of a most exemplary clergyman, now perfectly recovered, who, among other fancies, believing the asylum in which he was placed to be his own private property, and having a peculiar distaste to spending money on it, made it a fixed rule to remain in bed on Saturdays, in order, as he intended, to escape all bills, and the inconvenience of weekly payments.[80]

Indeed, within a few short years the numbers of insane professed religious had increased sharply. Between 1843 and 1856, the proportion of insane religious was believed to have grown threefold.[81] By 1856, the inspectors estimated that one in 220 professed religious were insane, as opposed to one in 750 of the remainder of the population.[82] Spiritual blessings could, it appear, bring some unexpected psychological consequences.

It is becoming increasingly clear that gender analysis is an important tool for historians of medicine, and indeed this volume of essays is evidence of a growing interest in the field. Emphasis within the discipline generally is shifting from an earlier preoccupation with the exercise of power by governments and institutions, to an examination of how factors such as class, race, and community responses, mediated the relationships between patient and practitioner. In the Irish case, gender analysis helps to situate the asylum within the narrative of political, economic and social change which characterised the nineteenth century. By incorporating gender as part of a critical response to psychiatric change, one is left with a more complex, but ultimately more satisfying, history.

Notes

1. Lord Russell introduced the Irish Poor Law, which was closely modelled on the English Poor Law Act of 1834, in a bill of 1837. For comment see H. Burke, *The People and the Poor Law in Nineteenth Century Ireland* (Dublin: Arlen House, 1987); R.B.

McDowell, *The Irish Administration 1801-1914* (London: Routledge & K. Paul, 1964), and G. O'Brien, 'The Establishment of Poor-Law Unions in Ireland, 1838-43', *Irish Historical Studies,* xxiii (1982), 97–120.

2. See D.H. Akenson, *The Irish Education Experiment: The National System of Education in the Nineteenth Century* (London: Routledge, 1970), and M. Daly, 'The Development of the National School System, 1831-40', in A. Cosgrove & D. McCartney (eds), *Studies in Irish History Presented to R. Dudley Edwards* (Dublin: University College Dublin Press, 1979).

3. J. Fleetwood, *A History of Medicine in Ireland* Dublin: 1951 and R. D. Cassell, *Medical Charities, Medical Politics: The Irish Dispensary System and the Poor Law, 1836-1872* (Suffolk: Boydell Press, 1997).

4. It is now believed that the famine accelerated existing trends rather than being the source of change. Nevertheless, the Great Irish Famine of 1845-50 had a dramatic impact upon Irish society, not least in reducing the population by half through starvation and emigration between 1850 and 1890. Historiography relating to the Famine is too vast to encompass here. However, for some discussion of the changes, see C. Kinealy, *This Great Calamity: The Irish Famine 1845-52* (Dublin: Gill and Macmillan, 1994); C. O'Grada, *The Great Irish Famine* (Basingstoke: Macmillan, 1989); J.M. Goldstrom, 'Irish Agriculture and the Great Famine', in J.M. Goldstrom and L.A. Clarkson (eds), *Irish Population, Economy and Society* (Oxford: Clarendon Press, 1981), 155–171, and D. Fitzpatrick, 'The Disappearance of the Irish Agricultural Labourer, 1841-1912', *Irish Economic and Social History,* 7 (1980), 66–92: 66.

5. Census of Ireland, 1896, *Vital Statistics.*

6. *6th Report on the District, Criminal and Private Lunatic Asylums in Ireland,* PP1852–3, XLI, 18.

7. St. Patrick's Hospital, known as 'Swift's' after its founder, Dean Jonathan Swift.

8. In Armagh. The title is suggestive of the more famous York Retreat, and was also run by the Society of Friends.

9. In Belfast for example there was great opposition to the appointment of religious ministers, because of fears of exciting religious tensions. In other asylums, where the majority of patients shared the same denomination, there was little difficulty.

10. There are many pitfalls associated with asylum records, not least of which is the difficulty in determining precisely who drove the admission process. David Wright has written of important role played by relatives of lunatics in admissions, which re-evaluates the

presumption that professionals determined access to institutions. 'Getting Out of the Asylum: Understanding the Confinement of the Insane in the Nineteenth Century' in *Social History of Medicine,* 10, 1 (April 1997), 137–55.

11. M. Finnane, *Insanity and the Insane in Post-Famine Ireland* (London: Croom Helm, 1981), 91.

12. For a discussion of cases inappropriately described as dangerous, see O. Walsh, '"The Designs of Providence": Race, Religion and Irish Insanity', in J. Melling and B. Forsythe (eds), *Insanity, Institutions and Society, 1800-1914: A Social History of Madness in Comparative Perspective* (London: Routledge, 1999), 223–42.

13. See David Dickson 'The Potato and Irish Diet Before the Great Famine', in C. O'Grada (ed.), *Famine 150: Commemorative Lecture Series* (Dublin: Teagasc, 1997), 1–27, for a discussion of the great impact of the potato upon Irish society.

14. My emphasis.

15. J.R. McCulloch, *Descriptive and Statistical Account*, quoted in C. O'Grada, *Ireland Before and After the Famine: Explorations in Economic History, 1800-1925* (Manchester, Manchester University Press, 1993), 181–2.

16. R.M. Rhodes, *Women and the Family in Post-Famine Ireland: Status and Opportunity in a Patriarchal Society* (New York, Garland, 1992), 85.

17. Rhodes notes an interesting development in female land ownership after the Famine, however. Irish marriage patterns changed so that men married later in life (partly as a result of delays in the surrender of the family farm by the father). Young women thus frequently married older men, and spent a good many years as 'directors of farms' in their widowhood. *Ibid.*, 192.

18. For an overview of emigration patterns, see D. Fitzpatrick, *Irish Emigration 1801-1921* (Dundalk, Economic and Social History Society of Ireland, 1984).

19. 'A 'typical' participant in Ireland's 'new' emigration at the end of the nineteenth century, then, was young (under 24 years), unmarried, from the west, and female'. Rhodes, *Women and the Family*, 250.

20. D. Fitzpatrick, 'A Share of the Honeycomb: Education, Emigration and Irishwomen', *Continuity and Change*, 1 (1986), 217–34.

21. The pioneering work on Irish family life (which has come in for criticism in recent years) was conducted by C.M. Arensberg and S.T. Kimball, *Family and Community in Ireland* (Cambridge: Harvard University Press, 1940), and K. H. Connell, *Irish Peasant Society: Four Historical Essays* (Oxford: Clarendon Press, 1968).

22. Rhodes, *op. cit.* (note 16), 190–1.

23. However, Showalter's conclusion – that greater numbers of female patients implied a gender bias within the asylum – is somewhat open to question. Recent research suggests that women were admitted to institutions in fewer numbers than men, but that they lived long within the asylum, producing over time a larger representation. *The Female Malady: Women, Madness and English Culture, 1830-1980* London: Virago, 1987, 51. See J. Busfield, 'The Female Malady?: Men, Women and Madness in Nineteenth Century Britain', *Sociology*, 28 (1994), 259–77, and N. Tomes, 'Feminist Histories of Psychiatry' in M. Micale and R. Porter (eds), *Discovering the History of Psychiatry* (New York: Oxford University Press, 1994), 348–83, for a response to Showalter's thesis.

24. Calculated from the *Register of Admissions*, CDLA, 1850-1880.

25. In her study of admissions in nineteenth-century France, Yanick Ripa suggests that women became the principal focus of attention by asylumdom. However, as she herself points out, their primary purpose was to remove potentially dangerous individuals from society, an agenda which embraced male as well as female deviance. *Women and Madness: The Incarceration of Women in Nineteenth-Century France* (Cambridge: Cambridge University Press, 1990), 3.

26. *Register of Admissions,* 1850–1880.

27. Arensberg and Kimball, *op. cit.* (note 21), 138.

28. *7th Annual Report*, PP1853–4, 22.

29. As the first and second generations produced by post-famine intermarriage matured.

30. Calculated from the forms of admission, 1870-1879.

31. There were for example 27 army and navy men, 25 clerics, 14 lawyers, 11 physicians, 36 merchants, 34 landowners, 17 students and 61 of other occupations.

32. See Oonagh Walsh, '"A Lightness of Mind": Gender and Insanity in Nineteenth-Century Ireland', in M. Kelleher and J. Murphy (eds.), *Gender Perspectives in Nineteenth-Century Ireland: Public and Private Spheres* (Dublin: Irish Academic Press, 1997), for figures relating to famine admissions, 160–2.

33. *6th Report*, PP1852–3, 18.

34. *8th Report*, PP1854–5, 22.

35. Diagnoses taken from the Forms of Admission, 1872. A total of 58 patients were admitted as Dangerous Lunatics (27 males and 31 females); of these 51 were ascribed a cause. The eight physiological causes were: hereditary (8); idiocy (3); epilepsy (2); uterine derangement (1); puerperal insanity (3); syphilis (1), sunstroke (1),

and head injury (2). The remainder were: unknown (19); shock (1); excitability of temper (1); domestic annoyance (1); religious excitement (3); disappointed ambition (1); disappointment in love (1); grief (1); fright (1), and a quarrel (1). These causes did not represent fixed medical categories, and they varied from year to year. They were an attempt to categorise and comprehend the causes of insanity in the population. A further 20 cases were admitted under Forms of Admission (11 men and 9 women).

36. *7th Report*, PP1853–4, 4.
37. See D. McLoughlin, 'Women and Workhouses', in M. Luddy and C. Murphy (eds), *Women Surviving* (Dublin: Poolbeg Press, 1990), 117–47.
38. There were some highly specific circumstances which encouraged admissions, such as the 'outbreak' of methylated spirits drinking in Tyrone in the 1860s, which increased admissions to northern asylums.
39. *8th Report*, PP1854–5, 13.
40. For a discussion of the associations between cultural expectations and health, see C. Russett, *Sexual Science: The Victorian Construction of Womanhood* (Cambridge Mass.: Harvard University Press, 1989).
41. The principal exceptions were 'climate', which was predominantly male, and applied in the majority of cases to former soldiers, and paralysis, which was also largely male, and associated with syphilis.
42. Elizabeth Malcolm, *Ireland Sober, Ireland Free: Drink and Temperance in Nineteenth-Century Ireland* (Dublin: Gill and Macmillan, 1986).
43. The 'snug', characteristic of Dublin pubs, was designed to allow women to have a drink in relative privacy.
44. See S. Payne, 'Outside the Walls of the Asylum?: Psychiatric Treatment in the 1980s and 1990s', in P. Bartlett and D. Wright (eds), *Outside the Walls of the Asylum: The History of Care in the Community 1750-2000* (London: Athlone Press, 1999), 244–65, for a discussion of some of the public anxieties regarding 'care in the community'.
45. I Vic., Cap. xxvii, 1838.
46. This is not to say that they were not violent prior to admission. As the inspectors noted, a change of environment could have a drastic effect upon patient behaviour, with previously maniacal patients becoming pacific on admission.
47. Including the county sheriffs, county constabulary, managers of gaols, masters of workhouses, and justices of the peace.
48. Admissions under the amended Act of 1867, which allowed Magistrates to commit directly to asylums instead of via gaols,

almost trebled the number of patients labelled 'dangerous' (351 in
1867; 979 in 1868). For commentary see the *18th Report*, 7–9.

49. Ann Goldberg's study of Eberbach asylum in Germany for example
indicates that in societies where marriage was the norm, women in
particular were most likely to assault their husbands. *Sex, Religion,
and the Making of Modern Madness: The Eberbach Asylum and
German Society, 1815-1849* (New York: Oxford University Press,
2001), 129–34.

50. For figures relating to 1871, see O. Walsh, 'Gendering the Asylum:
Ireland and Scotland, 1847-1877', in T. Brotherstone, D. Simonton
and O. Walsh (eds), *Gendering Scottish History: An International
Approach* (Glasgow: Cruithne Press, 1999), 199–215.

51. Warrant no. 47, admitted 22 May, 1872.

52. Warrant no. 50, admitted 5 June, 1872.

53. Warrant no. 8, admitted 14 January, 1872.

54. Lunatic Asylums (Ireland) Act: 8 and 9 Vict. C 107, Sect. 9.

55. 'The Library has been materially increased, and in addition to ball-
playing, hand and foot, other sources of amusement, bagatelle ad
croquet, have been introduced, as well as the cultivation of flowers
by the inmates... the general aspect... has been much improved
during the past year... by the introduction of flowering plants, birds,
and cheap and suitable decorations to the corridors'. *23rd Report*,
106–7.

56. In Ballinasloe for example in 1855 each patient cost approximately
£15 per annum to keep, compared with £25 in the Criminal
Asylum.

57. In 1872, two criminals from Castlebar attempted to feign insanity in
the belief that if they were transferred to the asylum and then
'recovered', they would be released. The Castlebar physician felt
obliged to warn them of the actual effects of an insanity plea: 'I told
them they were not insane, and that they would have to finish the
full term of their imprisonment after leaving the asylum'. *21st
Report*, 30.

58. Under the Lunatic Asylums (Ireland) Act of 1875, a prisoner
deemed insane, but not guilty of an offence which warranted
admission to the Criminal Asylum, was to be sent to the appropriate
district asylum. On the expiration of their sentence, they were to be
treated as an ordinary patient. Those sent to the Criminal Asylum
were transferred, once their time had been served, to their district
asylum. 38 & 39 Vict, Sect. 10 & 12.

59. In the *6th Report*, the inspectors recommended the release of two
recovered patients, because they were both 'under the certainty of

emigration'. They noted that they planned to recommend four more in the coming year, three of whom intended to emigrate to Australia. 16.

60. All of six cases above were men.

61. *45th Report*

62. This was also the case in England. See H. Marland, '"Destined to a Perfect Recovery": The Confinement of Puerperal Insanity in the Nineteenth Century', in Melling and Forsythe (eds), *Insanity, Institutions and Society, op. cit.*, note 12, 137–56: 146–7.

63. Based on figures in *7th* and *8th Reports*, PP1853–4 and PP1854–5, 16 and 20.

64. *7th Report*, PP1853-4, 18.

65. *Ibid.*

66. *9th Report,* PP1855–6.

67. M. Reber, 'Moral Management and the "Unseen Eye": Public Lunatic Asylums in Ireland, 1800-1845', in E. Malcolm and G. Jones (eds), *Medicine, Disease and the State in Ireland, 1650-1940* (Cork: Cork University Press, 1999), ch. 12, 227–8.

68. P. Prior, 'Mad, not Bad: Crime, Mental Disorder and Gender in Nineteenth Century Ireland', *History of Psychiatry*, 8 (1997), 501–16: 502.

69. Male Case Notes, no. 3729, 129–132.

70. Male Case Notes, no. 3743, 169–172.

71. Including a belief that he had 'saved all the Royal Family from horrible deaths'.

72. Male Case Notes, no. 3681, 17–18, and 31–32.

73. Male Case Notes, no. 3719, 109–112.

74. Provided dowries for them.

75. There are however many instances of spousal loyalty and affection, when husands and wives repeatedly removed their partners from the asylum, despite acts of violence, in order to care for them at home. In one such case, a wife removed her husband eight times in six years, he being readmitted each time for assaulting her, before she finally agreed with the physician that his delusions regarding her fidelity were incurable. Male Case Notes, no. 3711, 89–94.

76. A. Jackson, *Ireland 1798-1998* (Oxford: Blackwells, 1999), 118-124.

77. For an account of the various forms of radical female activity in Ireland, see M. Luddy, 'Women and Politics in Nineteenth-Century Ireland', in M.G. Valiulis and M. O'Dowd (eds), *Women and Irish History* ((Dublin: Wolfhound Press, 1997), 89–108.

78. V. Crossman, *Politics, Law and Order in Nineteenth-Century Ireland* (Dublin: Gill and Macmillan, 1996), 142–3.

79. *6th Report*, PP1852–3, 18.
80. *Ibid.*, 19.
81. This must be set against an increase in the professed religious in Ireland during this period, the number of whom trebled in the latter half of the nineteenth century.
82. *7th Report*, PP1853–4, 23.

4

Class, Gender and Insanity
in Nineteenth-Century Wales[1]

Pamela Michael

This chapter shows how class and gender defined the
experiences of patients admitted to the North Wales Lunatic
Asylum during the late-nineteenth and early-twentieth centuries.
Although not lending support to the notion that the asylum was
predominantly an instrument of class and gender oppression, it
does illustrate how threats of banishment to the asylum could be
utilised to reinforce norms of social behaviour outside the
institution in far-flung communities across north Wales. It
suggests that lay rather than professional encounters were
critical in the social construction of madness and the
enforcement of social control.

Introduction

The establishment of a comprehensive network of publicly funded
pauper lunatic asylums across the length and breadth of the United
Kingdom during the nineteenth century has long been the subject of
conflicting interpretations. Emerging in parallel with the New Poor
Law system which provided support for the indigent poor within a
corresponding network of workhouses or 'pauper palaces',[2] the vast
public asylums or 'warehouses of the insane' have been portrayed as
an integral part of the capitalist system.[3] They mushroomed
alongside a proliferation of mines, iron works and factories, and a
burgeoning market economy, and together with prisons and
workhouses they formed a ubiquitous disciplinary phenomenon of
the modern world – the 'total institution'.[4] The asylum system has
been characterised as an instrument of class oppression, essential for
the maintenance of social control, and the containment and
regimentation of the deviant and unmanageable poor. [5]

But why, if these remarkable edifices were the inevitable outcome
of the structural needs of the capitalist system, was there no resistance

to them by the working classes? Michael Ignatieff has argued that for too long there was an unquestioned assumption about the centrality of the state in the making of a social order, and that 'the progressive institutionalization of the deviant and dependent poor in the nineteenth century' was represented as 'a process in which the state was the hammer, and the working class only and always the anvil'.[6] Just as Anne Crowther has shown that the history of the workhouse was in part shaped by working-class demands,[7] and the readiness of the working classes to avail themselves of the refuge provided for their dependent sick and elderly relatives, so John Walton has demonstrated that the working classes willingly utilised the facilities offered by asylums. Families, he argued, took advantage of publicly funded provision for the relief of their insane relatives, often viewing the asylum not as permanent incarceration, but as an opportunity for a suffering member to regain health, or as a source of respite care for relatives burdened with constant caring.[8] In this, asylums could claim a reasonable success rate, for about a third of the patients admitted each year were discharged recovered within less than twelve months.[9] However, the difficulty of identifying the asylum as a progressive innovation, forming part of a nascent 'welfare state' reflects the duality of the asylum in constituting simultaneously both therapeutic site and custodial institution. Was the asylum a component of the hospital system, or was it part of the punitive and disciplinary structure of the modern state? Was it progressive or repressive?

Feminist critics have contributed a further strand to the debate, arguing within a structuralist framework that the asylum was an instrument that a patriarchal society used to subjugate women.[10] In terms of gender analyses, structuralist explanations have been fused with social constructionist arguments, focusing on the labelling of deviant behaviour as a form of madness within the context of the changing norms and expectations associated with 'womanhood'.[11] Psychiatrists, it has been argued, played a role in both the manufacture of madness, and in the prescription of appropriate feminine behaviour, and so were effectively agents of sexual oppression.[12]

The way in which the character of the asylum is cast is relevant to a consideration of both the class nature of the custodial institution and the gendered characteristics of captivity. There has been a tendency either to portray the asylum as basically a patriarchal institution, or to view it in class terms. Few studies have attempted to incorporate both dimensions.[13] However, historians in diverse areas of historical enquiry are increasingly seeking to explore both class and gender, and to understand how these two structural fault lines intersect and shape the lives of men and women.[14] This chapter will attempt to show how within a Welsh setting, class characteristics shaped the experience of gender, whilst at the same time the experience of class was filtered according to gender. In addressing the juxtaposition of class and gender a related and similarly challenging question will be posed. Did the asylum represent a microcosm of society, or did it reflect heirarchical structures of oppression, only imprisoning society's poorest and most deviant sections?

Perhaps more so than England, Wales is a land of diversity and of contrasts, often dubbed elusive and an enigma.[15] Historically it has comprised of many distinctive localities, dialects and idioms, customs and religions. These cultural characteristics intersect with material differences, shaped by physical geography. The mountainous core segments the country into regions and sub-regions of north and south, east and west, industrial and rural, predominantly Welsh speaking and predominantly English speaking.[16] There has been considerable debate over the class nature of Welsh society, with a strong populist belief in the idea that it has been something of a 'classless' society.[17] Compared to England, Wales had a fairly small middle class. Landholding and wealth were concentrated into very few hands. Most working people were dependent on selling their labour power and had few capital reserves to fall back on in times of hardship. Tenant farmers in nineteenth-century Wales were often little better off than their labourers. The notion of a Welsh 'people' (gwerin) undifferentiated by class therefore gained considerable currency. Such a superficial impression remains a vibrant ideological myth, the very reiteration of which seems to serve some purpose within the pursuit of an elusive Welsh identity.[18]

North Wales was an important region of early industrialisation, with its natural resources of copper and slate in the north-west, iron and coal in the north-east, and adjacent pools of surplus rural labour. Trade and commerce developed as the base of the economy grew, and shipping and railways, markets and manufactures created new opportunities for both profit and exploitation.[19] New class formations emerged, and a Welsh proletariat was forged.[20] Industrialisation and domesticity went hand in hand. Quarrying and mining, steel-making and railway building required energetic workmen, whose lives were improved if they could rely on the womenfolk to shoulder the burden of domestic chores. Employment opportunities for women were few, and confined mainly to paid work associated with the domestic sphere.[21] Old allegiances, to an ancient language, to extended kinship networks, and to a multiplicity of rival religious denominations gave north Wales a unique culture, which demanded of its members a high degree of conformity. Deviation from class solidarity, filial loyalties, religious observance or narrowly prescribed gender and sexual roles, carried heavy sanctions. The ultimate penalty was exclusion from its closely-knit communities.[22]

No private madhouses were opened in north Wales, perhaps due to lack of demand, reflecting the low purchasing power of the middle classes within the region.[23] The insane were mainly cared for at home, and regarded as the responsibility of their families. Although generally tended in a benign manner they were sometimes to be found locked in outhouses and restrained with cords. Seclusion and custody could occur at home. Prior to the opening of the North Wales Lunatic Asylum, in 1848, most lunatics and idiots were cared for in a domestic setting by relatives or paid carers, a few were placed in workhouses, and only rarely would they be sent away to lunatic asylums in England.[24]

When the committee to establish the North Wales Lunatic Asylum was founded in 1842, the project was carried forward by a group of predominantly male, middle-class subscribers, comprising local gentry, clergy and professional men. They were a local elite inspired by examples of 'moral treatment' pioneered by Tuke and Connolly in England. Eager to introduce more civilised and therapeutic forms of treatment to north Wales, the subscribers united with the magistrates of five counties to found a public/private asylum.[25] Following the model of Gloucester and other asylums the committee adopted the policy of segregating patients according to class, so that the building was designed to accommodate first class, second class and pauper patients.[26] The physical structure and organisational functioning of the asylum were also strictly segregated along gender lines. The internal arrangement of the asylum reflected in exaggerated form the class and gender divisions of the society beyond its walls.

But what of the people who came to inhabit these walls? How did they come to be segregated and confined, and what were their prospects for returning to the society from which they came? To what extent was their fate determined by class or gender?

The North Wales Lunatic Asylum

An almost complete set of admission records and case notes have survived for the North Wales Asylum covering the entire period of its history, from its opening in 1848 to closure in 1995. Placed alongside a complete run of annual reports and extensive administrative records, this rich collection of texts has facilitated an extensive and in-depth historical investigation of the institutional treatment of insanity in north Wales.[27] For the purposes of this chapter, the analysis of the social composition of the patient population of the North Wales Asylum will begin with an examination of the gender and class profile of patients admitted during the years 1848-1900 and will explore the evidence for uneven sex ratios, or the over-representation of either the working-classes or the 'lumpen-proletariat'. It will then move on to look at some of the class and gender patterns associated with the life stories of a sample of patients.

Proportion of male to female patients

Elaine Showalter has suggested that the disproportionate ratio of women in asylum care during the latter half of the nineteenth century reflected the increasing identification of insanity with womanhood. She claimed that the growth of the asylum, and of a professional agenda, led to the 'domestication of insanity', and to its construction as a 'female malady'.[28] Showalter's basic contention has not gone unchallenged, and Busfield has pointed to the flimsiness of the statistical evidence for such a sweeping claim.[29] Recent scholarship has focused upon the more nuanced differences facilitated by an analysis of the patterns of insanity from a 'gender' rather than a 'feminist' perspective.[30]

In order to locate the gendered profile of insanity in north Wales within this debate, patterns of incarceration will be examined firstly from a quantitative perspective. The Denbigh Asylum was opened in 1848 with a capacity of 200 patients. Within ten years it was over-full, with 107 male and 101 female patients remaining in custody at the end of 1858. A series of extensions increased the capacity of the asylum, so that by the turn of the century 721 patients were in residence. By 1900 a total of 6,253 patients had been admitted since opening, with the number of male admissions (3,200) slightly exceeding the number of female admissions (3,053). During that fifty-one year period a slightly higher proportion of the female patients had been discharged recovered (1,230) as compared to the male patients (1,003). Of the 2,159 patients who had died 'in custody' during that time 1,212 were male, and only 947 were female.[31] Therefore, during the first half century of the asylum's history, more men than women were admitted to the asylum, and once admitted male patients were more likely than female patients to die in the asylum. A markedly divergent pattern has been identified by one other study of a private asylum.[32] However, women tended to stay longer in the asylum. The average length of stay of patients admitted between 1875 and 1914 was slightly longer for women than for men. A ten per cent sample of patients admitted to the Denbigh Asylum between 1875 and 1914 showed that the average length of stay of patients who were discharged was 498 days for women and 471 days for men; the average length of stay for those who stayed in the asylum until they died was 2,258 days for women and 2,226 days for men.[33]

At the turn of the twentieth century there were 721 patients in residence in the North Wales Asylum, 44 of whom were private patients and 677 pauper patients. There were no criminal patients. Amongst the private class there were more males than females, the number being twenty-six males and eighteen females. Amongst the pauper class there was a very slight preponderance of females (341 as opposed to 336 males).[34] However, taking the whole of the second half of the nineteenth century, the proportion of male to female patients had been more or less evenly balanced, with a small excess of male patients. As one side of the asylum or the other filled up, then restrictions had to be placed on the number of admissions of either male or female patients, until such time as additional accommodation could be provided. The strategic decisions of the Visiting Committee determined hospital expansion, and whilst the Committee responded to demand, it also to some extent determined the rate of uptake of accommodation. During periods when the accommodation was full, a backlog of cases built up, and sometimes trade-offs were made, as workhouses agreed to readmit cases which had stabilised in exchange for sending unmanageable patients.

In order to obtain a fuller impression of any inherent gender bias in the statistics of recorded insanity, it is therefore necessary to look beyond the asylum, at the number of pauper patients registered under the Poor Law returns as being cared for either in workhouses or in accommodation with friends or family. Here it is possible to observe a pronounced excess of female over male patients. In the workhouses of north Wales there were 120 female, as opposed to 76 male lunatics and idiots, whereas in accommodation with friends, or in lodgings, the number of females was 159 as opposed to 103 males.[35] This may suggest that female 'lunatics' or 'idiots' were easier to manage in the workhouse, or in a non-institutional setting. There is much evidence to suggest that when men threatened harm to others or to themselves, the workhouse nurses, or the relatives caring for them at home (often female) found the task of constraining them too difficult. Within the seclusion of the asylum male patients were cared for by male attendants. To conclude then, more women than men were recorded as suffering from insanity in north Wales, but less of them were confined in the asylum.

It must be remembered that these figures do not represent what psychiatrists might refer to as the 'prevalence' of insanity or mental illness within the community, for they simply show the number of people registered as being in receipt of Poor Law assistance, and therefore labelled as 'paupers', whilst at the same time categorised as being either 'lunatic', 'idiot' or of 'unsound mind'. The figures are purely a social construct.

To understand more about the people who were incorporated within this construct, and to explore the class and gendered patterns of custodial care of the insane, it is necessary to analyse the social composition of the patients incarcerated within the institution, and explore their differential experiences of custody and seclusion. The admission details of all patients admitted to the Denbigh Asylum in each decennial year of the national census were entered into a database, so that the profile of patient admissions could be compared to the total census population of the asylum's catchment area in north Wales.

A comparison of the occupational profile of all patients admitted in 1891 with the occupational census of that year for the five contributing counties, (Anglesey, Carnarvon, Merioneth, Flint and Denbighshire) reveals not only that most sectors of the labour force were represented in the asylum, but also that the patients constituted a fair cross-section of society in north Wales.[36] There is a clear under-representation of professional occupations, and an over-representation of those employed in building and works of construction. For the purposes of this analysis patients were allocated to occupational groups according to the criteria of the census. Matching the two sets of information could be problematic, as in some cases the medical certificates only recorded the designation 'labourer', with no way of knowing whether these were employed in mines or quarries, in agriculture, or in construction. Apparent over-representation of men recorded as being employed in building and works of construction, could merely signify that men employed as labourers in other sectors have been wrongly entered under this category. It is notable that there is an under-representation of patients employed in mines and quarries, and it may be that quarry labourers, as opposed to skilled quarrymen, were recorded on asylum admission papers simply as 'labourers'. Nonetheless, the pattern revealed by this profile of the 1891 admissions confirms what the ten per cent sample of all admissions for the years 1848-1900 also indicated – that men employed as labourers were more likely to become pauper lunatics than other categories of workers. Two other sectors of male employment which are clearly over-represented are firstly 'commercial occupations', and secondly 'conveyance of men, goods and messages', which includes sailors. Both these areas of employment can be regarded as having high levels of associated 'risks', the first because of associated financial worries and the latter as will be shown below.

The domination of the Welsh economy by heavy industry and extractive industries resulted in an extremely narrow range of waged employment opportunities for women. Both the unwaged and waged female labour force was required to domestically service the male labour force, and carry out reproductive functions, essential to the needs of a rapidly expanding capitalist economy. The demand for male labour was multiplying as mines and quarries, foundries and factories, railways and roads, all sought strong and vigorous male workers. In Wales the dominant industrial pattern and the early displacement of women workers in the woollen industry, and from the mines, meant that female employment opportunities were considerably less than in England. The female participation rate in Wales fell from 28.9% in 1871 to 22.2% in 1911, as compared to a decline in England from 38.3% in 1871 to 32.8% in 1911.[37] This partly mirrored the shift in the economy from agriculture towards manufacturing and extractive industries. Whereas in 1851 agriculture was the second largest source of female employment, by 1911 it had fallen to fifth position. Domestic service was the main source of employment for women throughout north Wales. 'Domestic offices and services' absorbed an ever increasing proportion of the female labour force during the second half of the nineteenth century, so that in Carnarvonshire for instance, the number of women employed in this sector rose from 3,500 in 1851 to nearly 10,000 in 1891, and in Denbighshire from 3,800 in 1851 to nearly 8,000 in 1891. (In addition, many women left to become maid-servants in Liverpool and London.) Next in importance came occupations categorised as 'dress' followed by 'food, drink and lodgings'. All were in areas of work associated with female domestic roles. By the beginning of the twentieth century a small number of women were beginning to appear in professional occupations, mainly teaching.

An analysis of patient admissions to the Denbigh Asylum, indicates that this pattern of female employment was closely replicated amongst the patients, with domestic servants predominating. Some had been dressmakers, or 'lodging-house keepers'. However, a majority of women were categorised according to their relationship to a male head of household (e.g. 'wife of carpenter' or 'daughter of miner'). Thereby women's class position was invariably defined in terms of the patriarchal division of labour.[38] On marriage a woman assumed a new identity, and henceforth acquired her status as a dependent of her husband. The appellation 'wife of' was also suggestive of male ownership. In terms of class position women derived their status from their husband's occupation.[39] Many women may have continued to do some paid work after marriage, but this might not be recorded in the employment census, or on their medical certificates at committal, even though their contribution may have been crucial to family survival. The reliability of census data in regard to women's employment patterns is seriously in doubt.[40] Similarly the information provided on the committal certificates when women were admitted to the asylum may not provide a comprehensive record of their occupations. The data available suggests that whereas women of most occupational groups and backgrounds are represented in the asylum there is a slight over-representation of women who were domestic servants or wives of labourers or manual workers. These findings broadly concur with those of David Wright's study of the Buckinghamshire Asylum, reported in this volume, which shows that most occupational groups were represented amongst inmates and Joseph Melling's study of governesses in this volume. Nevertheless, the detailed evidence from the Denbigh Asylum does suggest that the representation of classes was not entirely equal and that the poorer classes and less skilled labourers were somewhat over-represented. The reasons for such 'inequalities' require further exploration.

Explanatory frameworks

Sociological analyses offer a range of alternative explanatory frameworks for inequalities of health according to social class and gender, most notably those of 'social causation', 'social drift' and 'social constructionism'.[41] In terms of class analysis the first of these perspectives, 'social causation', argues that social and economic hardships and pressures give rise to a higher incidence of mental illness amongst the poorest sections of the community. It also acknowledges the occupational hazards faced by members of the lower classes. The second perspective 'social drift' or 'natural selection' argues that those who suffer from mental illness are more likely to drift downward toward the lower end of the social stratum, a consequence of their inability to fulfill their work-roles, or survive in a competitive economy. The third explanation posits that class norms inform the labelling processes by which certain individuals are 'constructed' as aberrant and designated mad – that members of the lower classes are inappropriately judged by the received standards of the middle classes. In gender terms, these three frameworks suggest that women are more economically and socially disadvantaged than men, suffering higher levels of stress and illness that are directly due to their oppression within a patriarchally structured society. Secondly, they argue that women's social position is likely to be determined by their illness, (although in so far as women's class position is contingent upon the occupation of their husband, this might be less direct). Thirdly, they imply that the application of masculine norms regarding acceptable female behaviour leads to many women being regarded as deviant and labelled as 'mad'.

The remainder of this chapter will attempt to explore the inter-relationships between class and gender in the patterns of insanity in north Wales, and by considering each of these explanatory frameworks in turn, examine too the role of the asylum. In this preliminary analysis both class and gender differences will be 'bundled' together under the three aforementioned approaches, in order to explore their usefulness. A 'case history' approach will be employed to investigate how broader economic and social processes may have impinged on the personal lives of patients, drawing upon a study of the entire case history of a ten per cent sample of patient admissions to the Denbigh Asylum during the second half of nineteenth century.

Social causation

As wage labourers men experienced the daily hazards of working under capitalist systems of production. Many occupations were extremely dangerous. Sailors were often injured at sea, and patients arrived in the asylum who had received head injuries from crashing masts, or falling down a ship's hold.[42] Others were shipwrecked and saw their comrades drowned, or becalmed in tropical seas, suffered sun-stroke, thirst and hunger. Captains lost cargo and vessels, their own and other people's investments, and returned home as broken men. Occasionally they were committed to asylums in foreign countries, and when they failed to make a speedy recovery were repatriated. The perils of working at sea were frequently identified as a source of insanity.[43] William Wright, a fisherman's son, admitted in 1893, was said to have been out in a heavy gale about eight days previously, and as a consequence was suffering from 'ordinary acute mania'. He was described by the asylum doctor as being 'not strongly built, and poorly nourished'. On hospital food his condition improved, and he began to 'put on flesh'. He was put to work with the asylum painter, and so learned another skill and was discharged within five months.[44]

Accidents were frequent in other trades, especially in mining, in agriculture, and in transportation. Robert Griffith was a 27-year-old man from Bangor, who at the age of about seventeen had suffered a railway accident. At that time he had been employed as a locomotive fireman on the Bethesda line, and when an engine was derailed he had sustained a fracture of the arm and leg. His leg had required amputation, so that he was obliged to take up work as a tailor. He had also received some injury to the head in the accident. Although it was not clear whether this was the cause of his difficulties at the time of his committal, the fact that he was experiencing delusions and aural hallucinations was grounds for concern, and those around him connected his insanity to his accident. Griffiths was said to have become unmanageable at home, and required constant watching, as he was apt to attack his imaginary enemies. Cases such as these illustrate why lay people frequently associated occupational risk with insanity.

There was a particularly high rate of accidents in the quarrying industry, and special quarry hospitals were established to cater for injured workmen.[45] Occasionally men were sent to the asylum with fractured skulls, and other head injuries which left them permanently impaired. More often men who had suffered fractures, or loss of fingers, or crushed feet, were committed when their mental health deteriorated in the months following the accident. David Wynne, a quarryman from Blaenau Ffestiniog, was admitted when soon after his discharge from the Oakley (Quarry) Hospital, his mind became affected. According to his asylum admission notes, Wynne had been 'labouring under the idea that his long residence in hospital would incapacitate him from further employment'.[46] Another quarryman from Blaenau Ffestiniog was sent to Denbigh because 'he does not sleep and will not go to work. He talks incoherently and at times gets violent'. David Lewis had experienced a compound fracture of the tibia on Christmas Eve, 1896. He had always been a 'steady and hardworking man' and, when he was admitted to the asylum the following August, the asylum doctor concluded that 'the injury is undoubtedly the cause of his mental disorder'.[47] Injuries could not only cause debilitation but also threaten the livelihood of a working man. Other illnesses too threatened men's wage-earning capacity. Some suffering from tuberculosis kept on working in order to support their families, even when their health was seriously in decline. Men with epilepsy went to the quarries, even when this could be dangerous both to themselves and to workmates.[48] Occasionally, following life-threatening behaviour they would be committed to the asylum, as when David Jones 'attempted to throw his fellow workmen to the bottom of the quarry' a drop of some 300 feet. The role of breadwinner was crucial to the welfare of the family, and many a man suffered acute anxiety following accidents at work.

The quarry industry was one of the most conflict-ridden industries in the U.K., and some of the greatest battles of the working-class movement in Wales were fought amidst the mountains of Carnarvonshire. Men who blacklegged were ostracised by their fellow workers, experiencing social isolation often for many years after the event. Thomas Morris was admitted to the asylum in 1875. He was unable to sleep, had attempted to commit suicide, and was 'under the impression that his neighbours and fellow workmen are against him'. As one of the few men who had kept working whilst the Penrhyn quarrymen were on strike, and being 'greatly annoyed' by them, it had 'preyed upon his mind and produced these attacks'. On admission he was 'extremely low and unhappy – moaning and shedding tears but perfectly rational and well aware of his condition'. Morris was the father of nine children, six of whom were living, so that he was under a considerable burden of responsibility and suffered great anxiety about his duty to fulfill his role as breadwinner.[49]

David Jones, another quarryman admitted in 1881, had not been sleeping, had been noisy and troublesome, and had assaulted his housekeeper. 'At the election of 1874 he was the only Conservative among the Quarrymen and was generally disliked by them after which he became low spirited'.[50] Social isolation was the concomitant of aberrant class behaviour. Men, rather than women, were at the sharp edge of class conflicts, and trade union and political battles. They experienced danger and violent accidents in their employment in ways which women rarely encountered. When women experienced violence it was usually within the domestic sphere.

Retrospectively we can see how uncertain were some of the apparent assumptions regarding cause and disease aetiology. During the nineteenth century many organic diseases which affected people's mental health were little understood. General Paralysis for instance had frightening manifestations, but few lay people appreciated the connection with syphilis. They looked for explanations in terms of life events, and often linked the disease to occupational hazards. Richard Williams, for instance, was a former ship's captain who was admitted to the asylum on 1st August, 1886, and died within three weeks. He was described by the asylum medical officer as 'a well marked case of General Paralysis of the Insane', but on the committal certificate the explanation of family and Poor Law doctor was recorded. It seems that the 'Patient used to command a sailing vessel and a little over three years ago she was lost. This seems to have been the exciting cause'.[51] It was as hazardous to affix a social aetiology at the time, as it is to make retrospective diagnoses today.

Irving Zola has drawn attention to the cultural dimensions of symptom perception, and has emphasised the role of 'triggers' – that is social events, such as interpersonal crises, occupational troubles, and conflicts, which lead people to seek help.[52] In attempting to evaluate the role of social causation in mental illness it is necessary to acknowledge the complex nature of the identification of symptoms and diseases. Even in looking at the apparent social causes recorded in the certification papers and case notes of patients, we need to acknowledge the extent to which these statements embodied particular health beliefs, and social representations of health and illness. Claudine Herzlich's work on health beliefs in urban and rural France has shown how deeply socially embedded are people's explanations of health and disease.[53] Therefore social causation, and social constructionism need not be mutually exclusive as explanations of class and gender bias in the identification of cases in psychiatry.

Poverty and suffering amongst women

Women's dependent status made them particularly vulnerable to poverty. In his study of admissions to the Lancaster Asylum, John Walton drew attention to the number of women who were suffering from poor nourishment, and the debilitating effects of child-bearing.[54] A similar pattern may be witnessed amongst the cases sent to the Denbigh Asylum. The health and nutritional status of the wives of working men admitted to the asylum was frequently low, and for them the period spent in custody could be transformative owing to the improved diet, and basic medications such as iron and digitalis. Women such as Margaret Pritchard, the 26-year-old wife of a farm servant, admitted to the asylum in September 1894, undoubtedly benefited from the more ample supply of food, and the rest which they obtained whilst they were in custody. Margaret had not been well since her confinement, eleven months prior to her admittance and on examination she was found to be very thin and poorly nourished. Six months later the medical officer reported that the 'change has done her much good, and she is now fat and well in every way...'. Margaret was discharged recovered within less than a year.[55]

In other cases women recuperated and were able to return home, their health improved. Elizabeth Evans,[56] a 'most respectable looking' woman from Ruabon, was forty years of age and the mother of six children, when she was admitted to the asylum in 1876. Described as 'somewhat emaciated', Elizabeth's mental condition was attributed to 'Debility from poor feeding and having a child suckling'. Elizabeth told the medical superintendent that her husband, who was a collier, had been on strike lately, and that she had not lived very well in consequence. She was detained for over six months, during which time the doctor regularly noted the improvement in her condition, and the fact that she was 'gaining strength'.

The burden of child-bearing could be especially detrimental to the health of women whose health status anyway was poor. Margaret Davies[57] a labourer's wife, had suffered three miscarriages when the pregnancies were at seven months, and had four children who were alive, when she was admitted at the age of twenty-nine, with her latest baby who was only three months old. She was described as 'never very strong' and as being subject to hepatic congestion, and 'very anaemic', and ever since the pregnancy she had complained of pains in the head. Admitted in October 1877, she was already gaining in strength by the middle of November and was soon reported to be 'in excellent bodily health'. Such cases feature significantly amongst the 'success stories' of the asylum, and testify to its therapeutic benefit.

Recurrent child-bearing was especially burdensome for women who were vulnerable to mental afflictions following pregnancies. In 1885, at the age of forty-six, Elizabeth Williams became ill once again following the birth of her thirteenth child.[58] She had been treated seventeen years previously, following the birth of an earlier child.

Whilst extremes of poverty may have driven more women suffering the effects of economic deprivation into the asylum, the number of female patients suffering from poverty and malnutrition may simply have reflected the health status of women more generally within these communities.

In analysing patient case records of the Edinburgh Infirmary, Gunter Risse found that many of the female cases labelled as suffering from 'hysteria' were suffering from poverty and 'great deprivation'.[59] A majority of these cases were admitted during the winter months. Risse suggests that their condition 'was perhaps an effect of widespread malnutrition', noting that menstruation had 'virtually ceased among the labouring women during the winter months'.[60] There is no evidence that cases of malnourished women admitted to the Denbigh asylum were clustered in the winter months, nor that there was any cessation of menstruation during the winter. Their extremes of poverty were usually linked to family circumstances, e.g. the birth of another child, or a husband unemployed or on strike. Such problems seem to have been more acute in the north-eastern regions of north Wales – in the mining and industrial areas of Wrexham, Bersham and Holywell – than in the less industrialised western counties. Perhaps access to the produce of smallholdings, or the more extended family ties prevailing in the western counties, helped to insulate women from such extremes of poverty as lack of food. Alternatively, it may simply be that these farming communities were less likely to refer such cases to the asylum.

Some elderly men were admitted whose condition seemed to be closely linked to deprivation and poor nutrition. In common with child-bearing women they were excluded from the labour market, and therefore more likely to be on the margins of poverty. However, although men were admitted to the asylum who were suffering from poor nourishment and poverty, they were not suffering from the dual burden of poverty added to the physical demands of child-bearing.

Social drift

To what extent was mental illness itself the cause of pauperism? There was extensive discussion during the course of the nineteenth century regarding the relationship between insanity and pauperism. There is evidence to suggest that in a significant number of cases patients committed to the Denbigh asylum had lost their employment, and exhausted their material resources, during periods of mental derangement.

Samuel Rhoden, a gardener, 'had to leave his situation on account of his increasing peculiarity of behaviour'. Sent to the workhouse he several times attempted to commit suicide by various methods. He made grandiose claims, was considered mad, and so was transferred to the asylum – 'He says he is a God able to do anything, to give life and destroy it and that keeping on a continual warfare with the Devil he is fighting night and day with him. He says he is above God, and the Devil has no power over him; he can do as he pleases, with any one, and whatever he does is right because he is a God'. Such opinions might have been awkwardly challenging to any employer! After a month or two in the asylum Samuel began to settle down, proving himself to be 'a most excellent gardener', and was discharged recovered after eleven months in custody.[61] The asylum offered greater tolerance, and a wider range of work opportunities than the workhouse, and so probably improved the prospects of recovery, and a chance to return to gainful employment.

Women could also lose their position if they behaved in unacceptable ways, especially if they were domestic servants and living in with their employers. About four years prior to her admission to the asylum, Emily Hughes had given birth to a child, and became 'addicted to habits of debauchery – and has for this reason lost place after place'.[62]

Occasionally women withdrew from their paid occupations when they were unable to cope due to their mental state. Ellen Jones was a 27-year-old domestic servant from Blaen y Cae Uchaf near Carnarvon, who had 'become low-spirited following a quarrel with her lover'. Although she had remained in service for nearly a year after this, in the end she had become 'so despondent that she had given up her position and returned to live with her father'.[63]

The evidence provided in the case histories is insufficient to ascertain whether loss of occupation preceded or followed the onset of mental illness, but there is a clear correlation between insanity and loss of occupation. Alice Davies of Capel Garmon, Llanrwst, was formerly a small shopkeeper, but in May 1880, aged thirty-nine, she was reported to be wandering about the country 'night and day'. Apprehended by a police officer, she told him 'that all she met on the road tried to take her life away and boil her for rats'. In the asylum she was described as 'a little thin woman of tidy appearance, but with a despondent look'. She had been admitted to the asylum once before and had a 'vague remembrance of being in a "big house" some time in her life'. Both her brother and her father suffered from 'some kind of fits' and had both been patients in the Denbigh asylum.

Differentiating the social from the biological influences in individual case histories is fraught with difficulty. Perhaps it is wrong to look for any linear cause, but better to acknowledge the complex interplay of the corporeal and the social.

So far these case studies have emphasised the welfare function of the asylum, and the degree to which families and communities sent their ailing relatives and neighbours to the institution with the hope of obtaining some relief. Given so many cases of recovery, recuperation and rehabilitation this suggests the possibility of a more benign interpretation of the function of the lunatic asylum. How can we reconcile this therapeutic role with the notion of a social control function? Are these two roles mutually exclusive? It might be argued that if the asylum was to enforce normative assumptions concerning behaviour, it needed to be seen to have a legitimacy, and that this role could not have been established so effectively had it not been that the asylum was seen by outsiders to have a therapeutic and benevolent function. The patients who recovered, and who were successfully treated, were the ones who reappeared in their communities, tangible proof of the potential benefits the institution offered for recovery. The patients who did not return gradually lost contact with their friends and relatives, to became part of a mysterious, socially invisible population. Amongst the patients who did not recover were many unable to conform to the normative assumptions concerning thoughts and behaviour patterns deemed acceptable by medical staff and asylum visitors and relatives, the 'gate-keepers' mainly responsible for taking the decisions regarding discharge. Signs of recovery were attached to specific criteria and expectations of behaviour. It is here that underlying judgements concerning appropriate behaviour become decisively important, and appear to embody critical assumptions concerning class and gender specific norms.

Social constructionism

The Denbigh patient case notes clearly reflect the extent to which women were judged by the norms and expectations of Victorian society. Women who were deemed mad had expressed their insanity by their bold defiance of custom and expectation. Some had taken off their clothes and gone naked into the street. Others had left the house at night for no reason, escaping through bedroom windows, had smashed windows, or leaned out of them shouting or singing at the tops of their voices. Elizabeth Roberts was adduced to be insane because she was 'wishful to go out of the house with no definite object'. [64] For women to leave the home 'without purpose' was such a clear contradiction of norms and expectations of respectable female behaviour that it was interpreted as a clear sign of insanity. Elizabeth H from Ralph Street in Bangor, daughter of a shoemaker, had been wandering about at night, escaping in her night-clothes through the window. She had attacked her father 'who is in charge of her' with a poker. Elizabeth was thirty-two years of age, and eighteen months prior to her committal her sister had died. She was admitted to the asylum in 1891 and died there in 1912. [65]

Women who were disorderly in their conduct, or defied their fathers and husbands, were labelled 'mad'. [66] It is not to say that they may not have been suffering from some form of 'mental illness' or even physical illness. It is simply a claim that the evidence adduced for their insanity related to their expressive behaviour in defiance of social norms specific to their gender, and in defiance of male authority.

Women were expected to be quiet, obedient, and definitely not sexually expressive. Once inside the asylum women's behaviour was judged harshly, and any betrayal of emotion, or behaviour suggestive of sexual interest or arousal, was regarded as further proof of insanity. Elizabeth Williams, a 17-year-old dressmaker from Portmadoc, was described as a 'very affectionate' girl who 'evidently has but little control over her passions'. [67] Women in custody were expected to act demurely and asexually. The slightest aberrations were magnified within the context of the institution. Confined to the female wing, the only opportunity for women patients to encounter men was when they attended chapel or went to the weekly dance. The only members of the male sex who would regularly appear on the female wing were the medical officers, who observed their patients with a 'clinical gaze'. A note would be made of any amorous or demonstrative behaviour. Following a ward visit in November 1882, for instance, the Medical Officer made a fresh entry in Grace Jones' case notes: 'Still knits contentedly. Casts significant glances at the Medical Officers and is always ready to embrace them if they approach her (not otherwise). Appears bashful in their presence and altogether appears as if her sexual instincts acted too freely owing to the abeyance of the controlling intellectual functions'. [68] Goffman has argued that people are labelled mad by other actors interpreting their behaviour as deviant, because in the view of the observer they have committed 'situational improprieties'. [69] The seclusionary practices of the asylum rendered the sexually suggestive glances of women patients towards their doctors as inappropriate, and as signs of madness.

Women who were unruly and shocking to their neighbours might find themselves consigned to the asylum, but once there could obtain their discharge if they then conformed to appropriate standards of behaviour. Mary Jones, a domestic servant from Llandeiniolen in Carnarvonshire outraged her employers and neighbours by her indecent behaviour. On the medical certificate confining her to the Denbigh asylum in February 1875, she was described as: 'Perfectly unreasonable, talks unruly and conducts herself in a highly unreasonable and disgusting conduct – and she can't talk without cursing and talking incoherently. She goes about raising her clothes and conducting herself in a very indecent manner as proved by her neighbours.' She was described as 'excessively stout' and of medium height.[70] Although at first she was noisy, excited and foul in her language, she settled down after being sent to work in the asylum laundry, and within a few weeks was employed in helping to put the new house which was being prepared for the medical superintendent in order. Here she began to converse 'in a fairly rational manner'. By April she was 'greatly improved', and described by the medical officer as 'Perfectly rational in her conversation and manner. Working industriously in the laundry where her conduct is very decorous – although she is somewhat too garrulous'. She continued to steadily improve, and was discharged recovered in May 1875, after exactly three months in the asylum. [71] Such loud women could be returned to the community, so long as they appeared to have quietened down, and were making an attempt to conform to the normative expectations of their sex.

Within the asylum women were categorised according to their behaviour, and were positioned along a continuum, from good ('nicely-conducted', 'tidy', 'industrious', 'well-spoken', 'decorous') to bad ('loud', 'abusive', 'foul-mouthed', 'filthy', 'vociferous', 'troublesome', 'noisy'). A study of medical case notes of patients at the Pen-y-Fal Asylum in Abergavenny, Monmouthshire, showed that noisiness was regularly noted as a sign of insanity, and that the ideal female patient was quiet and obedient.[72] Laziness and idleness were viewed negatively, and consistently featured as attributes of insanity. Recovery was indicated when patients proved to be 'industrious' or 'hard-working', or when a man or woman proved themselves to be skilled workers, e.g. 'a fine carpenter', 'a very useful farmhand', 'an excellent seamstress', or 'a great help in the kitchens'.

The social constructionist model can be applied to some of the male cases in terms of class norms and behaviour, as when labourers left their positions, or failed to carry out their work properly, or when they imagined themselves to be important when society regarded them as inferior or unimportant.[73] Men would claim to be other famous men, or to have property, or power, to be in direct communication with God, or to be fantastically rich. Rule-breaking was what set them apart.

However, it is in regard to gender norms and expectations that the social constructionist model is most salient, and the role of the asylum as a rule enforcer becomes most apparent. It was not simply that the asylum itself was capable of enforcing rules. It was rather that the threat of the asylum played a disciplinary role within the society.

The threat of being cast out was incorporated into the language of everyday encounters, and became a tool of discipline used amongst friends, neighbours and families. A series of stories by the distinguished Welsh author Kate Roberts is set around the childhood of Begw, a girl growing up in a poor quarrying/smallholding community in north Wales. When Begw is sent with a basket of food up the mountainside to visit the isolated home of an elderly neighbour, she finds Nanw Sian disappointed that the weather has turned so cold. It means the old lady will be unable to venture out, for fear of slipping on the ice, and will spend Christmas alone. But Begw is excited at the thought that snow may fall by Christmas, and dreaming of the sort of Christmas which she has only ever seen on Christmas cards. Old Nanw Sian, who has lived long enough to know that there is no such thing as a 'good old-fashioned Christmas', but that life is hard, and that the only ones who prosper are those who tell lies which other people are foolish enough to believe, offers little Begw a salutary warning: 'Paid a mwydro dy ben blentyn. Felna mae pobl yn mynd i'r Seilam'.[74]

As Foucault might have argued, disciplinary power is dispersed throughout society in a multiplicity of sites.[75] It can be elusive, but all pervasive. Not only do the solid walls of the asylum enforce custody and seclusion, but the very idea of exclusion can be wielded as a weapon in communities far beyond the physical location of the total institution to enforce discipline and conformity. It can even be used by women themselves to warn little girls against the dangers of fancy, and flights of imagination. The asylum became the threatened destiny of those with unrealistic expectations, who fancied that they could go beyond the prescribed boundaries of their class, their gender, their home and their locality.[76]

Both English speakers and Welsh speakers were equally complicit in consolidating the power of the total institution and its representations of madness, as instruments of social control. Whilst working-class men and women may have felt oppressed by the institution, nonetheless without the willing co-operation and agency of working people, male and female, the asylum could never have attained the hegemonic power which it achieved. Only by being a welfare provider as well as a custodial regime could it obtain the collusion of its Welsh subjects, and exert so powerful an influence, thereby fulfilling a social control role in enforcing normative behaviour. It was in these more subtle ways that the asylum upheld class and gender boundaries, rather than by systematically confining to custody members of the lumpen-proletariat, or secluding a disproportionate number of the female sex. By virtue of its benign as well as its disciplinary role the asylum's influence extended far beyond the confines of the total institution and permeated throughout the Welsh communities from which it drew its clientele.

Conclusion

This chapter has shown that the patient community of the north Wales Asylum represented a cross-section of class and occupational backgrounds and that men and women were committed to the asylum in fairly even numbers. In this respect the findings accord with those of Wright and Melling in this volume. A detailed analysis of the occupational profile of patients suggests, however, a slight but significant over-representation of poor and unskilled workers in the asylum population and of some specific occupational groups. The examination of patient case histories demonstrates a link between certain occupational risks and the onset of insanity. Contemporary witnesses and medical staff often drew a direct link between poverty and insanity, and women often experienced in a more acute way the effects of class oppression. The close association between poverty and mental health problems associated with female reproduction has also been highlighted by Levine-Clark in this volume. In another chapter, Anne Shepherd has shown that amongst the women admitted to Surrey Asylums, the period of 'custody' could offer positive relief. The evidence from the Denbigh asylum confirms such an interpretation regarding the role of the asylum. Committal to the asylum was instigated by lay people. Patients were considered to be insane in the first instance because of their behaviour outside of the asylum. The boundaries of normal behaviour differed sharply for men and women, and as Houston has shown, the evidence adduced for female insanity was different to that applied to males. This chapter has shown how women were considered mad if they attempted to leave the house after dark, or without 'proper purpose', or if they neglected their household chores. Fear of the asylum reinforced customary rules and the asylum was often named by lay people in their exhortations to children and women to obey strict codes of conduct. It was lay people rather than professional psychiatrists who wielded the threat of the asylum as an instrument of social control. In a recent paper, Chris Philo has noted that the presence of Craig Dunain, the district lunatic asylum for Inverness, was felt in far-flung areas of the Highlands and Islands.[77] So too, the Denbigh Asylum cast a long shadow across the five counties of north Wales, reinforcing norms of behaviour and class and gender boundaries amongst communities that lay far beyond the asylum.

Notes

1. The research upon which this chapter is based was funded by the Wellcome Trust.
2. D. Fraser (ed.), *The New Poor Law in the Nineteenth Century* (London: Macmillan, 1976); A. Digby, *Pauper Palaces* (London: Routledge & Kegan Paul, 1982); P. Bartlett, *The Poor Law of Lunacy* (London: Leicester University Press, 1999). For a Whiggish view, portraying the growth of custodial care as a humanitarian project see: K. Jones, *Lunacy, Law and Conscience 1744-1845: The Social History of the Care of the Insane* (London: Routledge, 1955) and Jones, *Asylums and After: A Revised History of the Mental Health Services* (London: Athlone, 1993).
3. A. Scull, *Museums of Madness,* (London: Allen Lane, 1979); Scull, *The Most Solitary of Afflictions,* (New Haven and London, Yale University Press, 1993); G. Grob, 'Marxian Analysis and Mental Illness', *History of Psychiatry,* 1 (1990), 223–32.
4. M. Ignatieff, *A Just Measure of Pain: The Penitentiary in the Industrial Revolution, 1750-1850* (reprinted London: Penguin, 1989, first published 1978); E. Goffman, *Asylums: Essays on the Social Situation of Mental Patients and Other Inmates* (Harmondsworth: Penguin, reprinted 1968, first published 1961).
5. A. Scull, 'Humanitarianism or Control? Some Observations on the Historiography of Anglo-American Psychiatry', in S. Cohen and A. Scull (eds), *Social Control and the State: Historical and Comparative Essays* (reprinted Oxford: Blackwell, 1985, first published 1981), 118–40; D. Ingleby, 'Mental Health and Social Order', in *ibid.,* 141–88.
6. M. Ignatieff, 'Total Institutions and the Working Classes', *History Workshop,* 15 (1988), 167–77: 173.
7. M.A. Crowther, *The Workhouse System, 1834-1929: The History of an*

English Social Institution, (London: Routledge, 1981).

8. J. Walton, 'Casting out and Bringing Back in Victorian England: Pauper Lunatics, 1840-1870' in W.F. Bynum, R. Porter and M. Shepherd (eds), *The Anatomy of Madness* (London: Tavistock, 1985), 3 vols, ii, 132–46; Walton, 'Lunacy in the Industrial Revolution: A Study of Admissions in Lancashire, 1848-1850', *Journal of Social History,* 13 (1979), 1–22.

9. M. Arieno, *Victorian Lunatics: A Social Epidemiology of Mental Illness in Mid-Nineteenth-Century England* (Selinsgrove: Susquihanna University Press, and London and Toronto, Associated University Presses, 1989).

10. Y. Ripa, *The Incarceration of Women in Nineteenth-Century France* (Cambridge: Polity Press, 1990).

11. This has drawn on a large literature which suggests that femininity was pathologised, and that medicine played a crucial role in the new constructions of womanhood, e.g. J. Ussher, *Women's Madness: Misogyny or Mental Illness?* (New York and London: Harvester Wheatsheaf, 1991). E. Malcolm 'Women and Madness in Ireland, 1600-1850', in M. MacCurtain and M. O'Dowd (eds), *Women in Early Modern Ireland* (Edinburgh: Edinburgh University Press, 1991); J. Matthews, *Good and Mad Women: The Historical Construction of Femininity in Twentieth Century Australia* (Sidney: Allen & Unwin, 1984).

12. P. Chesler, *Women and Madness* (New York: Doubleday, 1972); T. Szasz, *The Manufacture of Madness* (London: Paladin, 1973); D. Russell, *Women, Madness and Medicine* (Cambridge: Polity Press, 1995).

13. A notable exception is J. Harsin 'Gender, Class and Madness in Nineteenth Century France, *French Historical Studies,* 17 (1992) 1048–70.

14. T. Dubbin, 'Gender, Class and Historical Analysis: A Commentary', *Gender and History,* 13 (2001), 21–3.

15. R. Pope (ed.), *Religion and National Identity* (Cardiff: University of Wales Press, 2001), see especially 1–13; R.M. Jones, *North Wales Quarrymen, 1874-1922* (Cardiff: University of Wales Press, 1981), chapter 3.

16. E.G. Bowen (ed.), *Wales: A Physical, Historical and Regional Geography* (London: Methuen, 1957).

17. This is captured well in the section entitled 'Gog and Magog Myths: Gwerin and Working Class', in G. A. Williams, *When Was Wales?* (Harmondsworth: Penguin, 1985), 234–41.

18. P. Morgan, 'Gwerin Cymru – y ffaith a'r ddelfryd', *Transactions of the*

Honourable Society of Cymmrodorion, Session (1967), 117–31; Morgan, 'The Gwerin of Wales: Myth and Reality', in I. Hume and W.T.R. Pryce (eds), *The Welsh and Their Country* (Llandysul: Gomer Press, 1986), 134–52; G. Day, *Making Sense of Wales* (Cardiff: University of Wales Press, 2002).

19. A.H. Dodd, *The Industrial Revolution in North Wales* (Wrexham: Bridge Books, 1990; 1st edition, 1933).

20. R.M. Jones 'Notes from the Margin: Class and Society in Nineteenth Century Gwynedd', in D. Smith (ed.), *A People and A Proletariat: Essays in the History of Wales 1780-1980* (London: Pluto Press, 1980), 199–214.

21. D. Beddoe, 'Images of Welsh Women', in T. Curtis (ed.), *Wales the Imagined Nation: Essays in Cultural and National Identity* (Bridgend: Poetry Wales Press, 1986); A. John (ed.), *Our Mother's Land: Essays in Welsh Women's History, 1830-1930* (Cardiff: University of Wales Press, 1991); J. Davies, *A History of Wales* (Harmondsworth: Penguin, 1993).

22. E. Davies and A. Rees (eds), *Welsh Rural Communities* (Cardiff: University of Wales Press, 1960); A.D. Rees, *Life in a Welsh Countryside* (Cardiff: University of Wales Press, 1950).

23. W. Parry-Jones, *The Trade in Lunacy: A Study of Private Madhouses in England in the Eighteenth and Nineteenth Centuries* (London: Routledge, 1972).

24. P. Michael and D. Hirst, 'Establishing the "Rule of Kindness": The Foundation of the North Wales Lunatic Asylum, Denbigh', in J. Melling and B. Forsythe (eds) *Insanity, Institutions and Society, 1800-1914* (London: Routledge, 1999), 159-79. D. Hirst and P. Michael, 'Family, Community and the Lunatic in Mid-Nineteenth-Century North Wales', in P. Bartlett and D. Wright (eds), *Outside the Walls of the Asylum: The History of Care in the Community, 1750-2000* (London: Athlone, 1999), 66–85; P. Michael, *Care and Treatment of the Mentally Ill in North Wales, 1800-2000* (Cardiff: University of Wales Press, 2003).

25. Michael and Hirst, 'Establishing the Rule of Kindness', *op. cit.* (note 24).

26. A similar pattern to that adopted in other voluntary or mixed asylums, see: L.D. Smith 'Levelled to the Same Common Standard?' Social Class in the Lunatic Asylum, 1780-1860', in O. Ashton, R. Fyson and S. Roberts (eds), *The Duty of Discontent* (London: Mansell, 1995), 142–66.

27. The records are retained at the Denbigh Record Office, series HD/1.

28. E. Showalter, 'Victorian Women and Insanity', in A. Scull (ed.),

Madhouses, Mad-Doctors and Madmen (London: Athlone Press,
1981); Showalter, *The Female Malady: Women, Madness and English
Culture, 1830-1980* (London: Virago, 1987).

29. J. Busfield, 'The Female Malady? Men, Women and Madness in
Nineteenth Century Britain, *Sociology,* 28 (1994), 259–77; Busfield,
*Men, Women and Madness: Understanding Gender and Mental
Disorder* (London: Macmillan,1996).

30. B. Labrum, '"Looking Beyond the Asylum": Gender and the Process
of Committal to Aukland, 1870-1910', *New Zealand Journal of
History, 26* (1992), 125–44; W. Ernst, 'European Madness and
Gender in Nineteenth-century British India', *Social History of
Medicine,* 9 (1996), 357–82.

31. *The Fifty-First Annual Report of the North Wales Counties Lunatic
Asylum for the Year 1899-1900* (Wrexham: 1900), 39.

32. A. Digby, *Madness, Morality and Medicine: A Study of the York
Retreat, 1796-1914* (London: Cambridge University Press, 1985),
288.

33. C. MacKenzie, 'Social Factors in the Admission, Discharge and
Continuing Stay of Patients at Ticehurst Asylum, 1845-1917', in
Bynum, Porter and Shepherd (eds), *op. cit.* (note 8), ii, 147–76.

34. *The Fifty-Second Annual Report of the North Wales Counties Lunatic
Asylum, Denbigh for the year 1900-1901* (Wrexham: 1901), 27.

35. *The Fifty-First Annual Report of the North Wales Counties Lunatic
Asylum, Denbigh for the year 1899-1900* (Wrexham: 1900), 71.

36. This finding is in accord with Marlene Arieno's study of patients
committed to Bethlem Hospital, London, Essex County Asylum,
Colchester, and Haydock Lodge Asylum, Lancashire, for the years
1845-62, where she found patients constituted a representative cross-
section of social classes as represented by occupations; Arieno, *op. cit.*
(note 9).

37. L.J. Williams and D. Jones, 'Women at Work in the Nineteenth
Century', *Llafur,* 3 (1983), 20–9: 23.

38. Some modern, radical feminists argue that women form a separate
and subordinate 'class', see C. Delphy, *The Main Enemy* (London:
Women's Research and Resource Centre, 1977), and Delphy, *Close to
Home: A Materialist Analysis of Women's Oppression* (London:
Hutchison, 1984).

39. Even in the late-twentieth century the use of the occupational tables
based on the male head of household as a surrogate for women's class
position can result in a very misleading picture, see P. Abbott and R.
Sapsford, *Women and Social Class* (London: Tavistock, 1987).

40. E. Higgs, 'Women, Occupations and Work in the Nineteenth

Century Censuses', *History Workshop Journal,* 23 (1987), 59–80; L. Tilly and J. Scott, *Women, Work, and Family,* (New York: Holt, Rinehart and Winston, 1978).

41. D. Pilgrim and A. Rogers, *A Sociology of Mental Health and Illness,* 2nd edition (Buckingham: Open University Press, 1999).

42. DRO HD/1/360, Admittance no. 2601, date of admission 17/08/1876.

43. There may have been other dangers associated with living at sea in close confinement, if crews were mixed. A.L. Lloyd reports that when he served on whaling vessels the vocal harmonising of hymn-singing sailors from Anglesey rarely ceased and 'some of the Englishmen went nearly scatty!'. (A.L. Lloyd, L.P. sleeve note, *Leviathan! Ballads and Songs of the Whaling Trade,* Topic Records, 12T174).

44. DRO HD/1/368, Admittance n. 4701, date of admission 18/12/1893.

45. J. Lindsay, *A History of the North Wales Slate Industry* (Newton Abbott: David and Charles, 1974); E. Jones, *Canrif y Chwarelwyr* (Denbigh: Gwasg Gee, 1964); R.M. Jones, *The North Wales Quarrymen 1874-1922* (Cardiff: University of Wales Press, 1981); *Report of Her Majesty's Principal Secretary of State for the Home Department on the conditions under which the quarrying of stone, limestone and clay is conducted, with the object of diminishing any proved dangers to the health of the workpeople engaged therein* (London: HMSO, 1894).

46. DRO HD/1/365, Admittance no. 4004, date of admission 13/9/1888. For fuller details of this and other cases see P. Michael 'Quarrymen and Insanity in North Wales: from the Denbigh Asylum Records', *Industrial Gwynedd,* 2 (1997), 34–43.

47. DRO HD/1/370 Admittance no. 5271, date of admission 23/8/1897.

48. See DRO HD/1/360, Admittance no. 2427, date of admission 20/2/1875.

49. DRO HD/1/360, Admittance no. 2441, date of admission 16/4/1875.

50. DRO HD/1/361, Case no. 3059, date of admission 5/2/1881.

51. DRO HD/1/363 Case no. 3731, date of admission 1/08/1886.

52. I. Zola, 'Pathways to the Doctor – From Person to Patient', *Social Science and Medicine,* 7 (1973), 677–89.

53. C. Herzlich, *Health and Illness: A Social Psychological Analysis* (London: Academic Press, 1973).

54. Walton, 'Lunacy in the Industrial Revolution', *op. cit.* (note 8), 12.

55. DRO HD/1/339, Admittance no. 4792, date of admission 15/9/1894.

56. DRO HD/1/331, Admittance no. 2551, date of admission 8/04/1876.

57. DRO HD/1/331, Admittance no. 2711, date of admission 9/10/1877.

58. DRO HD/1/334, Admittance no. 3571, date of admission 29/01/1885.

59. G.B. Risse, 'Hysteria at the Edinburgh Infirmary: The Construction and Treatment of a Disease, 1770-1880', *Medical History*, 32 (1988), 1–22: 17.

60. *Ibid.*, 16.

61. DRO HD/1/360, Admittance no. 2571, date of admission 2/06/1876.

62. DRO HD/1/342, Admittance no. 5701, date of admission 14/06/1900.

63. DRO HD/1/333, Admittance no. 3201, date of admission 15/11/1881.

64. DRO HD/1/340, Admittance no 4901, date of admission 8/15/1895.

65. DRO HD/1/338, Admittance no. 4364.

66. C. Smith-Rosenberg, *Disorderly Conduct* (New York: Alfred A. Knopf, 1985).

67. DRO HD/1/ 333, Admittance no. 3249, date of admission 20/03/1882.

68. DRO HD/1/333, Admittance no. 3211, date of admission 14/12/1881.

69. E. Goffman, *Interaction Ritual* (New York: Anchor Books, 1967), 141–7.

70. Bodily norms were regularly applied, so that women would be described as excessively thin, or overly fat. At the time there was no women's opposition to the stigmatising of size, as there would be today, see S. Orbach, *Fat is a Feminist Issue* (New York: Berkeley).

71. DRO HD/1/331, Admittance no. 2430, date of admission 26/02/1875.

72. K. Davies, '"Sexing the Mind" Women, Gender and Madness in Nineteenth-Century Welsh Asylums', *Llafur: Journal of Welsh Labour History*, 7 (1996), 29–40.

73. E.g. H. Hugh, a quarryman from Bethesda, had 'exaggerated ideas of himself', which led to his committal in 1906; HD/1/ Admittance no. 6777, date of admission 11/7/1906.

74. K. Toberts, 'Nadolig y Cerdyn', in *Te yn y Grug: Cyfrol o Storiau*

Byrion gan Kate Roberts (Denbigh: Gwasg Gee, 1959), 86–95: 93. Translated means 'Don't fuss your head child – that is how people end up in the asylum'. During the course of my research, I have lost count of the number of elderly people who have said to me that as children they were warned by their mothers not to misbehave or they would go to the asylum.

75. M. Foucault, *Madness and Civilization: A History of Insanity in the Age of Reason* (London: Routledge, 1965, reprinted 1992), 259, where he claims: 'In one and the same movement, the asylum becomes... an instrument of moral uniformity and of social denunciation. The problem is to impose, in a universal form, a morality that will prevail from within upon those who are strangers to it and in whom insanity is already present before it has made itself manifest'. See also Foucault, *Discipline and Punish: The Birth of the Prison* (New York: Random House, 1977).

76. As a little girl I remember that the women in our locality of Surrey who were sent to Nethern, the local mental hospital, were often described by my grandmother as those who had 'ideas above their station'. This was a salutary warning.

77. C. Philo, 'Scaling the Asylum: Three Different Geographies of the Inverness District Lunatic Asylum (Craig Dunain)', paper delivered to a conference entitled 'Space, Psyche and Psychiatry', Oxford Brookes University, December 2002.

5

'Embarrassed Circumstances':
Gender, Poverty, and Insanity in the West Riding of England in the Early-Victorian Years

Marjorie Levine-Clark

Gender assumptions in early-Victorian England held that men derived their identities from work, while women were dependent beings for whom employment was not a central component of identity. Yet just as the New Poor Law positioned women ambiguously, sometimes emphasising women's dependency and other times stressing women's ability to work, so too do asylum records reveal complicated relationships between gender, poverty, and employment. Patient case notes from the West Riding Pauper Lunatic Asylum suggest that employment was a central component of poor women's identities. Female insanity was sometimes attributed to a lack of work, and both medical practitioners and female patients expected poor women to be employed.

Susannah Oter, a 31-year-old single servant from Hunshelf in the West Riding, tried to hang herself in February of 1852. She was then admitted to the West Riding Pauper Lunatic Asylum. Susannah's case history reveals that after her mother's death in the early 1830s, her father remarried and threw Susannah out of the house. Susannah wound up living with the family of the Reverend Mance, apparently acting as their domestic servant. Six weeks before her admission to the asylum, she was reprimanded by the daughter of the house, who felt Susannah had been out too late attending a wedding. Susannah opted to leave immediately, taking her wages, aiming to go to her sister's home at Green Moor. At the Sheffield railway station, her money was stolen, leaving her with nothing: 'She raves about having lost her situation abruptly and having no money no home no Friends'.[1] Susannah Oter is typical of women of the nineteenth-century working class whose struggles with poverty sent them on one of two paths. Most – with or without families – applied to Poor Law authorities and either entered the workhouse or received an allowance. For others like Susannah, the pressures of poverty and unemployment led to a county asylum for pauper lunatics.

In early-Victorian England, ideas about poverty were intimately connected to ideas about work, and both were informed by gender assumptions. The Poor Law Amendment Act of 1834 wedded these concepts together by refusing welfare assistance outside a workhouse to any man who was physically able to be employed, whether or not he actually had employment or this employment could provide a subsistence wage.[2] The Poor Law has played a prominent part in several recent studies in the history of insanity and its institutions in nineteenth-century England, which emphasise the relationships between the Poor Law and the county asylum. Most of this work has explored institutional and administrative intersections, often challenging explanations of the growth of asylums that focus on psychiatric medicine. In their study of pauper lunacy in Devon, for example, Bill Forsythe, Joseph Melling, and Richard Adair contend that 'institutional factors were often as important as medical discourses in determining the disposal of the pauper lunatic. Our evidence indicates that the micro-politics of Poor Law administration was of much more significance and much more complex than historians of medicine have usually acknowledged'.[3] Other studies, such as those by Peter Bartlett, have compared and contrasted the ideological and legal frameworks of the county asylum and the Poor Law.[4] Increasingly, we are seeing a coming together of the histories of the Poor Law and of insanity in nineteenth-century England.[5]

My aim in this chapter is to examine the relationships between gender, poverty, and employment in the early Victorian county pauper asylum against the background of the New Poor Law. A focus on poor women as workers in this context highlights the themes of respectability and dependency as constructed by the gender and class assumptions of the early Victorians. There are obvious class and gender issues when looking at the connections between lunacy and poverty. As John Walton pointed out in 1986, 'For the better off, lunacy clearly often "caused" poverty, just as lower down the scale poverty, expressed through stress and malnutrition, "caused" lunacy, especially among hard-pressed working-class wives and mothers'.[6] This essay takes up Walton's call to 'explore such issues further',[7] focussing on the differential understandings of gender, work and poverty in Poor Law and pauper asylum practice. By gender I mean the socio-cultural assumptions and expectations attached to being a man or a woman. The New Poor Law assumed a male subject; it was unemployed able-bodied men who were seen as the key to the problem of pauperism and on whom Poor Law authorities focussed in their efforts to abolish assistance outside the workhouse. The causes named for women's insanity in pauper asylums, however, reveal that women, too, were identified as workers and felt the pressures connected with the scarcity of employment and poverty, as was the case for Susannah Oter.

My analysis is based primarily on records from the West Riding Pauper Lunatic Asylum in Wakefield, specifically on the six large volumes of female patient case notes that cover the period from 1834 to 1852, containing the records of 1489 admissions.[8] These case notes hold a wealth of information on patients' social and medical histories, as well as not-so-regular comments on a patient's progress during her asylum stay. Dr. Corsellis, the early-Victorian director of the asylum, probably was the author of the majority of the case notes,[9] but it is possible that the clinical clerk who was mentioned in the Annual Reports after 1842 might have become responsible for taking the cases at this time. Most patients came to the asylum with an order of admission from a Poor Law relieving officer or medical attendant, who recorded the patient's social and medical history. Slightly more than half of the female cases (760) register the causes to which a patient's insanity was attributed, thus providing a tool for analysing the ways in which poverty and work were conceptualised in relation to mental illness. Poverty, in addition to things like grief, religion, domestic violence, and jealousy, was considered a moral cause of insanity, in contrast to things like illness and injury, which were physical causes.[10] For the West Riding cases, the causes of insanity seem to have been constructed by the asylum director in conjunction with the information provided by a patient's family and friends, or alternatively, by a previous medical attendant. Even where cause is not indicated, or where the primary cause is not poverty related, other material in the case book can reveal a preoccupation with basic survival issues.

The case notes, however, cannot be read as transparent depictions of a patient's experience with poverty or insanity, for the stories of these patients' lives and illnesses were obviously filtered by their medical caretakers, as well as those supplying additional details. Jonathan Andrews has argued for the fruitfulness of using case histories, but with care, for 'there are numerous deficiencies in the comprehensiveness and integrity of the case record, including intertextual inconsistencies and sins of omission, and areas of bias and censorship. These problems were profoundly mediated by social proprieties and medical ideologies'.[11] The thorny question of how we hear a patient's voice through the case is one that applies to all patient records, but is especially difficult with the insane, whose rational ability to represent themselves is itself an issue. As Michael MacDonald has pointed out, 'historians of insanity do not in the first instance study the insane at all: they study observations of the insane'.[12] Most often it is the voices of medical attendants that come through in a patient case, but 'in some instances it is possible to detect in [these records] the beliefs and concerns of the patients' families and sometimes of the patients themselves'.[13] Taking these issues of representation into account, I am nevertheless convinced of the value of these records in exploring the relationships between gender, poverty, and work in the context of poor women's insanity.

The West Riding Pauper Lunatic Asylum in Wakefield opened in 1818, being established on the basis of the 1808 (Wynn) Act that urged but did not require the foundation of county asylums for paupers. The first director of the asylum was William Charles Ellis, a great proponent of moral management, emphasising the cure and reintegration into society of the insane, rather than their restraint and custody.[14] C.C. Corsellis, who succeeded him, extended Ellis's vision for the asylum. With increasing numbers of patients to cater for, however, this vision of cure through individual attention and care became difficult to sustain. In its beginnings, the asylum was designed to accommodate seventy-five men and seventy-five women.[15] By January 1844, there were 433 patients; by January 1855, there were 762; by 1866, there were 1,128.[16]

Gender and work

In the gender order of early-Victorian England, dominated by the newly enfranchised middle classes, it would have surprised no one to hear that men became insane as a result of poverty or a lack of work. Middle- and working-class men alike were expected to stand on their own two feet and provide sufficiently for a family as well.[17] Unemployment was regarded as the fault of the worker, not something integral to the capitalist system. A man without work was somehow less than a man – no matter to what class he belonged. A man with work who could not earn enough to support self and family simply had to work harder. Anna Clark and Sonya Rose, among others, have shown how industrialisation and the accompanying process of deskilling put stress on masculine identity for men of the working poor, many of whom lost the status associated with pre-industrial craftsmanship.[18] Independence and respectability were linked with skill and the ability to provide, and the masculinity of the unskilled and unemployed was put in doubt.[19]

This ideal of respectability connected to work was encoded in the 1834 Poor Law Amendment Act. While certain parishes in the eighteenth-century had tried to make Poor Law relief contingent upon entering a workhouse, the New Poor Law of 1834 legislated this process for able-bodied men. Being able-bodied was equated with the ability to find employment and to work. A man could be poor and respectable, but once reduced to pauperism and reliance on the Poor Law for relief, respectability – at least as imagined by the New Poor Law – would vanish.[20] Pauperism denoted dependence and stripped a man of the masculine independence associated with occupation. The fact that a married man's wife and children had to follow him into the workhouse is evidence that the ability to provide was identified as the responsibility of the male head of the household. This was the case even though most people acknowledged the need for wives and children alike to contribute to family survival.[21]

Social and legal structures presented very different expectations for women, especially married women, who were considered dependent by nature. Moreover, being without work did not hold the same meanings for women in the middle and working classes. For middle-class women, work connoted a certain independence that went against women's supposed domestic nature.[22] Work lacked respectability. It could even, as Elaine Showalter has written, be taken as a sign of insanity.[23] For poor women, work meant survival. Men of the labouring classes were pleased to marry an industrious wife, as women's work – both paid and unpaid – was valued for its contribution to the family economy. Yet already by the 1830s, women's work outside the labouring man's home was marked with a questionable respectability, both by middle-class observers and by many working people themselves who hoped to live up to a male breadwinner ideal.[24]

This lack of connection between women and work is evident in the New Poor Law, which has almost nothing to say about pauper women (with the exception of single mothers), for policy makers assumed that most women would be provided for by the men in their lives, whether husbands or fathers. There was some recognition that single women and widows had to work and find ways to maintain themselves, but married women were expected to have husbands to take care of them. In light of these principles, in some cases, it could be assumed that poverty and lack of work would take on the same meanings for poor women as they had for poor men and would cause mental distress; in other cases, the lack of work could be seen as natural, as it was for middle-class women. The cases from the West Riding Pauper Lunatic Asylum show that the causes named for poor women's insanity reflect this ambiguity regarding gender and class.

Class and women's insanity

Most studies of British women's insanity in the nineteenth century have focussed on middle-class women and the connections between ideas surrounding women's bodies and insanity. Scholars stress an increasing medicalisation of women's mental illness that relied on the assumption that women's ailments were predominantly internally induced as a consequence of their reproductive functions.[25] As Ornella Moscucci has written, 'Not only did woman's biological functions blur into disease; they were also the source of a host of psychological disorders from strange moods and feelings to hysteria and insanity'.[26] Nancy Theriot has found that nineteenth-century American women relied on reproductive explanations for insanity just as much as their doctors: 'With and without prompting about the cause of their symptoms, women most often related their [mental] illness to their female bodies'.[27] This emphasis on the reproductive body accompanies the more general Victorian medical dictum that women's physical and mental health were ruled by their biology and their social roles should follow the constraints imposed by their delicate bodies.[28]

This medical construction, however, was complicated by class. Medical practitioners, like others of their class, expected poor women to work to stay out of pauperism, while still believing in the inherent fragility of the female body and the ideal of domesticity. This conflict is present in the New Poor Law's assumptions about being able-bodied. Women, according to medical theory, were really never able-bodied; their reproductive functions precluded them from being so and made them dependent on others for survival. Poor Law authorities were quite inconsistent in their application of the able-bodied standard to women; sometimes female applicants were treated as workers, and if able-bodied, condemned to the harsh rules of the New Poor Law. At other times, women were treated as persons who were not expected to work, and thus granted the benefits of assistance outside the workhouse.[29] In general, it was single women and widows without young children who were measured by the able-bodied model, whereas married women were regarded predominantly as dependents, even if their husbands did not take responsibility for them.

The West Riding cases show that questions about poverty and employment in relation to insanity for working-class women most often privileged class rather than gender associations. In the context of Victorian gender norms, one would expect to find a number of female cases of insanity linked to reproductive causes such as pregnancy and menstruation, as well as to causes like a husband's inability to keep a family afloat. It is less likely that one would anticipate women's – especially married women's – internalisation of their own unemployment as a central cause of female insanity. The case books, however, reveal an expectation that poor women would work, and suggest that poverty and unemployment had as much of an impact on women's sense of identity as they did on men's.[30]

Poverty, work, and the causes of insanity

In the world of early-Victorian psychiatry, poverty and unemployment were significant moral causes of insanity. John Conolly, a major figure in mid-Victorian asylum work, lectured that

> A neglected infancy, an uninstructed childhood, scanty food, thin clothing, and all the pinching wants of those who depend on the labour of the day for the food of the day, prevent the healthy development of the body, of the brain, and of the mind... [and] bring numerous victims to an asylum – for them the only worldly refuge from want and care.[31]

William Ellis, the first director of the West Riding Asylum, wrote in 1838, 'as the [asylum at Wakefield was] established solely for the reception of the poor, it will not be a matter of surprise that a greater number of its inmates, both male and female, are sent thither through distressed circumstances, than from any other moral cause'.[32] Poverty, according to Ellis, was both a 'source from which [insanity] first originates... [and] the cause of relapses'.[33] The county asylums were set up to address the incidence of insanity among the poor, and the numbers of patients by the mid-Victorian period certainly seemed to contemporaries to attest to the causal connections between poverty and insanity. In her critique of the social control aspects of asylum historiography, Wendy Mitchinson argues that the 'asylum was not being used as a place to hide away the deviant or the idle... except to the extent that mental illness was defined as deviancy and led to an inability to work'.[34] Not only could the deprivation of work lead to insanity, but insanity itself would often preclude a person from earning her living. The Victorian physician A.J. Sutherland stated in an 1855 lecture, 'the maniac cannot work because of the multiplicity of new ideas which every moment distract his mind; the monomaniac is too much engrossed with the contemplation of one subject to be able to pursue external objects, either of pleasure or of profit'. Thus, the insane become improvident: 'all their wants must be supplied, or they would suffer under the severest privations'.[35]

Part of the asylum plan was to take people away from the causes of their insanity. For those suffering from poverty and lack of work, this meant providing basic necessities and occupation. Ellis was convinced of the benefits of this approach: 'Removal from the scenes of misery which have been so painfully felt, and occupying the mind with other objects, aided by the influence of a good diet, have often produced very salutary effects in a short time, and ultimately restored the patient to sanity'.[36] Asylum directors stressed the domestic worldview of the middle classes and attempted to recreate this world in class-specific ways for their impoverished patients. Whereas the New Poor Law operated through the logic of 'less eligibility' – meaning that the standard of living in the workhouse would be worse than anything on the outside – the asylums of the early-nineteenth century were organised around the concept of moral management, not punishment, and were supposed to, in the words of Corsellis, the Victorian director of the West Riding Asylum, 'afford the comforts of a home'.[37] As I have argued elsewhere, it is possible that the conditions in county asylums were even preferable to some patients, who desired to remain in the asylum rather than return home.[38]

Work was central to this class-based domestic vision. Indeed, the West Riding Asylum was famous for its institution of employment as therapy for the insane under Ellis and continued under Corsellis.[39] This employment was fundamentally gendered, based on assumptions about male and female roles and abilities. In his report for 1846, Corsellis was happy to communicate that

> The [male] Patients have been extensively occupied throughout the summer in the cultivation of the land and gardens, nor has there been any diminution in the diligence of the convalescent and orderly females in the domestic business of the wards, kitchen, and laundry, the fancy works of the sale room, and of those employed in the various trades as tailors, joiners, shoemakers, &c., to which they had previously been accustomed.[40]

While the ideal of middle-class domesticity encompassed the separate spheres of (feminine) home and (masculine) work, the practice of domesticity for the insane poor meant appropriate work for both men and women, but work that was separated spatially. The outdoor occupations, deemed 'infinitely preferable' by Corsellis[41] were apparently considered only for men, while women's 'domestic' habits kept them inside in the less salubrious atmosphere of laundry and kitchen.[42] In addition to its therapeutic value, employment 'also constituted practical preparation for a return to society after discharge', as Leonard Smith has argued; 'for the pauper lunatic, work was to become a primary means for keeping the asylum patient in touch with the key role of a member of his class in society – that of worker'.[43] It should be no surprise that men and women were assigned different tasks, as the expectation in society at large was that work itself was gender- as well as class-specific.

Being poor, female, and insane

In the remainder of this chapter, I will examine the West Riding female patients' relationships to poverty in the context of their insanity, exploring the meaning of employment in these women's lives and the way that employment was interpreted by their middle-class observers in the asylum. I am particularly concerned with issues of causation and the ways the case books represent the female patients' experiences of poverty and unemployment. This analysis of the connections between gender, poverty, and work in the asylum case records contributes to our understanding of early-Victorian perceptions of women's work and dependency, and can help shed light on the ambiguity through which Poor Law authorities approached assistance to women. The West Riding cases suggest that the associations between poverty and insanity in the context of female pauper lunacy parallel the complicated expectations regarding women, work, and dependency encoded in the New Poor Law. The causes to which their insanity was attributed illustrate that poor women were both dependent on others for survival (like their middle-class counterparts) and independently responsible for earning their own livelihoods (like the men of their class). The fact that they inhabited female bodies, however, seems less of an issue than the fact that they were poor, while the reverse was true in the case of the Poor Law.

The cases suggest that whether they had contact with the Poor Law or not, the female patients experienced poverty as central to their lives. Many expressed concerns about poverty, or 'raved' on the theme of poverty. Ann Reynard, a 52-year-old married woman, 'raves chiefly on the fear of poverty and destitution, not being able to pay for the necessaries of life'.[44] One has to wonder what role her husband chose to play in her support, or whether he had abandoned her altogether. Mary Dockray, a 37-year-old widow from Leeds, 'raves chiefly on coming to poverty and want'.[45] Both these women's case notes recorded 'no employment' under occupation, suggesting that the difficulty in obtaining paid work might be at the root of their destitution. On her readmission to the asylum in May of 1847, Hannah Hall, a waterman's wife with twelve children, 'imagines she is to live for ever; but is sadly afraid of not getting sufficient to eat'.[46] The widow Rachel Abson 'chiefly talks about her debts, and wants to pay them but is unable: her privations weigh heavily on her mind'.[47] Some 'ravings' make clear the importance of family in women's survival strategies. The widowed weaver Sarah Lapish, for instance, 'raves on the embarrassed state of her pecuniary circumstances, her son having gone for a soldier and her daughter leaving her to be married'.[48] The single Elizabeth Mitchell 'frequently raves on the misfortunes of her own family'.[49] Perhaps articulating the politics of the majority of the West Riding poor in the 1840s, the 50-year-old knitter Ann Shepherd 'supposes the rich are combined to oppress the poor'.[50]

The case notes frequently exhibit the view that poverty predisposed a person to insanity, manifested both emotionally and physically. The notes on Mary Lancaster, a 28-year-old married woman with three children, observe that 'poverty may have assisted to induce the Melancholy'.[51] Similarly, Ann Walker suffered from 'depressed circumstances ending in Inflammation of the Brain'.[52] This woman continued to worry throughout her asylum stay about financial issues, such as her inability to pay for the food she was served.[53] Moreover, a physical illness could bring about poverty that might end in insanity. This seems to have been the case for Mary Mason, who suffered from 'pecuniary distress after an attack of Influenza'.[54]

Out of the 760 female cases in my sample where cause was recorded, the 101 (13.3 per cent) that note poverty, unemployment and related factors as key causes for insanity suggest their significance in the psychiatry of the day [see Table 5.1]. The cases that record 'embarrassed' circumstances and the like [see note *i* in Table 5.1] as causes are not all explicit as to the financial character of the circumstances. Some terms used to describe circumstances, such as 'reduced' or 'straitened' are more obviously poverty-related than the more vague 'distressed' or 'embarrassed'. Yet these held specifically pecuniary meanings in the mid-nineteenth century,[55] and it seems clear from the context that they can be read as examples of financial

Table 5.1
Poverty/Employment-Related Causes

Cause	Primary	Secondary	Total
Business failure	1	0	1
Circumstances (pecuniary)[i]	24	6	30
Employment - lack of	4	4	8
Employment - fear of losing	1	0	1
Employment - leaving	2	0	2
Family circumstances (pecuniary)[i]	3	3	6
Food – want of	0	3	3
Hard times	1	1	2
Husband: business failure/bankruptcy	1	1	2
Husband: circumstances (pecuniary)[i]	3	0	3
Husband: employment - lack of	4	0	4
Money/worldlymatters: disappointments/anxieties	5	0	5
Money/property losses/misfortune	5	1	6
Poverty: dread/fear of	6	7	13
Poverty/destitution/want	15	5	20
Total	75	31	106[ii]

[i] described variously as embarrassed, distressed, depressed, reduced, changed, troubled, straitened, narrow, poor, difficult

[ii] this total of 106 reflects the fact that in some cases both primary and secondary causes were both poverty-related; overall 101 cases were poverty related.

difficulties. As Ellis argued, 'the consequences of severe poverty could include lack of food and over-exposure to cold... The physical effects were compounded by the emotional distress associated with the inability to escape from poverty'.[56] Both material and emotional 'circumstances' resulted from poverty and unemployment, and the language in the notes I have included in the 101 poverty-related cases is strongly suggestive of this point.

While poverty shows up clearly in the West Riding female case records themselves, it is not so clear in the compilation of causes for the annual reports. The West Riding Pauper Lunatic Asylum Annual Report for 1839, published in the *Lancet*, for example, did not include 'poverty' or 'pecuniary disappointment' as categories causing women's insanity, whereas they were included for men. Perhaps the female poverty cases were incorporated within the category 'domestic affliction',[57] although this category appears as well under male causes.[58] Of the 673 male cases I sampled, 366 (54.4 per cent) noted cause. Of these, 100 (27.3 per cent) were related to financial or work issues. This is proportionately over twice as many as the female cases, which would be expected in the context of Victorian gender roles. More surprisingly in this regard, specifically 'female' causes made up a relatively small number of the total of 760 primary causes for women. Eighteen cases (2.4 per cent) were said to be directly caused by pregnancy, while fifty-eight (7.6 per cent) were attributed to some form of irregular menstruation. There were a number of cases, however, in which reproduction-related causes were secondary, or where there were comments concerning a female patient's reproductive functions.

In this context, eleven of the women's cases whose insanity was attributed to poverty and related causes also had notes about reproduction – either as an additional contributing cause or as a significant aspect of the mental health history. Three of these were connected to childbirth, one to nursing, four to menstruation, and two to menopause. For example, 26-year-old Ann Burkinshaw was admitted in March 1840. Her insanity was attributed both to poverty and 'suckling'.[59] While Hannah Wadsworth's insanity was blamed on poverty, 'the attack is said to have come on at the birth of one of her children'.[60] Similarly, although 'bad circumstances' were the assigned cause of Mary Browne's illness in May 1844, the case history indicates that the 'attack came on after childbirth'.[61] In other cases reproduction was the primary cause, but poverty also played a role. The insanity of Ann Wood, a single 24-year-old, for example, was attributed to 'obstruction of the Menses on the first onset', but it was important enough to note that she 'considers the pecuniary matters in a state of embarrassment'.[62] While the reeler Mary Wilcock's second admission for insanity was blamed on the 'bad treatment of her husband', her case notes comment both that she 'raves on poverty' and that her 'menstrual discharge [is] doubtful'. Additionally, 'the first attack [came] three weeks after confinement, the second immediately after delivery'.[63] These observations concerning a patient's reproductive state fit in with the medical and social wisdom of the day which emphasised the dominance of the reproductive functions in women's overall physical and mental health.

Another way in which the cases support Victorian gender norms is in suggesting that women's fears of poverty were often linked to the inability or refusal of their husbands to provide for them.[64] This would be anticipated in a gender order that stressed women's dependence on men and a Poor Law that joined married women's fates directly to their husbands'.[65] Indeed, Ellis believed that most insanity related to poverty occurred among married people – parents who were unable to support their children, and particularly industrious husbands and fathers who could not provide sufficient material necessities: 'A poor man who has been in the habit of maintaining his family in respectability, has been, from depression in trade or some untoward circumstances, thrown out of employment, or not able with his utmost exertions to earn what has been sufficient for the bare sustenance of his wife and children'. The stress attached to this reality, according to Ellis, would inevitably weaken the brain.[66]

The cases I have been discussing suggest that many among the labouring poor believed that men should be the primary providers, and wives became anxious when their husbands did not live up to the ideal. Of the 101 female cases where cause was attributed to poverty and related factors, sixty-four involved married women.[67] Mary Slater, a 25-year-old straw bonnet maker, was distressed because her husband had run away to Canada. The secondary cause was fear of poverty, most likely deriving from the absence of a husband to support her and her child.[68] The husband of Susannah Spence had drowned himself a month before her admission to the asylum in April 1835, and her insanity was attributed to 'distress from pecuniary circumstances and want of Food'.[69] Presumably she was also affected emotionally by the loss of her husband. The case notes on 44-year-old Mary Stott state that 'the attack is supposed to arise from her Husband being in great pecuniary difficulties and taken to York Castle for Debt'.[70] Martha Brook was separated from her husband and feared poverty would be the result, having six children for whom to care.[71]

The causes to which the female asylum patients' insanity were attributed stress women's dependency on their husbands' employment status. Her 'Husband not having sufficient employment' was listed as the cause of Hannah Hall's insanity.[72] Mary Black of Huddersfield cut her throat because of 'domestic troubles and the unexpected Bankruptcy of her Husband'.[73] The 33-year-old Jane Rawson of Halifax 'has been depressed in her mind for some time past on account of her Husband's adverse circumstances.[74] 'Upon inquiry' into Edith Batty's situation, 'it is stated that her Husband is childish, unable to work, and the Family are much reduced in circumstances'.[75] One presumes this information did not come from the patient but rather from someone else who was acquainted with the family. All of these cases demonstrate women's reliance on their husbands' earnings for their own survival. Ideas about male responsibility, the low wages paid to women, and the limited opportunities for married women's work in the West Riding shaped this situation.

These kinds of financial pressures also contributed to domestic violence. As Anna Clark, among others, has shown, the inability of working-class men to live up to the expectations of being the breadwinner put strains on marriages that sometimes led to violence. While the domestic ideal that positioned men as the primary earners and women as their dependents was supposed to create harmony within families, it engendered tensions when the reality was that men could not provide and women had to work. Additionally, the ideal of domesticity itself could 'excuse violence against those wives whom their husbands perceived as failing to fulfill their domestic responsibilities'.[76] Seven of the poverty-caused cases contain evidence of husbands beating wives. The primary cause listed for Sarah Smith's insanity was that her husband was out of work; the secondary cause, however, was his 'bad treatment' of her.[77] Hannah Dixon's family had to rely on Poor Law relief for survival; Hannah was in and out of the asylum in the early 1840s, suffering from poverty and 'the extreme distress of her family'. Upon her first admission, her insanity was blamed on 'her husband who often beats and abuses her'.[78] The historical justification for wife-beating in common law and *couverture*, and a husband's frustration with not being able to live up to the expectations of the masculine role, thus combined to exacerbate poor married women's mental and material worries.

Similarly, the West Riding Asylum cases suggest that pressures associated with socio-economic status contributed to women's insanity. Susannah Houson's husband 'was at one time a wealthy confector, but is now in poverty from unfortunate speculation in trade: this probably the cause of her insanity'.[79] The September 1852 case of Lydia Johnson, a 19-year-old millhand who was recently orphaned, reveals status concerns combined with economic issues: 'Her Father was a Master Stonemason in good circumstances, and at his death the family were much reduced, and this with the grief attending the death of her mother seems to have been the cause of the malady'.[80] The barmaid Ann Yates had a father who 'was once an Innkeeper in Bradford, and in comfortable circumstances: he was intemperate, eccentric, extravagant: eventually he became insane, and was twice in confinement... His business lost, and being much reduced in circumstances, he became despondent, and committed suicide by cutting his throat three weeks since' in April 1843. Ann's insanity was attributed variously to 'change of circumstances', 'hereditary disposition', 'destitution, the painful feelings arising from the mode of her father's death, and an attachment to a man who is now abroad'.[81] In addition to the emotional difficulties of being separated from a potential marriage partner, this woman probably also worried about the economic stresses of remaining unmarried.

Other women had something to lose in the way of their own business or position. Many of these women were single or widowed, and were likely to have their insanity attributed to fear – either a fear of poverty itself or the loss of employment. The unmarried dressmaker Mary Brown was first admitted to the asylum in March 1840 and 'pecuniary difficulties' was the assigned cause of her insanity. On her readmission in August 1841, her insanity was attributed to 'losses in business and falling into poorer circumstances'.[82] The 41-year-old single shoemaker, Esther Bottomley of Leeds, had her insanity attributed to 'failure in business and fear of poverty'.[83] The illness of Harriet Hall, a single drawer in a cotton factory, also was blamed on fear of poverty. She 'raves chiefly about poverty; begs of anybody that comes to the house... Attack supposed to be caused partly from... her fears, that as she cannot earn so much as other young women who are weavers, that she could not earn sufficient'.[84] Ann Walker was a schoolmistress whose 'fear of losing her situation' was the cause assigned for her insanity.[85] While it could be expected that single and widowed women would worry about their work status, married women also were concerned with employment. The married Hannah Rider was admitted to the asylum twice in the late 1840s. Both times her illness was attributed to a lack of work.[86]

Work was obviously central to many of these poor women's identities, and they connected employment to their overall well being. Sarah Sharp, a 21-year-old weaver, 'talks incoherently about not having worked for a long time past', while Ellen Gledhill, a 33-year-old labourer's wife, 'wishes to be working as then she feels better'.[87] Sarah Rose became depressed 'partly from the distress caused by want of work'.[88] Hannah Auckland was a 73-year-old widow who had been in the workhouse for several years before being admitted to the asylum in November 1851. Her age most likely precluded her from continuing her occupation, for 'previous to the attack [of insanity] there was great depression of spirits approaching melancholy, regretting that she could not do her work'.[89] The single

33-year-old washerwoman Elizabeth Aveyard was disturbed by a 'lowness of spirits brought on by the hardness of Times' in 1834.[90] Sally Pickles, a married factory operative in her thirties, 'is low from being without work'.[91] Many of these women were certainly under pressure to find ways to maintain themselves or contribute to their family economies. The alternative would be reliance on the Poor Law, whose stigma the majority of the labouring poor wished to avoid, even if they felt entitled to assistance.

In fact, for some women it was a direct encounter with the Poor Law itself which was blamed for their mental distress. Fears of having to rely on the Poor Law for maintenance contributed to poor people's anxieties. The asylum director William Ellis was sensitive to this, noting that the respectable poor were 'unwilling to apply to the parish for assistance', and that the tensions surrounding being forced to apply to the Poor Law could cause insanity.[92] 'The supposed cause' of the widow Rachel Abson's insanity, for example, 'is the fact of her being about to be removed to the place of her settlement'[93] from her home once her circumstances forced her to apply for Poor Law assistance. The 68-year-old widow Mary Wooffenden 'raves chiefly on having her furniture sold and being sent to the Workhouse'.[94]

The issue of respectability comes through clearly in the language of these cases. Anxieties about having to rely on the Poor Law for survival is one way in which women expressed their concerns with remaining respectable. Their 'embarrassed circumstances' also caused women to worry about respectability. Sarah Mills, a single 19-year-old mill worker, was overtly concerned with status and respectability: 'An extreme anxiety to better her condition in life: anything approaching poverty seemed to distress her very much'.[95] Alice Wright, a 50-year-old handloom weaver, had her insanity attributed to 'offended pride' because she could not maintain what she believed was a respectable standard of living: 'She has always been a striving ambitious woman, desirous of improving her worldly circumstances, but trade has lately been poor, and wages small; and these disappointments probably predisposed [her] to the attack'.[96] This assessment clearly comes from someone other than the patient herself. Additionally, the language exhibits the class biases of the case taker. Other case language reflects an acknowledgment of, and even sympathy towards, the difficulties poor women negotiated in order to remain respectable. Mary Hutton, a married 50-year-old housekeeper from Sheffield, obviously struck the case writer as someone unusual for her class: 'from what can be learned of her past life, and present appearance, she seems to possess a peculiarly sensitive mind: she is highly intelligent for her sphere in life, and is an Authoress, but her sensitive nature subjects her to poignant suffering from the privations and hardships of life'.[97] This comment implies that others of her class somehow suffered less from their impoverishment.

Conclusions

While gender and class as categories of analysis have played large roles in understanding the history of insanity in the nineteenth century, the interaction between them has not been explored fully. A focus on gender has tended to emphasise the centrality of the female reproductive body in conceptualisations of insanity, while a focus on class has demonstrated the economic and political dynamics of pauper lunacy. This project has attempted to bring these categories together in an examination of female pauper lunatics and the intersections of gender, poverty, and employment in their social and medical histories. By analysing these themes concurrently, it has highlighted the centrality of the female patients' dependency with reference to both official Poor Law policy and their experiences as poor, insane women.

The West Riding female pauper lunacy cases demonstrate, not surprisingly, that poverty was a basic fact of working-class women's experiences. Many of these women seem to have lived on the edge of subsistence and struggled in various ways to make ends meet. A central aspect of that struggle was paid employment. Social, medical, and legal norms held that women were dependent beings and that work was not an integral component of their identities or experiences. The West Riding Asylum patient records show this was not the case for poor women, suggesting the class-based nature of these norms. Assumptions about the fragility of women's reproductive functions are present as causes of insanity, but to no more of an extent than poverty and work issues. This echoes the interaction of gender and class assumptions in the New Poor Law, in which women were positioned both as dependent women and independent workers.

Acknowledgements

This chapter could not have been completed without the tremendous assistance of Tracey A. Limbaugh. Jonathan Andrews and Anne Digby offered very useful suggestions throughout. I would also like to thank Jeff Cox, Stacy Salz, Lorraine Walsh, David Atwill, R.A. Houston, Mark Jackson, and Michael Levine-Clark for their comments, and the archivists and staff at the Wakefield Headquarters of the West Yorkshire Record Office for their help during the research process.

Notes

1. West Yorkshire Record Office, Wakefield Headquarters (WYRO), West Riding Pauper Lunatic Asylum (WRPLA), C85/851, Female Case Book F11, 382.

2. There is an enormous historiography on the New Poor Law. For an introduction to key issues, see D. Englander, *Poverty and Poor Law Reform in Britain: from Chadwick to Booth* (New York: Longman, 1998); D. Fraser (ed.), *The New Poor Law in the Nineteenth Century* (New York: St. Martin's Press, 1976); A. Digby, *The Poor Law in Nineteenth-Century England and Wales* (London: The Historical Association, 1982); and M. Rose, *The Relief of Poverty, 1834–1914*, 2nd ed. (London: Macmillan, 1986).

3. 'The New Poor Law and the County Pauper Lunatic Asylum – The Devon Experience, 1834–1884', *Social History of Medicine,* 9, 3 (December 1996), 35. J. Melling, R. Adair, and B. Forsythe have undertaken a detailed study of pauper lunacy in Devon in a series of articles: '"A Proper Lunatic for Two Years": Pauper Lunatic Children in Victorian and Edwardian England. Child Admissions to the Devon County Asylum', *Journal of Social History*, 31 (1997), 371–405; Adair, Melling and Forsythe, 'Migration, Family Structure and Pauper Lunacy in Victorian England: Admissions to the Devon Country Pauper Lunatic Asylum, 1845–1900', *Continuity and Change,* 12 (1997), 373–401; and Adair, Forsythe and Melling, 'A Danger to the Public? Disposing of Pauper Lunatics in late-Victorian and Edwardian England: Plympton St. Mary Union and the Devon County Asylum, 1867–1914', *Medical History*, 42 (1998), 1–25.

4. P. Bartlett, *The Poor Law of Lunacy: The Administration of Pauper Lunatics in Mid-Nineteenth-Century England* (London: Leicester University Press, 1999), and 'The Asylum and the Poor Law: The Productive Alliance', in J. Melling and B. Forsythe (eds), *Insanity, Institutions and Society, 1800–1914: A Social History of Madness in Comparative Perspective* (London: Routledge, 1999), 48–67. See also L.D. Smith, *'Cure, Comfort and Safe Custody': Public Lunatic Asylums in Early Nineteenth-Century England* (New York: Cassell Academic, 1999), and Smith, 'The County Asylum in the Mixed Economy of Care', in Melling and Forsythe (eds), *Insanity, Institutions and Society,* 33–47.

5. For earlier work that addresses pauper lunacy, see A. Digby, *Pauper Palaces* (London: Routledge and Kegan Paul, 1978); J. Walton, 'The Treatment of Pauper Lunatics in Victorian England: The Case of Lancaster Asylum, 1816–1870', in A. Scull (ed.), *Madhouses, Mad-Doctors, and Madmen: The Social History of Psychiatry in the Victorian Era* (Philadelphia: University of Pennsylvania Press, 1981), 166–97; Walton, 'Lunacy in the Industrial Revolution: A Study of Asylum Admissions in Lancashire, 1848–1850', *Journal of Social History*, 13 (1979), 2–22; Walton, 'Casting Out and Bringing Back in Victorian England: Pauper Lunatics, 1840–1970', in W.F. Bynum, R. Porter, and M. Shepherd (eds), *The Anatomy of Madness: Essays in the History of Psychiatry. Volume II: Institutions and Society*, (New York: Tavistock, 1985), 132–46; R. Hunter and I. Macalpine, *Psychiatry for the Poor: 1851 Colney Hatch Asylum–Friern Hospital 1973. A Medical and Social History* (London: William Dawsons and Sons, 1974); and D.J. Mellett, *The Prerogative of Asylumdom: Social, Cultural, and Administrative Aspects of the Institutional Treatment of the Insane in Nineteenth-Century Britain* (New York: Garland Publishing, 1982), especially chapter seven, 'Commissioners, Workhouses, and Pauper Lunatics, 1845–90', 134–58.
6. Walton, 'Poverty and Lunacy: Some Thoughts on Directions for Future Research', *The Society for the Social History of Medicine Bulletin*, 38 (June 1986), 64–7: 65.
7. *Ibid.*
8. WYRO, WRPLA, C85/846-C85/851, Female Case Books F6-F11. This chronological boundary reflectsthe concern of my forthcoming study *Beyond the Reproductive Body: The Politics of Women's Health and Work in Early-Victorian England* (Columbus:Ohio State University Press, 2004). I examined all the new admissionss to the West Riding Pauper Lunatic Asylum during these years. In most entries, notes on patients readmitted to the Asylum were included under the heading of the original case. In this essay, readmissions are not counted separately unless they were recorded as a new case.
9. In an 1841 publication, Pliny Earle noted that the Director kept a 'medical journal, in which he places a history of every case admitted to the Asylum'. *A Visit to 13 Asylums for the Insane* (Philadelphia: J. Dobson, 1841), 11.
10. Both moral and physical causes were 'exciting' causes of insanity that could be coupled with 'predisposing' causes, like heredity or gender. See, for example, J.C. Bucknill and D.H. Tuke, *A Manual of Psychological Medicine: Containing the History, Nosology, Description, Statistics, Diagnosis, Pathology, and Treatment of Insanity, with an*

Appendix of Cases (Philadelphia: Blanchard and Lea, 1858), 240.

11. J. Andrews, 'Case Notes, Case Histories, and the Patient's Experience of Insanity at Gartnavel Royal Asylum, Glasgow, in the Nineteenth Century', *Social History of Medicine*, 11 (1998), 255–81: 280. For further discussion of historians' use of case notes, see G.B. Risse and J.H. Warner, 'Reconstructing Clinical Activities: Patient Records in Medical History', *Social History of Medicine*, 5 (1992), 183–205. Some recent studies of asylums have made extensive use of case notes and discuss the methodological issues connected to them. See, especially, Bartlett, *The Poor Law of Lunacy, op. cit.* (note 4); and Smith, '*Cure Comfort and Safe Custody*', *op. cit.* (note 4). For other examples of the use of case records in the history of psychiatry, see A. Digby, *Madness, Morality, and Medicine: A Study of the York Retreat, 1796–1914* (New York: Cambridge University Press, 1985); E. Lunbeck, *The Psychiatric Persuasion: Knowledge, Gender, and Power in Modern America* (Princeton: Princeton University Press, 1994); and N.M. Theriot, 'Women's Voices in Nineteenth-Century Medical Discourse: A Step Toward Deconstructing Science', *Signs*, 19 (1993), 1–31.

12. M. MacDonald, 'Madness, Suicide, and the Computer', in R. Porter and A. Wear (eds), *Problems and Methods in the History of Medicine* (New York: Croom Helm, 1987), 207–29: 210.

13. *Ibid.*, 211.

14. For specific discussions of the issues surrounding moral management, see, for example, A. Scull, 'The Domestication of Madness', *Medical History*, 27 (1983), 233–48; R. Porter, *Mind-Forg'd Manacles: A History of Madness in England from the Restoration to the Regency* (Cambridge, Mass.: Harvard University Press, 1987), 222–8; and E. Showalter, *The Female Malady: Women, Madness, and English Culture, 1830–1980* (New York: Penguin, 1985), chapter 1 'Domesticating Insanity: John Conolly and Moral Management', 23–50.

15. For histories of the Asylum, see J.S. Bolton, 'The Evolution of a Mental Hospital–Wakefield, 1818–1928', *Journal of Mental Science*, 74, 307 (1928), 587–633; A.L. Ashworth, *Stanley Royd Hospital Wakefield. One Hundred and Fifty Years. A History* (London: Berrico Publicity Co. Ltd., 1975); and J. Todd and L. Ashworth, 'The West Riding Asylum and James Crichton-Browne, 1818–76', in G.E. Berrios and H. Freeman (eds), *150 Years of British Psychiatry, 1841–1991* (London: Gaskell, 1991), 389–418.

16. Todd and Ashworth, *ibid.*, 390; 'Annual Reports of the County Lunatic Asylums and Hospitals for the Insane in England and Wales,

published during the year 1855', *Asylum Journal of Mental Science,* 2 (1855), 285; Smith, *'Cure Comfort and Safe Custody', op. cit.* (note 4), 174.

17. On constructions of masculinity in Victorian Britain, see J. Tosh, *A Man's Place: Masculinity and the Middle-Class Home in Victorian England* (New Haven: Yale University Press, 1999); M. Turner, *Reform and Respectability: The Making of a Middle-Class Liberalism in Early Nineteenth-Century Manchester* (Manchester: University of Manchester Press, 1995); L. Davidoff and C. Hall, *Family Fortunes: Men and Women of the English Middle Class, 1780–1850* (Chicago: University of Chicago Press, 1987); and M. Roper and J. Tosh (eds) *Manful Assertions: Masculinities in Britain since 1800* (London: Routledge, 1991).

18. A. Clark, *The Struggle for the Breeches: Gender and the Making of the British Working Class* (Berkeley: University of California Press, 1995); and S. Rose, *Limited Livelihoods: Class and Gender in Nineteenth-Century England* (Berkeley: University of California Press, 1992).

19. Respectability is a key concept in L. Walsh's study in this volume of the patient population at the Dundee Royal Asylum.

20. By contrast, L.H. Lees has shown that poor people felt entitled to relief and did not necessarily internalise the unrespectable status authorities associated with Poor Law assistance. See *The Solidarities of Strangers: The English Poor Laws and the People, 1700–1948* (Cambridge: Cambridge University Press, 1998), especially chapter five, '"Though Poor, I'm a Gentleman Still"', 153–78.

21. For discussions of gender and the Poor Law, see P. Thane, 'Women and the Poor Law in Victorian and Edwardian England', *History Workshop,* 6 (1978), 29–51; Lees, *op. cit.* (note 20); M. Levine-Clark, 'Engendering Relief: Women, Ablebodiedness, and the New Poor Law in Early-Victorian England', *Journal of Women's History,* 11 (2000), 107–30; and A. Clark, 'The New Poor Law and the Breadwinner Wage: Contrasting Assumptions', *Journal of Social History,* 34 (2001), 261–81.

22. The question of middle-class women, respectability, and work has been addressed most specifically in relation to single women. See, for example, M. Vicinus, *Independent Women: Work and Community for Single Women, 1850–1920* (Chicago: University of Chicago Press, 1985); and J. Perkin, 'Making Their Own Way: The Lives of Unmarried Middle-Class Women', in *Victorian Women* (New York: New York University Press, 1993), 153–68. See also M. J. Peterson, *Family, Love, and Work in the Lives of Victorian Gentlewomen* (Bloomington: Indiana University Press, 1989); and E. Langland,

Nobody's Angels: Middle-Class Women and Domestic Ideology in Victorian Culture (Ithaca, N.Y.: Cornell University Press, 1995).

23. Showalter, *op. cit.* (note 14), 121.

24. There is a large literature on the relationship between separate spheres ideology, respectability, and poor women's work. For example, see Clark, *op. cit.* (note 18); Rose, *op. cit.* (note 18); D. Valenze, *The First Industrial Woman* (New York: Oxford University Press, 1995); A. August, *Poor Women's Lives: Gender, Work, and Poverty in Late-Victorian London* (Madison, N.J.: Fairleigh Dickinson University Press, 1999); S. Alexander, *Women's Work in Nineteenth-Century London: A Study of The Years 1820-50* (London: Journeyman, 1983); J. Long, *Conversations in Cold Rooms: Women, Work and Poverty in Nineteenth-Century Northumberland* (London: Royal Historical Society, 1999); and J. Lown, *Women and Industrialisation: Gender at Work in Nineteenth-Century England* (Minneapolis : University of Minnesota Press, 1990).

25. See most obviously, Showalter, *op. cit.* (note 14). For a critique of Showalter's thesis, see J. Busfield, 'The Female Malady? Men, Women, And Madness in Nineteenth Century Britain', *Sociology,* 28, 1 (1994), 259–77. For an example of more literary approaches toward British women's insanity, see H. Small, *Love's Madness: Medicine, the Novel, and Female Insanity, 1800–1865* (New York: Oxford University Press, 1996).

26. O. Moscucci, *The Science of Woman: Gynaecology and Gender in England, 1800–1929* (New York: Cambridge University Press, 1990), 102.

27. Theriot, *op. cit.* (note 11), 20.

28. See M. Levine-Clark, 'Testing the Reproductive Hypothesis: Or What Made Working-Class Women Sick in Early Victorian London', *Women's History Review,* 11, 2 (2002), 175–200. A. Digby explicitly connects gynaecological and psychiatric ideas in 'Woman's Biological Straitjacket', in S. Mendus and J. Rendall (eds), *Sexuality and Subordination: Interdisciplinary Studies of Gender in the Nineteenth Century* (New York: Routledge, 1989), 192–220.

29. Levine-Clark, *op. cit.* (note 21).

30. August also argues that poor women self-identified as workers in *Poor Women's Lives,* see especially 118–9 and 139–40; also see Clark, *op. cit.* (note 18), 36.

31. J. Conolly, 'On the Principle Forms of Insanity', *Lancet* (29 November 1845), 584.

32. W. C. Ellis, *A Treatise on the Nature, Symptoms, Causes, and Treatment of Insanity* (New York: Arno Press, 1976; original London,

1838), 60.

33. *Ibid.*, 64.

34. W. Mitchinson, 'Gender and Insanity as Characteristics of the
    Insane: A Nineteenth-Century Case', *Canadian Bulletin of Medical
    History*, 4 (1987), 99.

35. A.J. Sutherland, 'Introductory Lecture to a Course of Lectures on
    the Pathology and Treatment of Insanity, delivered at St. Luke's
    Hospital, in the Months of May and June, 1855', *Asylum Journal of
    Mental Science*, II (1855), 150.

36. Ellis, *op. cit.* (note 32), 64.

37. WYRO, WRPLA, C85/108, Annual Report for 1844. Smith makes
    this contrast explicit in his study of early nineteenth-century
    asylums: 'The new model asylum offered the opportunity to provide
    an alternative to the "less eligibility" philosophy of the workhouse
    for at least one section of the disadvantaged poor. These asylums
    were constructed, furnished and equipped with the intention of
    providing standards well above what most of the inmates had been
    used to in their own homes'. Smith, '*Cure, Comfort and Safe
    Custody*', *op. cit.* (note 4), 162. Also see Bartlett, *op. cit.* (note 4).

38. M. Levine-Clark, 'Dysfunctional Domesticity: Female Insanity and
    Family Relationships Among the West Riding Poor in the mid-
    Nineteenth Century', *Journal of Family History*, 25 (2000), 341–61.
    C. McGovern also makes this point in her study of Pennsylvania
    State Lunatic Hospital. See, 'The Community, The Hospital, and
    the Working-Class Patient: The Multiple Uses of Asylum in
    Nineteenth-Century America', *Pennsylvania History*, 54, 1 (1987),
    24–25.

39. Smith, '*Cure, Comfort and Safe Custody*', *op. cit.* (note 4), 228–36.

40. WYRO, WRPLA, C85/108, *Annual Reports*, 1846, 7.

41. WYRO, WRPLA, C85/108, *Annual Reports*, 1844, 10.

42. Several asylum physicians of the period stressed that active
    occupations were much better than sedentary ones. R. G. Hill of
    Lincoln Asylum stated simply that 'sedentary employments are not
    good', pointing particularly to things like needlework, which was
    considered women's work, in *Lancet* (6 July 1839), 554. Conolly
    explicitly indicated that 'more women get well who are employed in
    the kitchens, laundries, and wards, than in the work-rooms'. Yet still
    women were for the most part deprived of employment out of doors
    and the 'advantage... of its being carried on in the open air'. 'On the
    Construction and Government of Lunatic Asylums', *Lancet* (15
    August 1846), 169.

43. Smith, '*Cure, Comfort and Safe Custody*', *op. cit.* (note 4), 209.

44. WYRO, WRPLA, C85/848, 436.
45. *Ibid.*, 512.
46. WYRO, WRPLA, C85/849, 331.
47. WYRO, WRPLA, C85/847, 158.
48. WYRO, WRPLA, C85/850, 70.
49. *Ibid.*, 316.
50. WYRO, WRPLA, C85/849, 214.
51. WYRO, WRPLA, C85/847, 21.
52. WYRO, WRPLA, C85/848, 118.
53. *Ibid.*, 119.
54. WYRO, WRPLA, C85/846, 414.
55. G. Crabb, *English Synonymes* (New York: Harper and Brothers, 1837).
56. Smith, *'Cure, Comfort and Saft Custody'*, *op. cit.* (note 4), 104.
57. *Lancet* (8 February 1840), 732.
58. R.A. Houston, in his contribution to this volume, finds that for Dundee Asylum in 1820-21, 'domestic affliction' was the cause of insanity attributed to three of the twenty-eight women admitted that year, but none of the men admitted had cause assigned to 'domestic affliction'. He argues that this shows an association between women's insanity and causes located in the domestic sphere.
59. WYRO, WRPLA, C85/847, 391.
60. WYRO, WRPLA, C85/848, 46.
61. *Ibid.*, 392.
62. *Ibid.*, 52.
63. *Ibid.*, 529.
64. I have discussed these issues with reference to women's applications for Poor Law relief in Levine-Clark, *op. cit.* (note 21), 119 and 122.
65. A. Clark offers an excellent discussion of the way in which the breadwinner wage was conceptualised in Poor Law policy, emphasising the ambiguities with which Poor Law authorities approached women in reference to their ideas about male breadwinning. Clark, *op. cit.* (note 21).
66. Ellis, *op. cit.* (note 32), 61.
67. This preponderance of married women is more present in the poverty-related cases than in the profile of my entire sample of West Riding cases. In the 760 cases where cause was noted, about fifty-one per cent of the patients were married, thirty-eight per cent were single, and about eleven per cent were widowed. This finding differs from other studies which show more single than married women in asylum admissions; see for example, Digby, *op. cit.* (note 11), 176; and M. Finnane, *Insanity and the Insane in Post-Famine Ireland*

(London: Croom Helm, 1981), 130–33. While Mitchinson found that unmarried patients predominated over married in her study of the Provincial Lunatic Asylum of Ontario, among the married patients, women exceeded men. Mitchinson, *op. cit.* (note 34), 104.

68. WYRO, WRPLA, C85/847, 173.
69. WYRO, WRPLA, C85/846, 136.
70. *Ibid.*, 7.
71. WYRO, WRPLA, C85/847, 135.
72. *Ibid.*, 331.
73. WYRO, WRPLA, C85/846, 78.
74. WYRO, WRPLA, C85/847, 1.
75. *Ibid.*, 159.
76. A. Clark, 'Domesticity and the Problem of Wifebeating in Nineteenth-Century Britain: Working-Class Culture, Law, and Politics', in S. D'Cruze (ed.), *Everyday Violence in Britain, 1850–1950* (New York: Pearson Education, 2000), 27–40: 28–9; and Clark, *op. cit.* (note 18), 71–87. On domestic violence in Victorian culture, also see N. Tomes, '"A Torrent of Abuse": Crimes of Violence between Working-Class Men and Women in London, 1840-1875', *Journal of Social History*, 12 (1978), 327–45; A.J. Hammerton, *Cruelty and Companionship: Conflict in Nineteenth-Century Married Life* (New York: Routledge, 1992); M. Doggett, *Marriage, Wife-Beating and the Law in Victorian England* (Columbia: University of South Carolina Press, 1993); S. D'Cruze, *Crimes of Outrage: Sex, Violence, and Victorian Working Women* (DeKalb, Ill.: Northern Illinois University Press, 1998); and M. Tromp, *The Private Rod: Marital Violence, Sensation, and the Law in Victorian Britain* (Charlottesville: University of Virginia Press, 2000).
77. WYRO, WRPLA, C85/847, 369.
78. WYRO, WRPLA, C85/848, 10-11.
79. WYRO, WRPLA, C85/ 849, 40.
80. WYRO, WRPLA, C85/851, 524.
81. WYRO, WRPLA, C85/848, 218.
82. WYRO, WRPLA, C85/847, 380.
83. *Ibid.*, 147.
84. WYRO, WRPLA, C85/850, 246.
85. WYRO, WRPLA, C85/849, 64.
86. *Ibid.*, 174.
87. *Ibid.*, 44, 62.
88. WYRO, WRPLA, C85/848, 98.
89. WYRO, WRPLA, C85/851, 330.
90. WYRO, WRPLA, C85/846, 108.

91. WYRO, WRPLA, C85/850, 228.

92. Ellis, *op. cit.* (note 32), 61.

93. WYRO, WRPLA, C85/848, 158.

94. WYRO, WRPLA, C85/851, 112.

95. WYRO, WRPLA, C85/850, 292, emphasis in original.

96. WYRO, WRPLA, C85/848, 252.

97. *Ibid.*, 314.

6

Delusions of Gender?:
Lay Identification and Clinical Diagnosis of Insanity in Victorian England[1]

David Wright

This chapter examines the lay identification and medical diagnosis of patients admitted to public mental hospitals in Victorian England through an analysis of over 1,500 admissions to the Buckinghamshire Lunatic Asylum. It demonstrates three things: women were institutionalised in numbers commensurate with their representation in the adult population; the certification of the insane was not dominated by male informants; and there is no empirical evidence to suggest that gender played a dominant role in the decision over the selection of particular psychiatric diagnoses. This chapter suggests future areas of research for a new historical epidemiology of mental symptoms.

Introduction

Ever since the publication of Phyllis Chesler's *Women and Madness*, a generation of Anglo-American feminist historians, and sociologists of health and illness, have looked critically at the role psychiatry performed in redefining and controlling women's 'public' and 'private' behaviour. Chesler proposed that, from the formation of psychiatry in the nineteenth century, women in the western world have borne the brunt of psychiatric classification and treatment: 'Women of all classes and races', Chesler affirmed, 'have always formed the majority of the psychiatrically involved population'.[2] According to her thesis, women moving outside of accepted Victorian norms of social behaviour, or displaying exaggerated sexual conduct, found their behaviour pathologised and incorporated into a new psychiatric nosology. Empowered with the control and confinement of the insane in purpose-built institutions, male psychiatrists allegedly acted as the vanguard of a new social and sexual order. Psychiatric classification and involuntary confinement, the argument insisted, were the professional and physical manifestations of coercion being played out more subtly in other arenas of Victorian society.

Several influential academics followed Chesler's identification of the Victorian epoch as the genesis of this medical enforcement of social and sexual conformity. Elaine Showalter, for example, suggested that the Victorian period witnessed not only the 'widespread incarceration of women' under the guise of insanity, but also the 'feminisation' of madness itself.[3] Denise Russell, drawing heavily on Chesler's research, sought to explore why a 'close relationship' developed between women and psychiatry in twentieth-century America. For her, the answer also lay in 'the changing social conditions and the narrowing views on a woman's role' commencing in Victorian society.[4] These researchers pointed to 'new' mental illnesses – hysteria, ovarian madness, puerperal mania and climacteric insanity – as manifestations of the pathologisation of women's behaviour, in particular, behaviour associated with women's reproductive cycle.[5] Psychiatrists were thus, according to this collective critique, drawing on new definitions of women's 'sex-role' to pathologise those who fell outside the norms of social etiquette. Jane Ussher, in a provocative, though not unrepresentative manner, sub-titled her book *Misogyny or Mental Illness?*, in order to convey the stereotypes which, according to her, have medicalised and marginalised women's challenging behaviour over the past 150 years.[6]

This feminist school of revisionism within the history of psychiatry has thus revolved around three related propositions: (1) that psychiatrists drew heavily on contemporary norms of femininity to diagnose culturally unacceptable behaviour of women; (2) that male superintendents of Victorian mental hospitals had the power, authority and inclination to play leading roles in the involuntary hospitalisation of women (and men); and (3) that women were disproportionately confined in asylums by the end of the nineteenth century. By the late 1980s, however, some academics, almost all centrally concerned with mapping the social history of institutions, began to challenge empirically the last proposition – that women were incarcerated disproportionately in Victorian asylums. Nancy Tomes, in her monograph on the Pennsylvania Asylum, for instance, illustrated that men outnumbered women in ante-bellum American asylums. It was only with the growing 'respectability' of the asylum that families felt willing to send their daughters and wives there, and in this way gender-equality of asylum inmates was eventually reached.[7] Similarly, Anne Digby, investigating the Quaker York

Retreat in England, further modified Showalter's thesis in the context of her study of patients admitted to that famous charitable institution.[8] Other researchers, such as Ellen Dwyer, reinforced the emerging consensus that there was little quantitative support for the disproportionate incarceration when it came to the asylums of New York State.[9] Joan Busfield summed up the view of many when, analysing evidence in the institutional returns made to the English Lunacy Commissioners, she confirmed that women were not disproportionately incarcerated in nineteenth-century England.[10]

The recognition that both women and men were incarcerated in numbers proportionate to their representation in the general adult population, combined with the new interest in cultural history in the 1990s, encouraged researchers to look at Victorian asylum records from a new 'gendered' perspective and to revisit the alleged 'feminisation' of madness. It is perhaps not surprising that the advantages of this new approach were quickly appropriated by scholars working on colonial asylums, which were notable for the heightened admission of *male* patients. Bronwyn Labrum, for instance, concluded that there was 'no evidence of the "feminisation" of madness in Victorian New Zealand, nor of the overwhelming existence of a prevailing perception of a fundamental alliance between woman and madness'.[11] Waltraud Ernst concurs: in the context of British India, the typical faces of madness which Showalter identified were constituents of a plurality of mad stereotypes, some of which were identified with social constructions of masculinity.[12] Research on nineteenth-century Canada, Australia, South Africa and Ireland, where police were central to the identification and confinement of the insane, has suggested that officers of the law were more concerned with controlling and redefining public displays of male violence, disorder and aggression.[13] Slowly, this new research on gender and madness has influenced research on the history of British institutional psychiatry. Mark Micale, for example, has illustrated how Charcot's ideas on hysteria involved constructions of masculinity as well as femininity enunciated by English alienists, while Janet Oppenheim has revealed that men as well as women frequented the private clinics of Victorian London for relief from their 'shattered nerves'.[14]

This chapter seeks to contribute to this new perspective in the history of psychiatry by investigating the gendering of confinement and diagnosis of patients admitted to one rural asylum in Victorian England, the Buckinghamshire County Pauper Lunatic Asylum. County asylums are important inasmuch as they constituted over eighty-five per cent of admissions to mental hospitals in Victorian England.[15] The chapter is divided into three parts. First, it will illustrate how male medical superintendents of asylums, the forerunners of the modern day psychiatric profession, had no control over the confinement process in England. Indeed, legislation was framed to guard against wrongful confinement and specifically forbade alienists from participating in the medical certification of patients. Decisions over confinement rested on a delicate negotiation between families, local medical practitioners and Poor Law officers. This first section will illustrate how female and male family members, neighbours and local poor law officials played significant roles in the determination of insanity through the process of certification. Rather than being a reflection of male power and female passivity, the certificates enshrined an interdependence between household and medical authority, wherein the next of kin took responsibility for defining the attributes of insane family members. Thus confinement produced a psychiatric profession, and provided, through certification, the basic data for the eventual production of 'psychiatric knowledge', not *vice versa*.

The second part of this chapter will investigate the interaction between the descriptions of insane behaviour in the certificates of insanity and the diagnosis of these same patients by the medical superintendents of the asylum. It will thus analyse the plurality of behaviours, moods and thought that constituted Victorian madness. Although the medical superintendents had no control over who were sent to their institutions, they were required by law to inscribe in the admission register a 'form of mental disorder'. This gave them unbridled authority to classify patients arriving at their institution. Contrary to revisionist assertions about the widespread diagnosis of 'women's disorders' during the Victorian era, the results of this case study reveal that, in the case of asylums for the poor insane, the classic examples of new 'gendered' diagnoses did not figure prominently at all. Mania, Melancholia, Dementia, and Idiocy – the standard psychiatric classifications in the mid-Victorian period – were applied to men and women using consistent criteria across the genders. That is, there is no evidence that the constellation of behaviours, moods and thoughts (embedded in the certificates of insanity) resulting in a particular diagnosis – say of Melancholia – varied significantly between men and women. However, the *incidence* of particular institutional diagnoses did. 'Mood' disorders were more widely described in female admissions to the asylum, leading to more common diagnoses of Mania with Depression, and Melancholia. By contrast, men were more often classified as suffering from Mania with General Paralysis (General Paralysis of the Insane) and Idiocy. Contrary to the tradition of taking, as axiomatic, that this reported difference was a function of a gendered perspective amongst the medical superintendents, this paper will contend that these classifications were a function not of changing psychiatric classification (by medical superintendents) but of the differential presentation of women and men with these symptoms at the gates of the asylum. That is, there were more women diagnosed with Melancholia at the Buckinghamshire asylum because more women than men with melancholic dispositions were identified, certified and sent to the asylum by family members, local medical practitioners and poor law officials. Evidence to support this alternative proposition lies in the comparison of identical diagnoses of men and women (made by asylum superintendents in the asylum) with the description of behaviours incorporated in the certificates of insanity (compiled by testimony from family members).

Lastly, in an exploratory final section, this chapter will examine the types and contents of delusions described in the certifications of insanity of all women and men diagnosed as suffering from Melancholia and Mania with Depression. Exhibiting delusions did not constitute a *diagnosis*, but rather a common symptom associated with different types of psychiatric classifications in Victorian England. Indeed more than one-half of all admissions to the Buckinghamshire asylum were identified as having some sort of fixed false belief. This last section will analyse the delusions to see whether there were discernible gender patterns by type or content. The tentative results suggest that, even here, women and men shared common types of delusions, such as persecution, grandeur, guilt and nihilism (though they differed in rank importance). As for content or theme, women's delusions tended to be associated with kinship, family and household, and personal health, a function of the cultural importance of these aspects to the changing social circumstances in which women's social role became increasingly associated with the domestic sphere. Male delusions, by contrast were most often associated with work, status and property. Thus the changing social and sexual role expectations of Victorian women and men mad were reflected and distorted in the content of their own false beliefs.

The mid-Victorian period, usually described as the era commencing with the 1851 Exhibition and terminated by the onset of the Great Depression in 1873, constitutes a crucial period to study the interplay between gender, class and psychiatry. First, the landmark lunacy legislation in England and Wales – the Asylums Act and Lunatics Act of 1845, and the Lunatics Amendment Act of 1853 – were in place at the beginning of this era. The 1845 Acts obliged all county and borough magistrates to construct asylums for their insane poor, prompting the construction of two dozen asylums by the early 1870s.[16] These asylums provided the loci for the expansion of the Association of Medical Officers of Hospitals and Asylums for the Insane (the forerunner to the Medico-Psychological Association and, later, the British Psychiatric Association). The mid-Victorian period thus represented the era of the formation and consolidation of modern British psychiatry. The second act, the Lunatics Amendment Act of 1853, established the structure of the two key admission documents – Certificates of Insanity and Reception Orders – which underpinned the legal process of confinement and constitute the principal sources for reconstructing the socio-demographics and psychiatric symptoms of patients. They thus represent a census of the institutionalised psychiatric population and a unique compendium of testimony about Victorian madness which crossed class and gender divides. Secondly, the mid-Victorian period has been identified by women historians as the crucial turning point in the redefinition of women's social roles within modern England. Thus the period under study, and the asylum's records discussed below, represent a unique opportunity to investigate historically the relationship between gender, class and psychiatry.

Certification and confinement in Victorian England

The legal regulation of the confinement of the insane in public[17] institutions in nineteenth-century England[18] derived from laws dating from the 1808 Asylums Act. Under the terms of this act, county magistrates could establish asylums and charge parishes for the maintenance of 'their' insane paupers who were received into these new institutions. The 1808 Act was permissive, and poor law parishes had the freedom to decide whether or not they would seek institutional confinement of their insane poor, board them out in the community or send them to local workhouses. The growth in the number of institutionalised patients, sent by parishes and received by magistrate-run asylums, however, was steady, reflecting the fact that purpose-built institutions for the insane poor were fulfilling a demand throughout the county for institutional accommodation. By 1842, there were seventeen county asylums accommodating over 6,000 patients from parishes within their county border and from parishes in neighbouring counties that had, as yet, no formal asylum accommodation.[19]

The county asylums were established amidst public concern about the possible wrongful confinement of sane individuals. Largely in response to these concerns, legislation dating from 1811 stated that each county asylum had to have a certificate of insanity for every admission. These certificates were completed by a community-based qualified medical practitioner, who testified that, at the time of admission, the allegedly insane person was either 'an idiot, lunatic or person of unsound mind', the statutory definition of insanity. Successive legislation between 1811 and 1853 refined and extended the requirements of this procedure, especially with regard to private (paying) patients. Certificates had to be completed within seven days of confinement or they were invalid, and any signing medical practitioner shown to have deliberately falsified a statement was guilty of a misdemeanour. Importantly, an asylum medical officer could not sign a certificate for an admission to his own institution. Under the 1853 Lunatics Amendment, the medical practitioner was required to validate his comments with testimony from other individuals and state from whom this corroboration was given.[20] The certification of the insane in Victorian England was, therefore, a process performed largely in the 'community' and from which those most experienced in observing the behaviour of the insane – medical officers of asylums – were barred from participating. Technically, of course, a medical superintendent could sign a certificate of insanity for a person destined to another county asylum. This was, however, comparatively rare. Indeed, the majority of the people admitted to county asylums after the 1853 Amendment Act were certified by medical practitioners with little or no formal education or institutional experience in the examination and treatment of insanity. Thus, in a rather unique manner, public concern over wrongful confinement encouraged legislators to severely restrict alienists from participating in the certification process and required local medical practitioners to validate their observations with the views of other, usually non-medical, individuals.

The testimony of this unusual legal and medical process has been enshrined in the certificates of insanity for those patients admitted to the Buckinghamshire County Pauper Lunatic Asylum. Constructed in 1853, in the parish of Stone, just outside the county capital of Aylesbury, the Buckinghamshire Asylum was remarkable for its ordinariness. The building, established to hold 200 inmates, was functional, though not palatial. County magistrates accepted patients from parishes in the seven Buckinghamshire poor law unions of Amersham, Aylesbury, Buckingham, Eton, Newport Pagnell, Winslow and Wycombe.[21] Like most other institutions, demand for accommodation outstripped supply, and the residential population rose steadily to over 400 patients by 1873. The annual rate of admissions to the county asylum approximated that of the national average; moreover, the socio-demographic characteristics of patients corresponded to the results of other large-scale asylum projects which reveal that patients were sent from a cross section of the lower two-thirds of society. In the case of Buckinghamshire, this resulted in a wave of agricultural labourers, women lacemakers and strawplaiters, skilled artisans and their wives, as well as shopkeepers and clerks. The relative absence of professional groups and farmers suggests that they could afford 'buying in' care in the household, or sending relatives to one of the many licensed (for profit) homes in and around the Metropolis.[22]

Following their statutory obligation, the Buckinghamshire county magistrates appointed a medical man, William Humphrey, to take responsibility as institutional superintendent in 1855. Like many of his contemporaries, Humphrey had no background whatever in the treatment of the insane. This, however, did not seem to prevent him from a long and stable career as medical superintendent, remaining in the position for a remarkable fifty-three years until his retirement in 1908. Unlike the famous superintendents of the Hanwell Asylum and the Devon County Asylum, John Conolly and John Bucknill respectively, Humphrey enjoyed his secure position in Buckinghamshire and carried out this superintendency without any major successes or scandals. He was a member of the Medico-Psychological Association and authored only a handful of uninfluential articles in the *Journal of Mental Science*. He was, in summary, the very model of a modern medical superintendent.[23]

Humphrey performed his administrative responsibility as required, completing and compiling dutifully the admission registers, certificates of insanity, reception orders, death certificates, medical case books and discharge and transfer orders for inspection twice a year by the Lunacy Commissioners and monthly by the county visiting committee of magistrates. Largely because of these inspections, the records for all patients in Buckinghamshire for the entire Victorian period (like many other Victorian asylums) were meticulously organised and have been preserved in the county archive. The results, upon which the arguments for this chapter rest, were derived from a database study of admission register data (including diagnosis) for all patients admitted between 1853 and 1874 (1,722 individuals). In addition, information for the certificates of insanity for those 210 patients admitted during the English decennial census years (1861, 1871, 1881) were also entered in separate linked tables for qualitative investigation. Finally, all the certificates of insanity for those women and men listed as suffering from Mania with Depression (n = 115) and Melancholia (n = 206) were entered into the same database and coded by delusion type and content.[24] This provides the basic nominal, ordinal and interval data across gender, class and age divides. Testimony in these certificates of insanity provides evidence to illustrate patterns of symptoms, and recent histories of patients. Combined they offer a unique opportunity to explore some of the themes concerning gender, class and psychiatry in the nineteenth century which inform this book and contribute new research into the historical epidemiology of mental symptoms.

Certification of the insane poor in Victorian Buckinghamshire

Only recently has systematic research been conducted into the social context of certification, and much more work remains to be done.[25] Results from the sample Buckinghamshire records, however, suggest three principal routes of patients[26] to the county asylum that determined both the locus of certification and its central participants. First, and most common, was confinement directly from the household. In these circumstances, families arranged with poor law authorities and county magistrates to secure a bed in the county institution. After this had been agreed, a local medical practitioner, who may or may not have attended to the lunatic in the previous weeks or months, was called to the household to complete the appropriate documentation. In the case of non-paying patients, confusingly referred to as 'paupers' in the admission registers (even though many had not ever been in receipt of poor law relief[27]), doctors met with household members and took testimony to be included as 'indications of insanity' given by 'others' – that is, by those other than the certifying doctor. Since the certificate of insanity instructed the doctor to state the identity of the testifier, one can get an accurate picture of who contributed to this lay discourse of insanity identification. Most often, the principal testifier was the next of kin. Wives described the insane behaviour of their husbands, just as husbands supplied important information about the recent history of their insane wives. In the case of co-residing unmarried daughters or sons, fathers and mothers contributed in equal measure. Similarly, the sons or daughters (whether married or not) of widowed men and women informed doctors about their dependent parents.[28] In an era when married women could not own property or sign most legal documents, it is worth appreciating the status afforded to women in the certification process. Women testified freely to local medical practitioners and to magistrates assenting to, and facilitating, the confinement of their husbands, sons and fathers.

The second route to the asylum was through the poor law Union workhouse, a journey which included patients who had been sent there for a brief period of time (as a secure place of control before certification and transfer to the asylum) and patients who had long been resident in the house, but had become progressively or suddenly too unruly for the workhouse officers and nurses. In both cases, workhouse certification drew together an unusual alliance of observers, often including the workhouse masters, nurses, and other pauper inmates. Almost without exception, workhouse certification was completed by the poor law medical officer as one of his many duties on behalf of the poor law Guardians. The precise proportion of inmates sent to the asylum who were certified in the Union workhouses is difficult to determine. Peter Bartlett estimates that one-quarter of admissions to the Leicestershire and Rutland county asylum in the 1860s had been previously resident in constituent Union workhouses.[29] More recent research on the Plymptom St Mary's Union in Devon suggests that approximately thirty-six per cent of admissions to the Devon county asylum were certified, and had resided in the workhouse.[30] Evidence from Buckinghamshire certificates supports these conclusions: that about one-quarter of patients admitted to the asylum were resident in a workhouse, whilst another quarter were taken to the workhouse for security (and certification) for a short period of time before being conveyed to the county asylum.

Thirdly, and less frequently, lunatics were certified in the local jail or county prison. Contrary to popular belief, English asylums did not warehouse the vagrant and footloose of Victorian society; the proportion of individuals 'rounded up' by the police, sent from jails, or directed from the criminal justice system, never exceeded five per cent of admissions to Buckinghamshire. Major offences were dealt with through the criminal courts where insane persons found not guilty by reason of insanity or unfit to be tried were sent primarily to the Broadmoor Criminal Lunatic Asylum. A very small number of individuals were also transferred from the county prison, after having been determined insane. In these minority cases of admissions, the arresting constable was most often the person who retold the details of the lunatic's strange behaviour in the certificates. Similarly, in the cases of prisons, it was the prison medical officer.[31] Although jails played a central role in confinement in a colonial context,[32] they were, relatively speaking, unimportant to the confinement of the insane in England after 1845.

Certification placed the local medical practitioner in the role of interviewer and cross-examiner. He compiled the evidence on insanity from the witnesses and edited testimony for the certificate of insanity. The analysis of the sample Buckinghamshire patients suggests that certification was performed by a range of medical practitioners, not all of whom were connected with the poor law. Over eighty separate practitioners certified 210 patients sent to the Bucks asylum in 1861, 1871 and 1881. Of these, approximately twenty-two doctors, most of whom were employed as poor law medical officers, certified fifty-five per cent of the patients in these three years. The other half of the patients were certified by another sixty practitioners. Thus medical practitioners charged with the legal responsibility of inscribing 'indications of insanity' came from a surprisingly broad cross-section of the Victorian medical community. Their role in the marshalling of evidence in the certificates of insanity, then, can not easily be described as the imposition of a new *psychiatric* order on social behaviour. Indeed, the impression left by these documents is how 'untechnical' they were, and the extent to which medical practitioners relied on the testimony of others (particularly family members) to form their own opinion.[33]

'Psychiatric' classification of pauper lunacy

Once patients were certified by local medical practitioners, they were immediately conveyed, with the certificates of insanity, to the county asylum. Pauper patients also arrived with an Order for the Reception of a Pauper Patient (Reception Order) which listed social and occupational data upon each individual. Reception Order entries included: 'name', 'sex and age', 'marital status', 'previous occupation' and 'religious persuasion'. In addition, these documents, completed by local clergyman or magistrates, detailed what might be considered 'medical' questions, including 'when previously under medical treatment', 'age on first attack', 'number of previous attacks', 'supposed cause', and whether the insane person was 'suicidal', 'epileptic' and 'dangerous'. Finally, the Reception Orders listed the name of the next of kin,[34] and were co-signed by the relieving officer of the poor law union in which the person had Settlement. Medical officers and asylum clerks transferred the socio-medical attributes of patients into the admission register. In addition, and in accordance with the lunacy laws, they transcribed the 'indications of insanity' from the certificates into a new page of the medical case books. In this way, community-based lay and medical knowledge was fused and incorporated into an institutional medical framework. At this time the medical superintendent had to perform a medical examination of the patient and assign a 'form of mental disorder' (classify the insane behaviour) in the admission register. Thus the classification of patients was one area in which these medical superintendents could impose their growing specialist knowledge on a patient population produced by a social process largely beyond their control.

Table 6.1 represents the diagnoses of 1,722 patients admitted to the Buckinghamshire asylum during its first twenty years of existence. They may be broadly divided into five main categories: Mania, Melancholia, Dementia, and Idiocy. Mania was further subdivided into Acute Mania, Chronic Mania, Mania with Depression, Mania with General Paralysis and Puerperal Mania (see below). Several findings are immediately clear. First, in agreement with other quantitative studies of admission registers, the ratio of admissions, by gender, reflected the ratio of women and men in the community population. Thus, in Buckinghamshire, fifty-three per cent of admissions were women, exactly the same proportion of adult women in the county at the time of the 1861 census.[35] Secondly, one sees the close similarity in the breakdown, by gender, of classification and sub-classification. This table challenges assertions as to the 'widespread' use of new female-oriented psychiatric classifications during this mid-Victorian period. But it cannot tell us whether specific diagnoses – such as Melancholia – represented the same cluster of symptoms in women Melancholics and men Melancholics. Perhaps Showalter and others were correct in implying that male medical superintendents applied different standards of classification to female and male insanity? To answer this question, we must turn to the descriptions of insanity of the local medical practitioners and 'others' listed in the certificates under study and compare descriptions of women and men with the same classification.

The Lunatics Act of 1845 defined the 'insane' as including 'idiots, lunatics, or persons of unsound mind'. Thus 'idiots' and 'congenital imbeciles' were included, if awkwardly, under the jurisdiction of the 'lunacy laws'. Idiocy itself, was the least contested category of Victorian psychiatry, referring to those from birth, or an

Table 6.1
Forms of Mental Disorder, Buckinghamshire County Lunatic Asylum
(first admissions only), 1853-1874

		Male		Female	
Mania		**(n)**		**(n)**	
	(General)	487		517	
	Puerperal	0		18	
	Hysterical	0		4	
	with General Paralysis	27		9	
	Erotic	1		0	
	with Depression	41		74	
	Sub-total	**556**	67.9%	622	69.0%
Dementia					
	(General)	67		61	
	with General Paralysis	9		11	
	Epileptic	16		14	
	Other	1		3	
	Senile Dementia	2		2	
	Sub-total	**95**	11.6%	91	10.1%
Idiocy and Imbecility					
	Idiot	27		19	
	Imbecile	42		36	
	Deaf and Dumb	0		1	
	Epileptic	4		6	
	of Old age	1		0	
	with General Paralysis	1		0	
	Sub-total	**75**	9.2%	62	6.9%
Melancholia					
	(General)	87		118	
	Melancholia with Paralysis	0		1	
	Sub-total	87	10.6%	119	13.2%
Other					
	Chronic Lunatic	1		0	
	Delerium Tremens	1		0	
	Dipsomania	0		1	
	Sub-total	**2**	0.2%	1	0.1%
	N/A	1	0.1%	1	0.1%
	Unknown or no entry	4	0.5%	6	0.7%
Total		**820**		**902**	

early age, who were incapable of managing their own affairs due to mental weakness. Congenital imbecility was a medical, though not legal, term referring to idiots of less impairment. Thus Isabella Wooton, a 16-year-old from the Newport Pagnell Union, had been cared for by her mother at home and subject to epileptic fits 'since the age of 3.5 years'. Her mother testified that her daughter exhibited decreasing mental ability and was 'increasing helplessness and unmanageable'. The increasingly dependent Isabella was conveyed to the asylum in 1881 and diagnosed as suffering from 'idiocy'.[36] As mentioned above, an important minority of admissions were transported from Union workhouses, having resided there for some time.[37] One Buckinghamshire example of this was Albert Price, an 18-year-old inmate of the Winslow Union workhouse. Described as suffering from idiocy 'from birth', Albert was, by the testimony of another pauper inmate, 'violent – wants to bite everyone he sees – that he wants to run away'. To which the medical practitioner added, unhelpfully: 'He is very violent – wants to bite every one, looks wild – screams out loudly & wants to run away'. It seems that Albert had transgressed the threshold of violence tolerated in the mixed workhouse, prompting his incarceration in the county institution.[38] For most idiots and congenital imbeciles who were not violent, however, poor law Guardians seem to have preferred finding extramural solutions to their care and control.[39] In the limited number of cases, it is clear, however that idiot boys and girls were both described as having 'vacant' stares', 'imbecile expressions' and 'screaming without cause'. There is no demonstrable difference in the description of those labelled idiots or imbeciles by medical superintendents. Rather, the gendered difference lay in the larger number of boys than girls presented to asylum authorities during the Victorian era.[40]

Idiocy and congenital imbecility represented two states of 'chronic' and 'incurable' insanity the presence of which vexed the medical superintendents of asylums who desired to see asylums as primarily curative institutions. The other major classification of incurable insanity was dementia, a general term used to describe a decline in cognitive functioning, usually, though not exclusively associated with old age. Here again one sees a consistency across genders. The common symptoms listed in the certificates of insanity were a progressive and deteriorating loss of mental ability, bordering on imbecility, memory loss, and, sometimes, delusions. Mary Goodson, for instance, was an 80-year-old woman was cared for by two domestic servants, Eliza Arnold and Martha Orchard. These two servants found that they could not care for her and control her tendency to wander out of doors at night. Even their administration of opiates, given by the visiting medical practitioner, did little good.[41] Care and supervision of demented elderly men was no easier. Charles Eyles, a 73-year-old, formerly an inmate of the Winslow workhouse, became so disruptive in his delusional behaviour, that the workhouse master sought to confine him in the county asylum.[42]

Patients classified as suffering from Melancholia, by contrast, were understood to have experienced episodic, rather than chronic, periods of unsoundness of mind and were, generally speaking, considered amenable to treatment. The symptoms described in the certificates of insanity point to three principal features in order of importance: a 'great despondency', usually resulting in a state of incapacity, or an inability to perform expected gender-specific household duties; a tendency to suicidal thoughts, threats or attempts; and the existence of mood congruent delusions. Sarah Wallduck was described as insane both for her melancholia, her inability to perform the household duties she used to do, and her brooding over a former attempt to commit suicide.[43] Mary Anne Slade, by contrast, had been in and out of asylums for 'acute melancholia'. The local certifying doctor state that, by December 1880, she was 'in a state of profound and persistent melancholy – weeping without apparent cause, wishing she was dead. Says she feels so strange and low [and] wants to do something to herself'.[44] The threat or attempt at self-harm features in two-thirds of these melancholic women and men. Two Melancholic men of this diagnosis, both admitted to the asylum in 1881, were in states of 'great despondency', having both cut their throats in recent suicide attempts. The frequency with which patients were described in their certificates of insanity as having attempted suicide, or threatened suicide, made asylum authorities vigilant in their observation and surveillance of these patients after admission.[45] Gender certainly played a role in the expectation of private and public social roles. Thus women who neglected children or domestic duties, or men who declined to work in the fields and provide for their families, warranted comment in the certificates of insanity by other family members and neighbours.

The 'great despondency' of patients was common not only to the diagnosis of Melancholia (discussed above) but also to Mania with Depression, an important sub-group of the 'Manias'. In this category, medical superintendents classified the 115 admissions whose states of despondency were punctuated by periods of great excitement and elevated mood. Catherine Frost, for instance, was certified at a Union Workhouse in 1881. The poor law medical doctor described her alternating cycles of excitement and depression thus:

> She is very miserable and cries bitterly and on being asked a question she answers, in a very excited manner, and says her soul is lost – that the lady told her to trust to her and she would give her soul back again. That she was brought to the Union unknown to her – She will not believe her soul will ever again be restored to her and that she must die soon – she grieves much about 'her child' (a lad of 16) as she calls him and that he will lose his soul as she [has].

Charlotte Parker, a fellow workhouse inmate, confirmed Catherine's state of great despondency and that she 'weeps and cries all night', and the workhouse nurse lamented that her behaviour was preventing the sick from getting any sleep.[46] Similarly, Samuel Sears was diagnosed as suffering from Mania with Depression in July of 1871, having exhibited states of depression and excitement resulting in threatened violence toward family members. His certificate of insanity stated that he... [was] threatening to cut his mother's throat with a knife he was brandishing. For weeks before he had been in a 'great and unaccountable depression', thinking, like Catherine Frost (above), that his 'soul was lost' and exhibiting strange behaviour such as 'wandering off' and 'lying in a farmer's field'.[47] In both cases, alternating moods of excitement and depression, combined with delusions warranted a similar diagnosis. Also common was the violence and disruption towards others which made carers, both institutional and domiciliary, seek the greater supervision and control that an asylum could afford.

Two-thirds of all women and men were classified as suffering from some sort of 'Mania'. Mania was the most loosely defined psychiatric classification, most easily understood as unsoundness of mind not easily classified as idiocy, dementia, or melancholia. It was typified by delusional and disordered thinking, and states of irrational excitement. Throughout the mid-Victorian period, as medicine sought greater specialisation[48] and more nuanced categories, medical superintendents sub-divided mania by onset (senile, puerperal), by degree (acute, sub-acute, or partial), by frequency (recurrent, chronic), and by physical and emotional correlates (with depression, with epilepsy).

These more nuanced definitions of mania did indeed include disorders specific to women alone. As Table 6.1 indicates, this period witnessed the introduction of mania with hysteria (hysterical mania, sometimes also referred to by shorthand as hysteria) and puerperal mania (also known more generally as the insanity of childbirth[49]). Showalter famously asserted that ten per cent of admissions to Victorian asylums in England were labelled hysterical, and that ovarian madness and climacteric insanity were 'common'.[50] Her assertions do not seem to be supported by any evidence from the county asylums that received the overwhelming proportion of patients during this time. In the case of Buckinghamshire in the period before 1874, there were no cases of ovarian madness, nor of climacteric insanity. Fewer than one per cent of admissions were diagnosed as suffering from Hysteria or Hysterical Mania. Puerperal insanity – whether in the form of depression (puerperal melancholia) or in the form of mania (puerperal mania) – was a category which, for the medical superintendents was more common. Seventeen women (two per cent of all women admissions) were classified as suffering from puerperal insanity had good prognoses and stayed in the asylums for very brief periods of time, often fewer than six months. Hilary Marland has explored the struggle between obstetricians and psychiatrists over purportedly insane mothers and suggested that many were not admitted to asylums at all. She has found rates as high as ten to fifteen per cent (of all female admissions) in some asylums in the late-Victorian period.[51]

In conclusion, this examination of the diagnoses of over 1,700 patients admitted to an ordinary county asylum in the mid-Victorian period can find no compelling evidence either to support the contention that new psychiatric classifications were used to herd women into psychiatric institutions, nor that the standard classifications of the time were used in gendered ways to differently classify women. Clusters of disordered behaviour, thoughts and moods were applied, as far as the evidence can reveal, in a similar manner for constructing the diagnosis of male and female lunatics. Far from representing a dominance of disorders controlling women's challenging behaviour, new women-specific classifications (with the exception of puerperal insanity) are conspicuous by their absence in mid-Victorian pauper institutions. Yes, gender was important in terms of defining social or familial expectations. However, the inability to perform sex-specific activities (women's desire to care for children; men's responsibility to work and earn a waged living) was not absolute: that is, it was not the *absence* of a desire to fulfil sex-specific roles that warranted attention in the certificates of insanity (often romantically portrayed by historians as a form of liberation) but rather the sudden and unexplained *cessation* of former sex-specific activities that alerted family members that something was wrong.

Delusions of gender

As mentioned above, delusions figured prominently in the social identification of pauper insanity in Victorian England. Although there has been little quantitative examination of the frequency and type of these symptoms in the context of the nineteenth century, one exceptional study has been carried out by Allan Beveridge, who found that 49.5 per cent of men and 52.9 per cent of women admitted to the Edinburgh asylum in the years 1873-1908 exhibited delusional thinking. In his hierarchy, he identified delusions of persecution, grandeur, and guilt as constituting the three most common types of delusion, regardless of gender. As for the general 'theme' of the delusions, he found that 'sex featured only occasionally, whereas religion and science were recurrent subjects'.[52] It is worth comparing the results of the delusions found in the Buckinghamshire certificates of insanity to his institutional findings. In Buckinghamshire, 56.2 per cent of men and 68.6 per cent of women of the Buckinghamshire sample were described in their certificates of insanity as exhibiting delusions of some kind. Some of these delusions do not easily fall into a standard taxonomy. Richard Hobley, a 71-year-old former grocer's assistant believed that the French had invaded England and that a relation of his had shot several people in London. The testifier was his landlady in London. By contrast, Jane Drake, a 50-year-old carpenter's wife, believed that 'she herself is a prayer & is part of the scriptures'. Most delusions, however, fall into Beveridge's categories of persecutory, grandiose and guilt-associated delusions.

Individuals certified as insane were described as fearing that family members, relatives or neighbours were plotting to kill them. When William Saunders arrived at the Amersham Union Workhouse, he was convinced that his friends had taken him there 'to be murdered'. Before being transported to the asylum, he threatened to murder other members of the workhouse. More common fixations of paranoia usually focussed on poisoning, leading some insane persons in Buckinghamshire to forego food altogether.[53] Maria Hall, a 22-year-old domestic servant was setting fire to wooden boxes which, she believed, had wires in them which were 'bewitching her'.[54] At times, delusions of persecution shaded into delusions of guilt, as patients feared imprisonment for some

Table 6.2

Patients with delusions, expressed in absolute numbers and as a percentage of all patients with an identical diagnosis, admitted to the Buckinghamshire Asylum (first admissions only), 1853-1873

Men			
Diagnosis	With Delusions (n)	All (n)	%
Melancholia	50	87	57.5
Mania with Depression	23	41	56.1
Total	73	128	57.0

Women			
Diagnosis	With Delusions (n)	All (n)	%
Melancholia	59	119	49.6
Mania with Depression	48	74	64.9
Total	107	183	58.5

Men and Women			
Diagnosis	With Delusions (n)	All (n)	%
Melancholia	109	206	52.9
Mania with Depression	71	115	61.7
Total	180	311	57.9

undisclosed crime, or that they were, or were going to be, punished for some 'unpardonable' sin. At other times, persecution was accompanied by nihilism: delusions that the world was going to come to an end, that their 'lives were lost', that their 'souls were destroyed' manifested a sense of helplessness which sometimes culminated in refusal to work, to eat, to enter into conversation, eventually precipitating confinement in the asylum. References to 'science' are entirely absent from the themes of Buckinghamshire delusional patients, whereas religion clearly haunted the mindset of this earlier period: one-quarter of all delusions described in these samples of mid-Victorian certificates include some reference to the Devil, almost always in a 'persecutory' role.

By exploring the delusions listed in the certificates of insanity of patients diagnosed at the Buckinghamshire Asylum with 'Melancholia' and 'Mania with depression' patients, Tables 6.2 (above) and 6.3 (overleaf) are produced. They lend some very tentative support to some of Beveridge's findings. First, delusions were a common manifestation of these disorders (across both sexes), and were identified repeatedly by lay and medical authorities in the

Table 6.3

Frequency of delusion type, patients diagnosed as suffering from Melancholia and Mania with Depression, Buckinghamshire County Asylum, 1853-1873

Type of Delusion	Melancholia		Mania with Depression	
	Males (n)	Females (n)	Males (n)	Females (n)
Nihilism	19	26	6	17
Persecution	17	11	9	10
Guilt	5	11	2	6
Control	5	9	2	2
Unspecified	4	7	3	3
Grandeur	3	4	1	4
Somatic	3	4	3	3
Poverty	5	2	2	3
Bizarre	2	2	2	4
Demon Possession	1	2	2	1
Ill-Health	0	2	0	1
Infestation	0	1	0	0
Infidelity	0	1	0	0
Unworthiness	3	0	0	0
Misidentification	1	0	1	1
Love	0	0	0	0
Reference	0	0	0	0
Thought Projection	0	0	0	1
Wealth	0	0	0	1
Other	0	0	1	2
Total	**68**	**82**	**34**	**59**

Note: Number may exceed total number of patients with these diagnoses, as some patients exhibit more than one discrete delusion.

social construction and identification of insanity. Secondly, there was an absence of delusions of sexuality in these pauper certificates, either for male or female patients. The Buckinghamshire certificates also reveal similar differences in relative importance of the type of delusion by gender as the Edinburgh results: men were more prone to delusions of grandeur, women were more likely to exhibit delusions of persecution and guilt. Unlike Edinburgh, however, the sample of Bucks certificates suggest a higher incidence of women displaying delusional thinking than men.

Conclusions

The results of this chapter inform several debates in the history of psychiatry. First, as this chapter has shown, the procedure governing the admission to asylums in Victorian England was enshrined in successive legislation framed to prevent wrongful confinement. Medical superintendents were barred from certifying patients sent to their own institutions. The process of identifying and certifying patients was left to a subtle and complex local interaction of family members, neighbours, Poor Law officials and Poor Law medical officers. As the data from the admission papers have illustrated, this process did not privilege medical over lay opinion, and did not lead to the widespread incarceration of women by men. Rather, family members of both genders were central participants in the confinement of their children, spouses, and parents and in testifying in the certification process.

Secondly, this chapter illustrates that the vast majority of women and men were diagnosed within the dominant psychiatric classifications of the Victorian era – Mania, Melancholia, Dementia, and Idiocy. There appears to be no compelling evidence from this case study to conclude that the behaviours, moods and thoughts that led to the diagnoses of idiocy, dementia, melancholia or mania differed in the male and female certificates of insanity. This paper has argued that the gender incidence of the specific diagnoses – like melancholia or mania with depression – did not reflect a gendering of *diagnosis*, but may have possibly reflected either a gendering of the confinement process or a 'real' gender difference in the presentation of symptoms leading to social identification. These alternative possibilities, however, cannot be addressed within the confines of this chapter, but deserves to receive sustained analysis by a historical community that seems too ready to believe that all mental disorders in the past were socially constructed, rather than to investigate to what extent biological or epidemiological reality of many mental disorders interacted with family imperatives, changing social and cultural values, and legal constraints, to lead to institutional confinement.

Thirdly, this case study provides little support for feminist revisionism within the history of psychiatry which suggests that psychiatry used a new 'sexist' nosology to classify women's aberrant behaviour in the mid-Victorian period. No doubt, there may have been some families who sought to abuse the asylum system and confine female members of their household in a mental institution.

But these represent a small minority of cases. As this study of a typical county asylum in rural England has shown, the diagnoses of 'hysteria' and 'climacteric insanity', 'ovarian madness' were not in widespread use before 1880. The sole example of these terms to be used regularly in the Buckinghamshire Asylum was puerperal mania, a classification that affected seventeen women in total, or only two per cent of all female admissions. There is fragmentary evidence to suggest, however, that these terms were more widely employed in asylums *after* 1880. If this was indeed the case, then historians should be more precise in their association of 'Victorian' psychiatry with the emergence of new gender-specific nosology. As this paper has argued, after forty years of the Victorian period, and twenty-five years of the rapid incarceration of the insane in England had already passed, the new allegedly 'misogynist' taxonomy of psychiatric classification had not yet, at the public asylum level at least, had any appreciable effect.

However, even if the use of these gender-specific terms of classification did become more widely used in the argot of alienists in the last two decades of the nineteenth century, there is a more general question as to the relationship between this new taxonomy and the social process of confinement. As this paper has shown, confinement was a *sine qua non* for classification, not the other way around. Thus the changing and more nuanced psychiatric classification system employed by medical superintendents was a function of a growing desire for greater specialisation in diagnosis and classification, rather than being used as a weapon to control women's challenging behaviour. Indeed, as this chapter has illustrated, 'psychiatric knowledge' was predicated upon the production of lay and non-specialist descriptions of mad behaviour encapsulated in the Victorian certificates of insanity. This suggests that the production of psychiatric knowledge cannot be considered independently of changing popular attitudes to madness but must be seen, as Michael MacDonald has proposed, in a dynamic relationship with lay knowledge and tradition.

Clearly, much more work is needed on the social identification of madness, the process of certification and the medical classification of patients arriving at asylums, in order to validate these findings.[55] It may well be the case that, because the asylum under study was a *county* asylum, the gender differences in descriptions of categories may have been less pronounced than in private asylums for the wealthy,[56] or charitable asylums receiving a greater proportion of patients from the middle classes. If the 'newer' classifications of hysterical mania were associated with wealthier, bourgeois clientele, they would not have shown up in the admission registers of the Buckinghamshire asylum. It is true that voluntary lunatic asylums such as the York Retreat and the Royal Holloway Asylum, accommodated a greater proportion of women than county institutions, suggesting that class may be indispensable to our understanding of the role of gender in the confinement of the insane in the Victorian era.[57] Ultimately, we may discover that the roots of Chesler and Showalter's influential critiques may lie not in the process of confinement, nor even empirical evidence in the diagnosis of the overwhelming number of women admitted to public asylums during the Victorian era, but rather in the changing medical discourses about women's bodies and minds articulated about, and relevant to, a relatively small group of upper middle-class women in the last two decades of the nineteenth century. A new history of the nineteenth-century asylum and the confinement of the insane thus needs to place the relatively few cases of wrongful confinement and hysteria – colourful as they are – within their appropriate context: amidst the hundreds of thousands of women and men admitted to public institutions in Western Europe, Britain, and the British colonies between 1800 and 1960. Their disorders and disabilities are no less worthy of historical scrutiny and analysis.

Notes

1. This paper was written with the assistance of a grant from the Wellcome Trust, London, and ongoing funding from Associated Medical Services (Hannah Institute), Toronto. I am grateful to Mona Gupta, James Moran, and two anonymous referees for their comments on earlier drafts of this chapter.

2. P. Chesler, *Women and Madness* (New York: Avon Books, 1973). For excellent summaries of feminist critiques of psychiatry and the approaches to the history of psychiatry, see J. Busfield, 'Sexism and Psychiatry', *Sociology*, 23 (1989), 343–64 and N. Tomes, 'Feminist Histories of Psychiatry', in M. Micale and R. Porter (eds.) *Discovering the History of Psychiatry* (Oxford: Oxford University Press, 1994), 348–83.

3. E. Showalter, *The Female Malady: Women, Madness and English Culture, 1830-1980* (New York: Pantheon Books, 1985), 53 and *passim*.

4. D. Russell, *Women, Madness and Medicine* (New York: Polity Press, 1995), 10 and *passim*.

5. W. Mitchinson, *The Nature of their Bodies: Women and their Doctors in Victorian Canada* (Toronto: University of Toronto Press, 1991),

ch. 10.

6. J. Ussher, *Women's Madness: Misogyny or Mental Illness?* (Amherst: University of Massachusetts Press, 1992), especially chapter 3.

7. N. Tomes, *A Generous Confidence: Thomas Story Kirkbride and the Art of Asylum Keeping, 1840–1883* (Cambridge, Cambridge University Press, 1985), 28, 190, and chapters 3 and 5.

8. A. Digby, *Madness, Morality and Medicine: A Study of the York Retreat* (Cambridge: Cambridge University Press, 1985), 174, table 8.2.

9. E. Dwyer, *Homes for the Mad: Life Inside Two Nineteenth-Century Asylums* (New Brunswick: Rutgers University Press, 1987).

10. J. Busfield, 'The Female Malady?: Men, Women and Madness in Nineteenth-Century Britain', *Sociology*, 28 (1994), 259–77.

11. B. Labrum, 'Looking beyond the Asylum: Gender and the Process of Committal to Auckland, 1870–1910', *New Zealand Journal of History*, 26 (1992), 125–44: 127–8.

12. W. Ernst, 'European Madness and Gender in Nineteenth-Century British India', *Social History of Medicine*, 9 (1996), 357–82: 370.

13. The history of colonial psychiatry and mental health is now immense. For seminal works on different colonial or quasi-colonial contexts see M. Finnane, *Insanity and the Insane in Post-Famine Ireland* (London: Croom Helm, 1981), 130; S. Garton, *Medicine and Madness: A Social History of Insanity in New South Wales, 1880–1940* (Kensington, Australia: New South Wales University Press, 1988), 22; S. Marks, '"Every Facility that Modern Science and Enlightened Humanity have Devised": Race and Progress in a Colonial Hospital, Valkenberg Mental Asylum, Cape Colony, 1894–1910', in J. Melling and W. Forsythe (eds), *Insanity, Institutions and Society: A Social History of Madness in Comparative Perspective* (London: Routledge, 1999); J. Moran, *Committed to the State Asylum: Insanity and Society in Nineteenth-Century Quebec and Ontario* (Montreal: McGill/Queen's University Press, 2000).

14. M. Micale, 'Charcot and the Idea of Hysteria in the Male: A Study of Gender, Mental Science, and Medical Diagnostics in late Nineteenth-Century France', *Medical History*, 34 (1990), 363–411; Micale, 'Hysteria Male/Hysteria Female: Reflections on Comparative Gender Construction in Nineteenth-Century France and Britain', in M. Benjamin (ed.), *Science and Sensibility: Gender and Scientific Enquiry, 1780–1945* (Cambridge: Basil Blackwell, 1991), 200–42; J. Oppenheim, *Shattered Nerves: Doctors, Patients and Depression in Victorian England* (New York: Oxford University Press, 1991).

15. A. Scull, *The Most Solitary of Afflictions: Madness and Society in Britain, 1700–1900* (London: Yale University Press, 1993), 362,

Table 10.

16. P. McCandless, 'Build! Build! The Controversy over the Care of the Chronically Insane in England, 1855-70', *Bulletin of the History of Medicine*, 53 (1979), 553–74.

17. This chapter will deal only with the 'county' asylums in England and Wales. It will not discuss admission to charitable asylums (unless they were charitable cases accepted in county asylums), private madhouses (licensed homes), Chancery cases, or the confinement of 'criminal lunatics'.

18. Scotland and Ireland both operated under different legislation, though the general arguments in this paper may well apply to asylums in those jurisdictions. Wales was governed by the same legislation as England, though this paper will concentrate on the English county asylums.

19. K. Jones, *Asylums and After: A Revised History of the Mental Health Services* (London: The Athlone Press, 1993), 64, 116, Table 7.2.

20. To provide for extra protection for private patients (who were considered to be at greater risk of wrongful confinement), two certificates of insanity were required. These two certificates had to be completed by medical men who were not in practice together, and these medical men could not complete the certificates at the same time. For a more extensive discussion of certification, see D. Wright 'The Certification of Insanity in Nineteenth-Century England', *History of Psychiatry*, 9 (1998), 267–90.

21. Sometimes Poor Law Unions included parishes in different counties. Thus Leighton Buzzard and Henley Unions and had some, though not all, of their constituent parishes in the county of Buckinghamshire.

22. C. MacKenzie, for instance, reveals that two patients from Buckinghamshire were admitted to the exclusive Ticehurst Asylum in West Sussex during this period. See MacKenzie, *Psychiatry for the Rich: A History of the Private Ticehurst Asylum, 1792–1917* (London, Routledge, 1992), 131, Fig. 5.1.

23. J. Crammer, *Asylum History: Buckinghamshire County Pauper Lunatic Asylum-St. John's* (London: Royal College of Psychiatrists, 1990), 55. Crammer is less than enthusiastic about Humphrey's reign, entitling the chapter covering this period 'Fifty inglorious years'. See *ibid.*, chapter 5.

24. I am grateful to Anne Shepherd and Mat Savelli for research assistance with these additional certificates of insanity and their coding.

25. See *inter alia*, J. Melling *et al.*, '"A Proper Lunatic for Two Years",

Pauper Lunatic Children in Victorian and Edwardian England: Child Admissions to the Devon Country Asylum, 1845-1914', *Journal of Science History,* 31, 2 (1997), 371–405; B. Forsythe *et al.,* 'The New Poor Law and the County Pauper Asylum – the Devon Experience 1834-1884',*Social History of Medicine,* 9, 3 (1996), 335–55; R. Adair *et al.,* 'A Danger to the Public? Disposing of Pauper Lunatics in late-Victorian and Edwardian England: Plympton St. Mary Union and the Devon County Asylum, 1867-1914', *Medical History,* 42 (1998), 1–25; P. Bartlett, *The Poor Law of Lunacy: The Administration of Pauper Lunatics in Mid-Nineteenth Century England* (London: Leicester University Press, 1999); and Wright, *op. cit.* (note 20).

26. Approximately ten per cent of admissions to the Buckinghamshire county asylum were transferred from other county asylums or private licensed homes. Under this system, the original certificate of insanity – that is, the one completed before confinement in the former institution – was still valid for the new admission, and was copied and sent (with the patient) to the second institution. Transfers were often conducted when it was discovered that the patient had settlement in a parish outside of the county boundaries, though magistrates sometimes arranged for special payments between visiting committees to pay for the housing of 'their' lunatics in other county magistrates' asylums.

27. There has been some confusion over the definition of what constituted a 'pauper lunatic'. Peter McCandless rightly point out that 'pauper' simply referred to those patients who had not contributed to the cost of asylum treatment, rather than those individuals who were destitute and in receipt of poor law relief. P. McCandless, 'A House of Cure: The Antebellum South Carolina Lunatic Asylum', *Bulletin of the History of Medicine,* 44 (1990), 220–42: 224. A team of researchers in Exeter have supported this interpretation: R. Adair *et al., op. cit.* (note 25), 1–25: 11.

28. This general pattern has also been found in research on the Denbigh county asylum in North Wales. See P. Michael, 'Occupations, Gender and Insanity in 19th and 20th century Wales', unpublished paper, 5.

29. P. Bartlett, 'The Poor Law of Lunacy: The Administration of Pauper Lunatics in mid-Nineteenth Century England with Special Reference to Leicestershire and Rutland' (unpublished Ph.D. thesis, University College London, 1993), 195.

30. The authors emphasise that up to sixty-two per cent went 'through' the workhouse en route to the asylum, but only thirty-six per cent

gave the workhouse as their previous place of abode. R. Adair *et al.*
op. cit. (note 25), 11 and *passim.*

31. For a study of the relationship between mental disorder, prisons and
asylums, see J. Saunders, 'Institutionalized Offenders – A Study of
the Victorian Institution and its Inmates, with Special Reference to
late-Nineteenth Century Warwickshire' (unpublished Ph.D. thesis,
University of Warwick, 1983).

32. Ernst, *op. cit.* (note 13).

33. For a similar finding regarding the certification of idiot children sent
to a charitable asylum, see Wright, 'Childlike in his Innocence: Lay
Attitudes to "Idiots" and "Imbeciles" in Victorian England', in D.
Wright and A. Digby (eds), *From Idiocy to Mental Deficiency:
Historical Perspectives on People with Learning Disabilities* (London:
Routledge, 1996), 118–39.

34. Technically, the person who should be contacted in case of the death
of the patient, though this was invariably the next of kin.

35. Since the asylum rarely accepted individuals under the age of sixteen,
the asylum population was compared to the adult census population.

36. Certificate for Isabella Wooton. All the certificates of insanity,
reception orders and admission registers used in this paper are part
of the archives of the Buckinghamshire County Pauper Lunatic
Asylum/St. John's Hospital, held at the Buckinghamshire County
Records Office, series AR100/89. Copies of the completed database
may be obtained by contacting the author, dwright@mcmaster.ca.

37. Research in the history of poor law have long established that that
longest serving inmates were idiots and imbeciles. See, for example,
M.A. Crowther, *The Workhouse System. 1834–1929: A History of an
English Social Institution* (Athens GA.: University of Georgia Press,
1981), 75, 164.

38. Certificate for Albert Price.

39. For an examination of boarding out that highlights this means of
caring for idiots and imbeciles, D. Hirst and P. Michael, 'Family,
Community and the Lunatic in mid-Nineteenth-Century North
Wales', in P. Bartlett and D. Wright (eds), *Outside the Walls of the
Asylum: The History of Care in the Community, 1750-1900* (London:
Athlone, 1999), 66–85.

40. D. Wright, *Mental Disability in Victorian England: The Earlswood
Asylum, 1847-1901* (Oxford: Clarendon Press, 2001).

41. Certificate for Mary Goodson.

42. Certificate for Charles Eyles.

43. Certificate for Sarah Wallduck.

44. Certificate for Mary Ann Slade.

45. A. Shepherd and D. Wright, 'Madness, Suicide and the Victorian Asylum: Attempted Self-Murder in the Age of Non-Restraint', *Medical History*, 46 (2002), 175–96.

46. Certificate for Catherine Frost, 1881.

47. Certificate for Samuel Sears, 1871.

48. R. Stevens, *Medical Practice in Modern England: The Impact of Specialisation on State Medicine* (New Haven: Yale University Press, 1966) and M. J. Peterson, *The Medical Profession in Mid-Victorian London* (Berkeley: University of California Press, 1978).

49. See H. Marland, 'At Home with Puerperal Mania: The Domestic Treatment of the Insanity of Childbirth in the Nineteenth Century', in Bartlett and Wright, *op. cit.* (note 39), 45–65.

50. Showalter, 'Victorian Women and Insanity', in Andrew Scull (ed.) *Mad-Houses, Mad-Doctors and Madmen: The Social History of Psychiatry in the Victorian Era* (Philadelphia, University of Pennsylvania Press, 1981), 313–36: 323.

51. Marland, *op. cit.* (note 49).

52. A. Beveridge, 'Madness in Victorian Edinburgh: A Study of Patients Admitted to the Royal Edinburgh Asylum under Thomas Clouston, 1873–1908 (part I)', *History of Psychiatry*, 6 (1995), 21–54: 37–8, Table 7.

53. Certificate for William Saunders.

54. Certificate for Maria Hall.

55. See, *inter alia*, P. Michael, 'Gender, Class and Insanity in Nineteenth-Century Wales', in this volume.

56. MacKenzie states that 'puerperal' and 'hysterical' sub-groups of manias were used in the private Ticehurst Asylum after 1850, but does not state how often they appear. MacKenzie, *op. cit.* (note 22), 153 and Table 5.5; see also 184, Table 6.2.

57. A. Digby, *op. cit.* (note 8), 174, Table 8.2 shows that 55.9 per cent of all admissions were women. The highest rate, during any tenure at the Retreat, was 61.3 per cent. *Ibid.* A. Shepherd, 'The Public and Private Institutionalisation of the Insane in the late Nineteenth Century', unpublished paper read to at the SSHM conference 'Insanity, Institutions and Society: New Research in the Social History of Madness', University of Exeter, 18-20/4/1997, conference proceedings, 38.

7

Sex and Sensibility in Cultural History:
The English Governess and the Lunatic Asylum,
1845–1914[1]

Joseph Melling

This chapter is concerned with the experience of the Victorian
governess and other female teachers in the lunatic asylum during
the Victorian period. There is now a formidable and complex
literature on the governess but little discussion of her experience
behind the walls of the asylum. The chapter offers two kinds of
comparison: the distinctive pattern of care of governesses in
three different institutions in Victorian Devon; and secondly, the
progress of those identified as 'governess' with other groups of
female teachers in the same period. A number of interesting
contrasts emerge. The evidence also indicates the importance of
cultural and social influences in the construction of the persona
of the female teacher.

Introduction

In the past two decades the claims of cultural history have made a
significant impression on the ways in which historians undertake
their work. Social historians who had previously been concerned to
map out the journey of human beings across the landscape of the
material world were compelled to acknowledge the importance of
perspective: that the historian as well as the subject were creating a
narrative of interpretation at a particular point in time and space.[2]
The impact of post-structural thinkers such as Michel Foucault on
the practice of writing history has been vividly apparent in the
debates on the history of insanity, where some recent research on
demography and family arrangements has re-asserted the importance
of the material world in the discovery and treatment of madness.[3]
Foucault's claims with regard to the growth of scientific rationalism
and its role in the history of the asylum has also remained the subject
of debate. Roy Porter argued, for example, that it was the rise of

sensibility and the romantic pleasures at the end of the eighteenth century, which legitimated the 'empire of the imagination' and opened the door to psychiatric interpretations of sexual dilemmas.[4]

There remains a deep interest among social historians of madness in retrieving the voice of the mad subject from the various textual sources available to us, restoring them to a rational narrative of history.[5] Feminist scholars have made a particularly important contribution to the understanding of gender relations in the construction of insanity. Elaine Showalter, Mary Poovey and Sally Shuttleworth amongst others have drawn on scientific as well as literary texts to explore the terms in which femininity and madness were represented in distinctive fields of knowledge and by different authors.[6] Such cultural historians offer an impressive analysis of the anatomy of feminine melancholy in Victorian society, showing how the conflicting expectations of work and domestic duty created an epidemic of mental maladies amongst educated women.[7] Showalter's particular contribution was to suggest that the feminisation of madness in the mid-nineteenth century was consolidated around the practice of male psychiatry and the institution of the new asylums founded in large numbers after 1845. In a brilliant discussion of the domestication of madness, Showalter suggested that the asylum was increasingly modelled around domestic imagery of comfort and behaviour, which associated recovery from insanity with a rediscovery of practical, home-making skills. The boundaries between what was regarded as a range of social institutions and conventions, including the lunatic asylum, policed the public and private spheres of feminine behaviour. Such institutions were also part of the political fabric of Victorian society and maintained the peculiar codes for recognising and attending to the needs of their clients.

A significant innovation in the mid-nineteenth-century period, as described by Showalter and Poovey amongst others, was the introduction of scientific methods and models, which provided a particular kind of factual rationale for social perception. The growth of psychiatry and other specialised branches of medicine offered an explanation for the working of the bodily economy within the political regime of commercial society. These comments are framed within a larger discussion of sanitary science and gendered practices within industrial societies, as states sought to irrigate the city and expand their scope for the control of disease and ignorance. Shuttleworth shows how the spread of anatomical realism influenced the development of literary character, as novelists used the language of social enquiry and scientific understanding to enlarge the interior life and capacities of their narrators.[8] Ermath has linked realism in Victorian literature to a scientific pre-occupation with the precise location of the action in real, measurable time.[9] Julia Swindells has suggested that scientific medicine functioned both to produce commodities for bodily consumption and as a locus of cultural or symbolic exchange.[10] Various writers have traced the parallel progress of sanitary and bodily control in contemporary society, assisted by the disciplinary models of the medical sciences, and the development of a Victorian literature in which social interrogation and self-analysis are brought within the gaze of the novelist. Male professionals were able to expand the empire of scientific knowledge available to the public whilst regulating their own labour markets and prescribing the terms of physical, mental and moral health that could be secured.[11]

There has been growing criticism of the interpretation of female insanity offered by Showalter and literary scholars, as well as medical historians and sociologists, who suggest that the evidence offered in *The Female Malady* can be contradicted by contemporary sources and that the chronology of creative and scientific writing provided by Showalter obscures an earlier tradition of writing as well as the important contribution of women to scientific understanding.[12] Yet the claims of cultural history have not themselves been subjected to critical scrutiny in this debate. Cultural history has undoubtedly provided us with a more sophisticated understanding of different kinds of texts and their readership at particular moments in history. The crude assumption that a selection or canon of materials can be taken as the true reflection of social attitudes has been effectively discredited. There is less evidence that the methods of cultural history have integrated an interrogation of different texts with a critical awareness of the techniques of social history. It may be argued that many of the practitioners of cultural history often rely on derivative and even materialist assumptions about the social context in which distinctive texts were produced and read. One consequence is that the documentary evidence, which informs historical analysis, is not subjected to the kind of scrutiny which guides the discussion of self-consciously literary and scientific material. The published and unpublished accounts of those who experienced the diagnosis of insanity may reveal rather different themes than fictional texts, though it is also possible that the perceptions of those suffering from madness may be influenced by the literary and scientific culture of the time. Their recollections and delusions may bear the impression of their reading.

The argument made in this essay is that we need to learn from the techniques of social, political and institutional history if we are to comprehend the experiences of those women and men who were classified as insane in the nineteenth century. The complexities of contemporary debate and the evolution of historical relationships can be more clearly understood by comparing a range of sources, from the selected work on insanity published at a specific period, to the evidence yielded from institutions and individuals. The argument made here is that the discussion of insanity was shaped by a range of contemporary struggles over the formation of class and domestic boundaries as well as the political liberation of women and their access to knowledge in Victorian society. These campaigns developed in ways that politicised and gendered insanity at particular moments and foreclosed the discussion of women's madness at others. It is also possible to contrast the engagement with the problem of insanity as a women's issue in the public domain during the mid-century years, with the distinctive continuities in the private world of the mad woman and her personal treatment in the institutions of the Victorian era. These contrasts between public controversy and the domestication of madness were, it is suggested here, rather different from those outlined in Showalter's work. For the private experience of insanity and the treatment of the insane continued to be influenced by the social boundaries of class and gender, echoing the living space and the life struggles of educated women even when the question slipped from the agenda of public controversy. The evidence from institutional and personal sources also provides material for some understanding of the mental furniture of those who were identified as insane during the nineteenth century, as well as broader trends in the patterns of admission to, and discharge from, the institutions built for their care and treatment.

These arguments are pursued in a discussion of insanity and the Victorian governess, including the ways in which the governess was represented in census sources, asylum records, and other contemporary materials. Many accounts have seen the governess as a bearer of particular social and cultural burdens, enacting a larger cultural and sexual drama. Comparison of different texts allows us to examine the choices available to them and the terms in which they expressed their own needs and desires. Whilst there has been much debate on the cultural construction of the domestic sphere and the role of the governess, there has been relatively little investigation of the distinctive narrative of the insane governess provided by the asylum records, or the significance of census materials for an understanding of her movements within contemporary society. The

Victorian asylums provided their own distinctive and varied accounts of the governess drama, which differed in important respects from the larger political and literary imagery of the time. The following section reviews some of the scholarship on the Victorian governess and her place within the evolving class structure of Victorian society. This survey is followed by a discussion of evidence drawn largely from asylum sources in southwest England, including an examination of the different ways in which the mental as well as material world of the governess was portrayed in unpublished sources.

Literary images of the Victorian governess

In the crowded world of Victorian literature there are few figures as striking as that of the youthful governess. *Jane Eyre* was only the most famous amongst a sizeable academy of fictional characters that were enrolled to perform the leading role in dramas of romantic attachment and domestic disorder. Gilbert and Gubar first identified the preternatural laughter of Bertha Mason as the suppressed voice, not only of the governess whom she shadowed, but also of Brontë herself as an author struggling against the limitations of contemporary society.[13] This thesis has been reworked numerous times, most recently in Mary Poovey's influential interpretation of gender relations in mid-Victorian England. In her discussion, Poovey cites Lady Eastlake's famous review of both *Jane Eyre* and Thackeray's *Vanity Fair*, including her assertion that 'the lunatic asylums of this country are supplied with a larger proportion of their inmates from the ranks of young governesses than from any other class of life'.[14] Poovey also followed Jeanne Petersen, Pamela Horn and others in using the archives of the Governesses Benevolent Institution to assess contemporary claims that the daughters of the commercial middle classes were overcrowding the labour market, driving down the wages of the formerly genteel calling of governess.[15]

The confinement of women to the domestic sphere is often taken to be the vital material and political context in which to understand the frustrations of the educated women for whom, and to whom, novels such as *Jane Eyre* speak. As an educated servant, the governess also occupied a sensitive position in the hierarchy of domestic employment; required to be a visible member of the family home and responsible for the training of the children, but liable to be excluded from the private society of her employer when her services were no longer required.[16] Poovey suggested that the potency of the governess as a cultural reference in the mid-Victorian era lay in the contradictory impulse of the affluent to exploit the talents of the governess for the rearing of children whilst deploring the threat which an unmarried woman posed to the wife's dominance over the domestic sphere.[17] Some scholars have argued that by the late-Victorian period the governess was distanced from the kind of physical dirt associated with domestic service but her role was highly eroticised in pornographic as well as respectable literature.[18]

One appeal of the governess novel in Victorian society may well have been the opportunity it provided to explore the boundaries of domestic obligation. The dramas of sexual role-play and transgression were necessarily private affairs in this setting, while the duties of social propriety could be linked to struggles over property and personal desire. Yet the social predicament of the governess was a familiar feature by the eighteenth century, as has been shown by Vickery. Many 'well-born' women were pressed into the ranks of the governess by family misfortune and personal obligation, with little prospect of improvement beyond a good marriage.[19] There were also important literary exchanges long before the Victorian years, even amongst the family circle of major authors, on the role of the literary genre in the representation of the female teacher and the moral instruction of children.[20] At least as important as the emergence of middle-class domesticity in literary and documentary representations of the governess was the translation of pre-capitalist ideals of personal service into the architecture and values of bourgeois society. One of the more important ways in which the class and status conventions of English society were embedded in domestic life can be seen in the arrangement of the interior geography of the wealthy household. Leonora Davidoff has illuminated the ways in which the roles of status and class power could fire erotic tensions between masters and servants in the Victorian decades, as strains between physical proximity and social distance in the respectable household helped to cultivate some of the exotic fantasies of contemporary literature.[21] The governess was the bearer of the cultural map, which marked out the territory of etiquette as well as the latitude to be given to servants. As a powerful female member of the aristocracy, Aclands noted in discussing the qualifications of a suitable governess, that it was essential that such a person should not 'throw' the children 'amongst the servants'.[22] It was even more vital to the reputation of the household that any governess maintained an impenetrable boundary between herself and the male members of the household, since any scandal would represent social disaster for even the most secluded and modest household.[23] The peculiar and restricted value of this intimate knowledge of complex social rules became apparent when governesses decided to emigrate to the colonies during the mid-century decades and found that many of their skills were irrelevant to the new frontier societies of an expanding British Empire.[24]

The vivid discussion of the proper breeding and duties of the governess which took place in the 1840s–50s, was also framed in a larger political discourse on political rights and the utility of scientific and literary knowledge. Middle-class challenges to aristocratic power drew on popular protest, appealing to the ideal of dignified labour in contrast to the principle of natural leadership by landed society. Such debates figured prominently in what Terry Eagleton terms 'rival mythologies of power', expressed in the popular movements of the Brontës' West Riding as well as many other regions of Britain.[25] The western counties of England as well as the northern heathlands were scarred by rural incendiaries and popular unrest in the Chartist era..[26] This was the larger social context in which the English governess was charged with translating social rules, as well as scientific and moral understanding to her pupils, enforcing proper conduct alongside intellectual and social training, thereby policing the domestic boundaries between the world of the servants and the society of her employers.[27] Feminist authors controversially and vigorously challenged the conservative vision of the governess within a pastoral ideal of country-house society over the 'surplus' of spinsters in mid-Victorian Britain.[28] Barbara Leigh Smith stressed the dual hazards of prostitution and hysteria confronting women who were offered genteel leisure rather than productive employment in commercial society.[29] Isa Craig adopted a more radical approach in suggesting the association of insanity with social deprivation and the predicament of females who were encouraged to display affection rather than rationality in everyday life.[30]

The political and cultural tensions in English class society during the 1840s are evident in Lady Eastlake's denunciation of *Jane Eyre* as the agent of a 'murmuring discontent' against the divinely appointed order of society. Her remarkable social commentary on the novel claimed that the genteel vocation of the governess was being degraded by the arrival of 'under-bred' women from the lower-middle and middle classes. The practical basis for her politics lay in the active endorsement, along with leading evangelists such as Lord Shaftesbury and many aristocratic ladies, of the Governesses Benevolent Institution as the expression of a traditional service relationship.[31] Read in this way, the exchanges which formed the public discussion of the 'governess problem' in the mid-Victorian years were framed within a larger discourse on the nature of civil obedience as well as the purpose of female education, including the relative value of genteel embellishment versus practical knowledge in the instruction of young ladies.[32] Recent studies of political rhetoric in England during the nineteenth century have argued that notions of domesticity were still contested in popular debates of the 1840s and 1850s, rather than being fixed boundaries of social obligation between the sexes.[33] Many of the leading authoresses of the day were concerned to find a public platform on which to voice domestic experience and virtue in the radical campaigns of the 1840s.[34] The language in which the governess was depicted and the accomplishments required of her, ensured that she was a necessary participant in the vocabulary of domestic virtue which many political reformers claimed as essentially English middle-class virtues and yet which clearly encompassed the aspirations to gentility and a knowledge of refined manners which derived from much older notions of Continental culture and refinement.[35]

The interpretation sketched above places the mid-century 'crisis' of the insane governess as the product of a political and class rhetoric in which different authors exploited the role of the private teacher as a device to make general moral claims about social progress. The significance of the feminist campaigns of the 1840s and 1850s was to create a platform from which women could publicly address the politics of health and moral choice in relation to the opportunities available for female labour. These movements also made an important contribution to the growing professionalisation of the female teacher, including the increasing reliance on certificates and other examination qualifications in the classroom. One consequence was to accentuate a divide between state-funded and private education in this period, probably increasing the dependence of the non-certificated female on the private market. Whilst the expansion of state schools in the later-nineteenth century offered women greater access to teaching and professional status, there remained a heavy market demand for both the residential and the day-governess, with at least a tacit promise of skills in genteel behaviour which were rooted in a conservative vision of society. The relative success of the movement to secure women access to teacher-training and elementary education in the second half of the nineteenth century may also have contributed to a declining interest amongst feminists and career women in the circumstances of the private unqualified teacher.[36] Within a decade of the publication of *Jane Eyre*, Harriet Martineau was expressing a growing impatience with tragic tales of the governess and, whilst the plight of the needlewoman continued to attract social concern in the 1860s, those interested in the position of the unmarried teacher directed their energies to assisting such women in finding a position in such colonies as Australia.

Having argued that the different social and political interests of Victorian society seized on the governess as a rhetorical device in the pursuit of their goals, there remains the interesting question of how the female teacher continued to function in a world where she had some opportunities to exploit her own value, even where her choices remained limited. More importantly for this essay, there is also the question of how the governess was diversely constructed in texts where the subject was more obscure and the audience less certain than the figures that dominated the feminist debates of the mid-nineteenth century. The following section briefly considers the social position of the governess and other female teachers in the later-nineteenth century, revealed in evidence from the census and other sources. This is followed by a discussion of the governess in the Victorian asylum.

Languages of vocation:
Employment status and the Victorian governess

The controversy which surrounded the publication of *Jane Eyre* formed part of a vigorous public debate on the role of female education in class society, including the importance of 'social breeding' in the qualification of private teachers. This debate was informed by struggles over the utility of knowledge, as well as the claims of women to equal citizenship with men. The intervention of commentators such as Eastlake was also a response to the undoubted expansion of the main labour market for educated women. By the 1850s there were at least 25,000 governesses employed in England and Wales, living and working in the more prosperous areas of southern England such as the fashionable bathing centres of Brighton and Bath.[37] Although most private teachers were found near to more affluent areas of agrarian, commercial and professional wealth, significant numbers could also be found in northern cities of England and even, more sparsely, in the central industrial region of Scotland.[38] At the height of the insanity debate in 1851, there were already more than twice as many female schoolteachers as governesses employed, even if the predicament of the classroom worker attracted much less literary and social interest.[39] In the prosperous county of Devon, for example, the occupation of schoolteacher was much more important as an employment than the 572 governesses recorded in

1851.[40]   The fashionable coastal resorts of Torbay, Exmouth and Budleigh Salterton, as well as the suburban districts of county towns, rather than the large city of Plymouth, attracted the governess, who was much more likely to be found in private residential employment than either 'teachers' or 'schoolmistresses'.[41]

It is important to note that the boundary between teacher and governess was not always strictly drawn, and the distinctions were as much a function of subtle social discrimination as a rigorous description of employment relations. Many teachers and mistresses were found in private colleges, and others offered private instruction in their own homes. Employees of private schools might claim the title of governess as a means of emphasising the exclusive character of their position.[42] There is little doubt that women in the market for educated labour faced serious struggles in the middle and later decades of the nineteenth century. The contemporary claims by Lady Eastlake and others that it was the competition of females from commercial families which drove the governess of sensibility out of business and into the asylum, should not, as Kathryn Hughes has shown, be taken as an accurate account of contemporary employment patterns.[43] In the 1880s the governess continued to be recruited from families of rank and status, as well as educationalists, though a sizeable number came from modest households without a servant in residence, as well as from a wide range of commercial and professional occupations.[44] The governess, in the southern counties of England at least, continued to originate in non-commercial families with connections to education, non-manual pursuits and the professions rather than the business community as such.[45]

About one half of the Devon females occupied as governesses were resident in the homes of non-relatives in the later-nineteenth century and a large majority of these were given the title of governess or servant in the household, undertaking duties directed by the employer.[46] Although the residential governess occupied a relatively privileged rank within the ranks of domestic servants at this period, the conditions and terms of her employment varied from the occupant of the aristocratic mansion, to the teacher who took a room at the local inn.[47] In rural counties such as Devon, the most common employer was a farmer, though 'people of rank' and clergy, as well as educationalists, figured prominently as householders where governesses resided.[48] These resident households were usually more prosperous than the families where the governess was not resident, and many women were finding work in the homes of substantial Devon farmers and clergymen in the 1880s.[49] More affluent employers could afford to recruit their governess from more distant counties of England or abroad, seeking out native French or German speakers, but with a cautious eye to their religious persuasion.[50] More modest households provided the bulk of the demand, not only for the residential teacher, but also for the massed ranks of the daily or 'day governess' who travelled to work or offered private tuition in their own dwellings. When all governesses are taken into account (resident and non-resident), including the large number living with their own families, then the single most common occupation of the head of the household was that of education. Since a number of such women appear to have been employed both as residents of a private school and as teachers with family members, it is again hazardous to draw a hard or fixed line between the working experience of the governess and that of the private schoolteacher.

The titles awarded to female teachers, and the social distinctions that they conveyed, do appear to have been slowly consolidated in the second half of the nineteenth century. The growing emphasis on formal certificates in state education appear to have widened the divide in expectations between the social graces and genteel polish required of the governess, and the formal knowledge conveyed by the qualified teacher.[51] It was rare for the governess to claim for herself, or be accorded the title of certificated teacher, even where qualifications were claimed. In 1851 there were relatively few women in education who were identified simply as teachers, the title being mainly associated with very young females.[52] The title of 'schoolmistress' was far more common than that of female teacher and their numbers were substantially greater than those of the governess.[53] The position of schoolmistress seems to have been associated with more mature and authoritative individuals. Possibly in response to the growing emphasis on the acquisition of school certificates, the private governess frequently appropriated the status of 'professional' or even 'professor' in advertising their more rarefied accomplishments.[54] They were more likely to rely on impeccable personal references and presentation as a means of emphasising the mystique of social graces as well as the linguistic and musical skills still commonly demanded for young ladies of affluent families. Reputation remained the most important and fragile aspect of the human capital carried by such women and connection with good families or academies was vital to successful employment.

The youthful residents of large houses who figured as the heroines of the Victorian governess novel were reasonably accurate reflections of contemporary experience, though the age and marital profile of female teachers in the later-nineteenth century suggest a number of contrasts in their relationship to the labour and marriage markets. The occupation of governess was overwhelmingly the calling of the unmarried, being also undertaken by relatively young women in the middle and later decades of the nineteenth century.[55] Less than five per cent of governesses were married in 1851 and even fewer were widowed. More than half of these single governesses were in their twenties and relatively few remained in post beyond the age of forty.[56] A significant number of governesses probably left on finding a marriage partner, though the Devon evidence suggests that women who remained spinsters usually retired by their fifties, sometimes to head their own household, though more often to live in the homes of relatives or in paid lodgings. It seems likely that the unmarried governess was required to exercise stringent economy to guard against sickness and the loss of employment, as well as provide for her own retirement.[57] A limited minority of governesses were able to head their own household in the 1880s, though these were largely confined to larger urban centres, and the majority of those who did not live with their employers were to be found in the homes of their parents or (more rarely) an unmarried or married sister.[58]

There is little contrast in the relative youth and inexperience of female teachers in the later-nineteenth century. The census group of female 'teacher' was even more starkly associated with younger women than the governess class in this period. Large numbers of teenage females were employed as pupil teachers, though in other respects the age profiles of the governess and teacher were remarkably similar.[59] Sharper contrasts can be detected in the marital status of the different groups, with female teachers more likely to be married or widowed than the governess.[60] This divergence becomes deeper when the 'schoolmistresses' are included in the analysis, since they were rather older on average and a much higher proportion of this group was married. A fair number of widows were also employed as schoolmistresses.[61] The calling of a private schoolteacher offered women such as Charlotte Brontë a rare opportunity for entrepreneurial independence, escaping the dependence on the good opinion of an employer and the dismal prospect of rented lodgings in later life.[62] The residential pattern of those variously identified as governess, teacher and schoolmistress also suggests some material differences in the employment of the different groups. In Devon, female teachers were more evenly spread across the county and were noticeably concentrated in the large city of Plymouth, whereas the governess was more prominent in older and more genteel county towns such as Exeter.[63] Female teachers were more likely to be wives and also householders than were governesses, even though they also included a very large constituency of pupil teachers. In comparison to the governess, a larger number of teachers were resident with their parents and only a tiny fraction lived with their employer.[64] This contrast is again more marked in the case of the schoolmistress, with a sizeable sprinkling of wives and substantially more women heading their own households. Whereas the status of 'servant' was applied to a minority of governesses, this connection was virtually unknown amongst the schoolmistresses.[65]

The evidence from the period 1851–81 suggests a number of important contrasts amongst those described variously as governesses, teachers or as schoolmistresses. It is important to distinguish the social experiences of the private teacher revealed in census and other documentary sources, from the particular rhetoric of libertarian feminism, which campaigners were developing as part of a platform for women's rights in the mid-nineteenth century. The education question was central to feminist concerns and for a period the governess problem formed a significant feature of debate. It is arguable that the governess question can also be read in the social context of professionalisation of employment and the continuing conversation between the virtues of practical knowledge and the values of gentility in English society, we can gain a fuller understanding of the social predicament of the governess. The decline of the governess debate may also reveal an important discontinuity in feminist politics in the Victorian era. One of the interesting absences in the British feminist writing of the later-nineteenth century is the rarity of confessional accounts of asylum life, not only in comparison to prison testaments, but also in considering the relative abundance of such confessions in American feminist literature of the period.[66] In contrast to the great crusade against the Contagious Diseases Acts, with their incisive discussions of medical orthodoxy in respect of syphilitic insanity, as well as the vigorous debates of the 1850s on the subject of feminine insanity, there appears to have been only limited discussion of the rights of women during and after the passage of the important 1890 Lunacy Act.

Although disturbing accounts of false imprisonment had surfaced during the 1850s, and Shaftesbury had bitterly attacked private madhouses in 1859, there was relatively little controversy until the sensational account of her own sinister incarceration was provided by Georgiana Weldon in the 1880s. The story of Mrs Weldon's escape from a private asylum dressed as a nun must have provoked comparisons with Wilkie Collins' *Woman in White* as well as Reade's *Hard Cash*, as a vociferous public campaign led by the Alleged Lunatic Friends' Society culminated in the 1890 legislative reforms.[67] A possible explanation for the limited role played by feminists in this public furore over the private certification of the insane may be found in Janet Oppenheimer's argument that female intellectuals made a significant contribution to the making of medical orthodoxy during the late-nineteenth century.[68] Whilst Mrs Weldon joined some other prominent libertarians in engaging frankly with the question of supernatural and non-rational forces in promoting their cause, many feminist educationalists appear to have strongly aligned with the rationalist politics in promoting the rights of women. Another possible explanation for the limited public debate on this aspect of women's health is that feminist writers and educationalists were divided between those who had become strongly identified with the cause of scientific rationalism and others who endorsed Ashley's model of compassionate public regulation which precluded the elaborate legalistic system for which the reformers were pressing in the 1880s.[69]

The evidence yielded by the census and other documents suggests that we need to carefully examine how contemporary rhetoric on female education and insanity was related to (and distinct from) the material relations by which the governess negotiated her world. The relationship between the changing role of the private teacher and the incidence of female insanity in these decades requires not only an exploration of the literary and scientific publications which figure in the scholarship of Showalter and Poovey, but also some critical examination of the massive textual legacy of the institutions primarily responsible for the maintenance and treatment of the insane. For the institutional market-place was itself shaped by cultural as well as political and commercial concerns. The private asylum sought to distance itself from the Poor Law institutions established in each county after 1845. The next part of the essay examines the fate of the governess and other teachers in such institutions during the later-nineteenth century and attempts to recover something of the relationship between public rhetoric and private conduct in the way that insanity was identified and treated.

The private and the public in the making of the insane governess: the public asylum in Victorian England

The vast array of official enquiries and reports which mapped out the expansion of British government activities in the nineteenth century were themselves part of the apparatus by which the 'public mind' was formed and informed during the Victorian decades. The prosaic descriptions of occupations and material activities which are drawn in the enumerators' books remained deceptively complete, rarely betraying signs of deeply political contests, overt gender bias, or ideological battles between compilers of the census and the people who were being portrayed.[70] The composition of the insane person was more obviously a complex affair, involving the passage of documents through many hands before the individual was secured in the asylum. The cameos of the insane found in asylum texts were formed as compound portraits, drawn by many hands as the individual moved from early sketches of eccentricity to the formal identification in legal documents. A final veneer was provided by the notes made in the asylums recording the institutional progress of the patient and inmate.

The range of sensitive calculations which were made in framing documents relating to the insane, especially the well-connected lunatics of Victorian England, mean that they remain complex and often elusive sources for the historian. The declining interest in the governess question during the 1850s, reflected in the impatient comments of Harriet Martineau cited above, was not a response to the disappearance of the insane governess from institutions during the later-nineteenth century. In her discussion of the asylum population in 1861, Kathryn Hughes finds 136 governesses amongst 13,000 inmates. This figure represented a larger proportion of the census group than the 121 schoolmistresses or even 2,695 female domestics.[71] Hughes concludes that many of the elderly governesses who entered the Victorian asylum were 'not so much mad as senile, consumptive or simply homeless'.[72] It is widely agreed that the published statistics on the occupational profile of female lunatics need to be handled with great care. The returns from the private asylums in particular were often incomplete and uneven. They usually originated as fee-paying or charitable institutions catering for the more affluent and respectable sections of British society after the reforms by Lord Ashley in the nineteenth century, to be clearly distinguished from the pauper asylums funded by the ratepayers.[73] The high standards imposed by a vigilant Lunacy Commission help to explain the relatively slow expansion of private places in the later-nineteenth century. By the 1880s, the Commissioners reluctantly acknowledged that the inmate population of the pauper (or public) asylums outnumbered the 'private class' of institutional lunatics by a ratio of almost ten to one, as Poor Law institutions failed to meet the needs of the modest middling sort of people in society.[74]

The relatives and friends of a stricken governess were faced with a peculiar difficulty. Her domestic means might be modest but it was vital that her confusion should not be well publicised lest her future employment prospects were blighted. Many private teachers who relied on connections with the 'best circles' were understandably anxious to maintain some proximity to the privileged world of their employers.[75] The prospect of prolonged madness could pose a more serious threat to the unmarried educated professional than the risk of physical illness or the loss of character references. Unless such women and men could recover their ability to teach and their connections, they were obviously dependent on the support of relatives and friends. Admission to a pauper institution was extremely difficult for such as the private tutor or governess. The shame of insanity could hardly be concealed or redeemed if the governess applied to the Relieving Officer of the Poor for a place in one of the public asylums established by each county. The exhaustion of family resources would dictate the movement of individuals back to the home of their relatives, or to a less expensive facility. It appears that only 'in extremis' was the governess sent to the public asylums catering for the broad mass of the population.

Even the census enumerators appear reluctant to have returned the insane as disabled or invalids.[76] The different ways in which the rights of the private and the public were exercised can be seen in the failure or refusal of the largest fee-paying asylum in Devon, Wonford House, to disclose to the 1881 census the occupational identities of the patients, which had been so laboriously entered on their admission to the institution. In comparison, we have a fairly full account of the occupations of those who were resident in the public asylum in Exminster at the same period.[77] A possible objection to linking census and institutional records to reconstruct the environment of the insane governess is that the usage of occupational and other titles remained notoriously ambiguous in the Victorian decades, and that females in particular were often deprived of an occupational status on the grounds that their labour was not recognised as valuable in its own right. Similarly, there is very little use made by census enumerators of the 'invalidity' column of the census, with only a tiny number of governesses in 1881 having an invalidity, four being resident in the County Pauper Asylum and the majority of the others scattered across Devon with mostly unspecified disabilities.

To frame these portraits of individual medical careers and to gain some understanding of the larger movement of groups of people through the procedures of certification and treatment, historians of insanity need to examine the peculiar structures of the Victorian asylum and the regimes of care which were designed to treat the individual. Even when the limitations noted above are recalled, it is possible to reconstruct a substantial part of the social and personal world in which the governess moved and some insights into her experience of asylum care in Victorian Devon. The rules of the private and the public domains of society were an essential feature of the re-enactment of respectability in an institutional culture that registered the necessity of difference. The patient's sense of self could hardly be redeemed if the 'educated classes' were allowed to descend into the babbling, foreign world of pauperism. The struggle between conservatism and commercialism did not, however, always deliver the individual to the bespoke institution of their choice.

Amongst the English counties in the nineteenth century, Devon offers a particularly interesting case for an examination of the treatment offered to the Victorian governess. Agriculture, commerce, trade and naval activities, with a declining industrial mining sector, dominated the economy of the county. The robust upper and middle classes drew their income from a range of sources, with the employment of governesses noticeably strong in the affluent coastal areas of east and south Devon. During the eighteenth and nineteenth centuries the county also saw a flourish of charitable and state-sponsored building of medical and educational institutions, often associated with the aristocratic and wealthy merchant groups that dominated Devon politics. These activities included a series of initiatives to make provision for those with mental disorders and deficiencies, including the public County Asylum in the village of Exminster, which was founded in 1845. This Poor Law institution was funded by the ratepayers of the county and was clearly distinguishable from Devon's charitable and private institutions, which had been in existence since the eighteenth century. By 1914 more than 13,000 admissions had passed though its gates and entered its records.

The admission registers of the County Asylum show governesses accounting for about one in every 200 females arriving at

Exminster.[78] Such a figure is very roughly proportionate to their numbers amongst employed women in such contemporary sources as the census for 1861, though it is impossible to make precise statements when women's employment is so poorly recorded in the Victorian census. Their appearance was not confined to any particular period, though they were absent from the admissions hall of the asylum during the 1890s. A high proportion of the women came from the Poor Law Union of Newton Abbot, which encompassed important resorts such as Dawlish, Teignmouth and Torbay. Only the very first governess recorded was identified as a private patient, arriving in the celebrated J.C. Bucknill's earliest years as Asylum Superintendent, though others arrived from private and subscription institutions and a number were re-admitted after a previous visit to the asylum.[79]

These women formed only a tiny fragment of the inmate population of the public asylum of Devon in these decades and it is difficult to make any sustained comparison with the larger mass of patients, still less with the wider inhabitants of the county. The females were, with one exception, unmarried, but in contrast to the occupation as a whole they were evenly distributed in age, with half of the twelve women younger than forty and the remaining females aged forty-eight to sixty-four. This profile suggests that the women were far from being elderly and infirm spinsters, though they were far removed from the youthful stereotype of *Jane Eyre*. There was more of a resemblance to the Brontë novel in the case of one governess who had been resident in Belgium, where the governess heroine of *Villette* faced insanity, and who came to Exminster after being placed in different institutions. In contrast to the turbulent struggle between Protestantism and Catholicism which figures in that novel, virtually all of the Devon Asylum entrants were simply identified as Anglicans.

The certificates of insanity and admission documents provide a common-sense narrative of observed behaviour rather than providing any clear diagnosis of the causes of insanity. A majority of the women was reported to have been suffering for only a matter of weeks, though a few had been insane for months or even several years within their home, with the care of relatives or a landlady. For example, Elizabeth L. had been in Exminster before returning to live with her sister at Teignmouth and had been visited by a local doctor each quarter for two and a half years before she was re-admitted in 1883. It was usually the decision of relatives or neighbours to report disturbing conduct that provided the cue for examination and certification. Violent behaviour was more often threatened than enacted, as when Susan L. of Brixham declared that she would, like *Jane Eyre's* Bertha Mason, burn down the house where she had lodged for six years until 1872, and added that she would also cut the throats of those living there. The conduct that brought these women to Exminster was usually less florid, though the first governess to arrive, Charlotte T., was troubled by powerful visions of being 'buried alive by her friends' before coming into Bucknill's care.[80] Their time at the asylum was varied but usually unremarkable. In common with most other patients, three out of ten cases examined recovered their senses and left within a year or so of their arrival. Six of the women died in the asylum, either very quickly or after lengthy stays of twenty or thirty years.

It is difficult to catch more than a glimpse of these women before they were admitted and after they were discharged, though two were in the Exminster Asylum when the 1881 census was taken. A comparison of asylum and census sources suggests that the status of the women admitted was sometimes uncertain, in particular whether some governesses should be described as schoolmistresses. There was much less uncertainty, however, in titles of governess versus female 'teacher', with asylum governesses rarely identified as 'teacher' in the census. The governesses usually came directly from fairly undistinguished or even modest family homes, with evidence of personal connections to the family. There is usually little sign in the admission documents of dramatic events or an immediate crisis connected with an employer's household prior to entry to the public institution at Exminster. The indication of a fluidity in the status of governess and schoolmistress is difficult to interpret, though it is noticeable that whereas very few female 'teachers' are identified in the admission registers of the public asylum, a fairly substantial sprinkling of twenty 'schoolmistresses' appears amongst a large sample of 2,000 women admitted in the seven decades after Exminster opened.[81] Almost twice as many schoolmistresses as governesses arrived at the institution, particularly in the years after 1890 when few governesses appeared in the registers.

Most of the governesses appear to have come from modest, respectable family households, though signs of domestic turbulence can be read in cases such as that of Ellen C. who appears in 1864, daughter of a schoolmaster in Exeter, who had himself been an inmate of the asylum for a few weeks in 1860. In contrast to the preponderance of working governesses who figure in the census as either daughters or residents of their employer's household, the most common relative to figure in the certificates of insanity of the

Exminster governesses was that of sister or sister-in-law. Perhaps in deference to the delicacy of their social position as well as to notions of feminine indisposition, a physician in their family home or lodgings rather than at the workhouse infirmary examined virtually all of these women, even though they were admitted at the ratepayers' expense. They were almost all diagnosed as 'of unsound mind' rather than as lunatics or imbeciles.

Further clues can be gleaned from the census for a handful of these women. A number appeared to possess only modest means. Elizabeth S. had been born in Somerset but was living as an unmarried woman of fifty-one with her sister Mary Ann C. and brother-in-law who was employed as a gardener, both older than Elizabeth. She was recorded in 1881 as an invalided lunatic, having been formerly a schoolmistress and an inmate at Exminster in 1874 before re-admission in 1883, where she remained until her death in 1909. Others recovered to head their own households. Mary J. was born in London and spent a relatively brief period in the Devon Asylum in 1861 when she was aged forty-eight. Two decades later she appears to have been living quietly in her own household at Lympstone on the banks of the Exe.

The impression given by such brief lives is that the governess who came to the public asylum in Devon was noticeably older than the average age of the teaching profession. There is again some similarity with the age-profile of schoolmistresses, since half of the schoolmistresses for whom ages are available, were in their forties.[82] Marital status does appear to have had some bearing, not only on the liability for admission, but also on the prospects for release from the public asylum in Devon. This appears to have been true of schoolmistresses as well as governesses in the Victorian and Edwardian decades. The former group were given rather better rates of improvement in the asylum records, with about half of the schoolmistresses leaving Exminster having recovered or their symptoms relieved (frequently after very short stays), and the remainder leaving 'not improved' or dying in the institution. This pattern was not only better than that for governesses, but wives and widows also seem to have enjoyed greater powers of recovery.[83] In terms of representation and high death rates, the unmarried schoolmistresses admitted to the county asylum were much closer to the experience of the asylum governess than their respective profile in the census returns would have predicted. One possible conclusion is that unmarried females who were identified as governesses or as schoolteachers (though not, it seems, as female teachers), had poorer prospects of recovery once admitted to the Devon County Asylum than their married and widowed counterparts.

Since the county institution drew primarily from the rural hinterland of Devon, it is worth briefly comparing the intake with that of the borough asylum established by Exeter at Digby Fields in 1886. The Digby Asylum was purposely designed by the Poor Law authorities of Exeter to accommodate fee-paying as well as pauper inmates and in this respect the institution competed directly with other establishments within and beyond the county. One of the most effective methods for raising revenue was to agree a contract with another urban or rural authority to care for a group of their paupers, although private individuals could also be housed for a fee. The new Exeter institution proved adept at attracting batches of patients from the overcrowded London asylums. During its first decade of activity, Digby recorded 312 female and 261 male pauper admissions as well as ninety-eight female and seventy-seven males on a private list.[84] Amongst the females on the private books, half were recorded as having no occupation, about a quarter of the total being simply described as wives or widows. There were two governesses admitted to Digby, both as pauper rather than private inmates. Each was a single woman in middle-age sent from a Greater London asylum in the early 1890s, and both were diagnosed as suffering from mania. Whilst London County Council paid for Isabel H.'s fees, Alice J. was chargeable to the Exeter Union. She was almost immediately transferred to the private class of patients and only after nine years of residence was she transferred back to the pauper group, presumably due to exhaustion of private funds.

These women may be compared with the two female teachers of music also admitted as paupers in the early 1890s. They were single women in their early twenties, one remaining little more than a year before her recovery, and the second staying for several years before being released without improvement. The only other case of note was a fairly elderly teacher of French admitted as a private patient in 1895 and only transferred to the pauper list a year before her apparent death in 1919.[85] In contrast to the notable presence of schoolmistresses in the County Asylum, where they clearly outnumbered the governesses, they are extremely scarce in the Digby admission registers. Two unmarried schoolmistresses aged twenty-eight and thirty-two were admitted as private patients in the decade surveyed, each suffering 'mental strain' and both dying within the institution, one within a few years and the other after a long residence.[86]

The limited comparison of the county and borough asylum in the late-nineteenth century suggests that the classification of patients as well as the character of intake may vary between establishments. The schoolmistress is prominent in the county institution where virtually no fee-paying inmates were admitted, whilst the same title is applied to a handful that were admitted as private rather than rate-funded patients at Digby. There also appear to be some parallels in the pattern of educated women admitted to the two public asylums. Although female 'teachers' were not unknown at Exeter's borough institution, it appears once again that elementary teachers were not prominent, and teachers of music and French were particularly identified. At Digby as well as Exminster the female educationalist was a relatively mature and disproportionately unmarried woman in comparison with her peers in her profession.

It was suggested earlier that the growing professionalisation of teaching in the later-nineteenth century might have led to a divergence in the working experience and social position of the publicly-employed teacher or schoolmistress and the privately-employed governess. This division within the profession of teaching was linked, it was argued, to a distinction between practical knowledge and social accomplishment. If this reading of the teaching environment of the governess has any weight, there may have been greater pressure on the governess, not only to defend her professional status, but also to avoid the dire threat to her future employment that the news of admission to a pauper asylum would represent. There would therefore be considerable advantage in avoiding institutional treatment or finding a place in a discreet private asylum, even though the resources of the governess may have been very limited. To assess the appeal of the private asylum for the governess compared to other female teachers in the later-nineteenth century, we can briefly consider the pattern of admission to the largest private asylum in Devon.

The private asylum and the Victorian social order: Wonford House, 1850-1914

The massive expansion of the public asylum system after 1845 has been more extensively documented than the parallel history of charitable and fee-paying institutions in the Victorian era. The growth of places in private institutions was far less rapid than the expansion of the state-funded institutions, as reformers complained in the 1860s, with a limited investment of charitable funds in such projects. Many of these establishments pre-dated their Poor Law counterparts by decades and, as Charlotte Mackenzie and Jonathan Andrews have shown, the charitable asylums tended to move up the insanity market-place during the nineteenth century. Mackenzie shows that the proportion of patients paying fees in charitable foundation and similar places rose from two-fifths of residents in 1850 to about three-quarters by 1880.[87] The strategic re-alignment of the non-state establishments was often forced on charitable governors as they sought to maintain standards under the vigilant eye of the Lunacy Commission, and also to increase their social distance from pauper institutions to attract the custom of the more affluent client. Lord Shaftesbury and his fellow Lunacy Commissioners were not always sympathetic inspectors of these private facilities, as they imposed standards of space and staffing which the public institutions were able to fund from ratepayers. In response, many of the private and charitable madhouses sought to increase their fee income whilst preserving a sliding scale of payments for deserving and needy cases. For the middle- and lower-middle-class families, the limited availability of places for their insane relatives posed a significant financial as well as social dilemma: there was often a fairly stark choice between an expensive private institution, a charitable asylum where respectable persons with few resources might offer more modest fees, or to gain entry to the public institutions which catered for the broad mass of the population in the Victorian period. This sensitivity of such families and the private asylums themselves towards the unwelcome gaze of the public helped to sustain the system of certification, whereby prior to 1890 a private patient could be admitted to a fee-paying asylum on the authority of two physicians and a relative, without the support of a magistrate or Poor Law authority that was required for entry to a public asylum.[88] It was the abuse of this system in the Weldon and other cases that provoked the furore of the 1880s. The female teacher with few means of support was an acute example of social distress. Governesses were occasionally housed in very small private asylums and convalescent homes, as well as being cared for in private residences. The precise nature of their illness and the conditions of their tenure are frequently difficult to discover.[89] The evidence suggests that even when relatives were hard-pressed to finance her residence at the private nursing home or asylum, family and friends usually struggled to avoid her admission to a pauper institution.

The private institution which served the city of Exeter was Wonford House. The asylum originated in the St Thomas district of the city, before moving to the more rural area of Wonford on the outskirts of Exeter in 1869. It is often difficult to establish details of the inmates from the census returns, which probably reflects a greater reticence of the private asylum to disclose personal details of their patients even to state officials. Their reluctance may have been guided not only by an anxiety to protect the friends and relatives of their clients, but also their attachment to a genteel world and its social descriptions which would have clashed with the more literal understanding of the census enumerator. Between 1853 and 1914 there were almost 1,700 admissions, fifty-three per cent of whom were female. This corresponds very closely to the pattern of gender admissions at the Devon County Asylum at Exminster, and to the distribution of the sexes in Devon itself.[90] Almost all of those admitted to Wonford paid fees on a scale which ranged from the modest to substantial. A clear majority of the male admissions was married, but single women outnumbered wives by almost two to one. More than a third of females admitted to Wonford were recorded in the registers as having no occupation, whilst another fourteen per cent were described in terms of their husband's occupation. Remarkably, almost a third were endowed with the occupational status of 'gentlewoman'.

Most of the 'gentlewomen' arrived at Wonford from south west England, with a dozen from London and the remainder thinly dispersed across a wide range of counties primarily in the southern and central area of England. Since a minute fraction of Devon's population was given such a title by the census enumerators there is a clear disparity in the description of patients and populace.[91] Even if the attic of every large country house in the county yielded up an insane resident it is doubtful that they could have equalled the Wonford returns.[92] It is more likely that the private asylum authorities were generous in allocating the status of gentility to their inmates, even though occupational descriptions provided by the public institutions appear to have been fairly consistent with census accounts.[93] The discretionary status accorded its female patients appears to have been one of the peculiar social functions of the Victorian madhouse. Even as the title of 'gentlewoman' was becoming something of a curiosity in the occupational returns of the Victorian census, the cultural power of genteel femininity seems to have been sustained in the fee-paying asylum.

The social credit of a private facility such as Wonford House was also an important reference point for the private governess whose own knowledge of social deportment and personal manners was an important skill in her appeal to employers. Amongst almost 900 female admissions to Wonford were more than thirty admissions involving governesses. Their arrival was fairly evenly distributed across the period, though with rather fewer entering in the years 1885-1900, a period when public controversy surrounded the question of private certification of women. The governess patients were again noticeably older than the profile of Devon governesses recorded in the census, none of the admitted being younger than twenty-one and most females at Wonford aged twenty-six to forty-seven. Elderly women were also uncommon at only seven, of whom one was retired, older than fifty.[94] There is little evidence to support Hughes' argument that private and charitable asylums were used mainly as a refuge for the elderly, exhausted governess with few other means of care. There was a rather higher proportion of married governesses at Wonford than at Exminster but their numbers remained very small. The overwhelming majority of the group was again, single females.[95]

Contrasts as well as some similarities can be found between Wonford and the public facilities at both Exminster and Digby. Only three schoolteachers are recorded at the private institution, all single women ranging in age from thirty-five to sixty, outnumbered by the seven schoolmistresses, one of whom was retired, and once again these mistresses were decidedly older, being evenly distributed between single, married and widowed.[96] In contrast to the pauper asylums, however, schoolmistresses were fewer in number than governesses, and teachers were virtually absent. There is some evidence that the educationalists were retitled on admission, and the concern of Wonford to appropriate the trappings of gentility is again indicated in the description of one patient as a 'gentlewoman governess', while another woman who was previously seen as a schoolmistress was identified as a governess. It is difficult to envisage the reclassification of entrants without at least the tacit agreement of their families, though this translation of titles may account for some of the contrasts between the public and the private in the Victorian asylum. The census information suggests that the title of 'governess' could be interchanged with 'schoolmistress' and even 'teacher', though in most cases the evidence indicates some consistency in the career of the private governess. The mysterious Julia S. was one patient who was given the title of gentlewoman on her return to the asylum after an earlier discharge, which may suggest that she was identified as the daughter of a gentleman or gentlewoman in addition to being a governess.

Some clues as to the mental as well as the social condition of the governess can be gained from the diagnoses entered in the asylum records. Whilst it is sometimes suggested that melancholy was a peculiarly female malady in the Victorian years, mania being far more commonly reserved as a diagnosis for males, the evidence of initial diagnoses at Wonford indicates a far more even balance of mania and melancholy being used for women entering the asylum, with rather more maniacs than melancholics being identified. This bias in favour of a diagnosis of mania was much more pronounced for the governess, with nineteen suffering from mania or acute mania and only four said to be melancholic.[97] The prospects for recovery were much better for this governess group of patients, with more than half of the governesses leaving recovered and another third being released 'relieved', whilst only three died in Wonford. In comparison, only a third of the larger female population of the asylum left recovered, almost a quarter relieved and more than fifteen per cent died within its walls. Given the relatively high number of single females who died in the asylum and the preponderance of spinsters amongst the governesses, this is an interesting finding.[98]

The passage of female educationalists into and from the private asylum may be partly explained in terms of their family connections and resources. Recent research into the history of asylum provision, such as that by David Wright, has drawn attention to the significance of household relationships and resources in the prospects for both admission and release amongst the inmates of such institutions.[99] This remains a complex question and little light can be thrown on the family backgrounds of many of the governesses who spent time at Wonford. Some of these women were members of households where a group of unmarried sisters and/or brothers lived together. Mary V. remained at the asylum for a few months in 1855, aged twenty-seven, and more than a quarter of a century later was still living in the family home at Whimple with her two sisters and brother, deriving income from the estate itself. Amelia Steele P. came to Wonford in 1862 and is recorded in 1881 as living at home with three unmarried sisters on private means. More remarkable was Susannah R. who entered Wonford three times in 1858-63 and made a fourth visit in 1869-70. Little more than a decade later she headed a household of four sisters, all described as 'annuitant housekeepers'. Both Mary Elizabeth G. and Eliza I. had connections with the famous textile village of Colyton, Mary living with her sister (another governess) and her brother at their parents' home a few years after returning from Wonford in 1877. Eliza came to the asylum from Colyton in 1881, having returned from the coastal resort of

Teignmouth (where she had been born) with an unmarried older sister.

Residence with one or more unmarried sisters in an established family home was a common feature in the background of the Wonford governesses, though some had more complex domestic arrangements. Julia S. first came to the institution in 1856 and returned in 1873 from her mother's house in Exeter. Departing in 1881 she remained out for a little more than two years and in autumn 1883 again returned to Wonford on the authority of a sister named Tozer. The latter appears to have been a lodging housekeeper in Exmouth, from where Julia was sent to Wonford, though the connections and household arrangements remain obscure. Evrell W. also arrived from Exmouth in 1901 on the authority of a sister, having previously lived with her sister Emma and a brother at the family home near Exmouth. Whilst both unmarried sisters were described in 1881 as schoolteachers, only Emma was clearly identified as a 'national' teacher. The circumstances of Eleanor A. were very different, coming to Wonford aged thirty-eight in 1884 as the wife of one engraver and the mother of another, with three more children awaiting her return. She was discharged after eighteen months but returned within a few weeks and remained until early 1886.[100]

Most of the women appear to have been dispatched from family households rather than the place of employment, again suggesting that even the resident governess would be returned to her own relatives before formal certification and admission. Such family households often possessed land or annuities which provided a steady income, and frequently employed servants. The most familiar relationship to emerge from the census is that of residence with an unmarried sister or sisters, though this was not necessarily the authority which appears on the admission documents. The capacity of the governess to depart from the private asylum may have reflected on a greater capacity of relatives and friends to influence the discharge as well as the admission of the fee-paying patient in the Victorian period. The fate of the unmarried governess in the public asylum appears to have been considerably bleaker than that recorded for those who entered the private institution. One possible interpretation is that the medical staffs of the charitable and commercial asylum were more willing to release the individual to the relatives, and even to record significant improvement in the condition of those discharged. Another interpretation may be that families who were willing to accept the governess back into the family home possessed resources to care for her, which may not have been available to those women who entered the public institutions. Public concern at the fate of those privately certified may also help to account for the slight decline in numbers of female educationalists appearing in 1885-1900, though it is difficult to detect that there was any serious resurgence of the 'governess problem' in this controversy.

Conclusions

The figure of the Victorian governess continues to exercise an important influence on the literary and cultural history of the nineteenth century. Contemporary commentators such as Lady Eastlake made the first steps in attempting to explain her prominence in the novels of the period by discussing the position of educated women in English society. After the period when the domestic governesses appeared in the 'sensation novels' of the 1860s and 1870s, she reappeared at the end of the nineteenth century in the work of Henry James.[101] A number of scholars have traced the 'governess problem' to the tensions inherent within the ideals of domesticity and the concern of the expanding empire of medical science to feminise insanity as well as to domesticate the asylum as a model for the orderly society. This view of the mid-century period was challenged by historians of insanity, sociologists as well as literary historians, who have traced the antecedents of Victorian literature in the eighteenth century and also noted the prominence of males in private as well as public asylums in the later-nineteenth century.

This essay has considered the methodology of cultural history as well as the rich variety of sources available for textual and quantitative analysis. It has been suggested here that many cultural historians continue to frame their discussion in terms of a larger material context of class, gender, racial imperialism, and so on, while privileging particular texts as the basis for exploring social attitudes and personal dilemmas. A more authentic perspective may be gained from a comparison of the different texts which were created to map out the boundaries of contemporary society, and the terms on which insanity could be recognised and regulated. Social historians have long been concerned with the problem of individual and collective agency in the making of personal identity and in the connections between the classification of the material world and the allocation of social status. The correspondence of aristocratic families as well as the categories deployed by different groups of enumerators and statisticians formed part of the distinctive ways in which English society was being reformed in the mid-century decades. The Eastlake review of *Jane Eyre* signalled both the broad and continuing struggle between traditionalist and radical versions of social justice in the post-Chartist era and the distinct voices claimed by women for their causes. Public debate served a complex range of social needs as well as contributing to the unprecedented stream of state reforms during the nineteenth century. It has even been argued that Victorian intellectuals were themselves driven to promote such public works as asylum building by the deep anxiety that they might relapse into a self-indulgent depression.[102]

The mid-century period was arguably an important moment in defining the relationship between the private and the public domains of English society. Such exchanges were drafted within a larger rhetoric of political and moral obligation rather than flowing directly from the material relationships of the household or a dominant ideology of domestic motherhood. The terms of domesticity were themselves being contested in a period of widespread popular protest and feminist demands for greater access to citizenship. Debates on the nature and extent of insanity were influenced by the larger platform of discussion on the purpose of female education. Feminist responses to the question of insanity in the mid-century years ranged from radical claims for equal citizenship, to the pledges of philanthropic activists who aligned with Shaftsbury's notion of Christian social compassion, to rationalists who seized on the new psychiatry and medical science to ground their arguments for human behaviour.[103] The campaigns for greater professional status for educated women in the later-nineteenth century contributed to the opening up of the ranks of the teaching profession to females. They also gave women some degree of choice, however limited, over the kind of teaching they wished to pursue and the status attached to it.

It has been argued above that the institutions of education as well as the asylums designed for the insane bore the imprint of the continuing struggle between traditional, commercial and rational virtue as England evolved into a recognisably 'professional society' in the later-nineteenth century.[104] The popular champion of factory and lunacy reform, Lord Ashley, later Lord Shaftsbury, retained a brooding dislike of both political economy and professional groups who extended their hold over public institutions in the second half of the century, weakening the moral and political authority of aristocratic 'natural rulers' such as himself.[105] Even he was forced to acknowledge that the public asylum system introduced after 1845 had not met all needs and that there remained an unfulfilled demand from the respectable middle classes for a private asylum charging moderate fees. Nor had the public asylum model prevented a major expansion of the institutional population in the second half of the century, casting doubts on its curative potential.

Women made an important contribution to the growing professionalisation of English society as well as its literary and scientific culture. The passage and repeal of the Contagious Diseases legislation provided an important moment at which the limits of moral authority and rationalist enquiry were discussed. The apparent absence of a robust feminist literature on the asylum and insanity in the years around the 1890 Lunacy Act, when private certification was fiercely contested, offers an interesting contrast with the discovery of the 'governess problem' in the mid-century decades. The association of Mrs Weldon with mysticism and non-scientific circles may have deprived her of the support of intellectuals and educationalists who were attached to the cause of rational psychiatry, including contemporaries of the Brontës. Perhaps the connection of the private asylum with personal and domestic crisis deprived the reformers of the kind of urgent support that mobilised at the time of public asylum legislation.

It is difficult to discern any clear echo of public debates on the insane governess in the detailed institutional records, which chart the progress of these women through their treatment in the Victorian decades. These materials do register the binary division between public and private provision, and the importance of social circumstance and assumptions in the compilation of the portraits of the certified governess. The vocabularies of rank and manners as well as variations in social position distinguish the classification of patients in the different Devon institutions during the later-nineteenth century. An important feature of the asylum records is the apparent absence of females from the fast-growing ranks of the teaching profession in the period, though there were a number of schoolmistresses and rather fewer governesses in our large sample. The female educationalists in the public asylums at Exminster and Digby were primarily married and unmarried schoolmistresses in their middle years, whilst the governesses were almost invariably unmarried, though again in mature adult life rather than in youth or advanced age. It would appear that women with strong family or marital connections had better prospects of release than more solitary females, though in many other respects these women appeared unremarkable. There were decidedly more governesses in the private asylum at Wonford, again primarily of unmarried women in middle or later life, though with much better prospects for recovery than either their counterparts in the public asylums or even the majority of females in the private institutions. In the uncertain circumstances of private teaching, the maintenance of strong household connections was possibly even more essential as a personal resource and perhaps as a constraint on the movement of the female governess. If the governess was required to maintain a visible distance from the broad mass of domestic servants, then reliance on an unmarried sister or family household would become more apparent in periods of mental illness.

Cultural history has made an important contribution to our understanding of the representation of gender and insanity in scientific as well as literary texts in the nineteenth century. Contemporary debates on the governess have been illuminated by references to the struggles to demarcate the boundaries of household obligation in the mid-Victorian period and the impact of psychiatric theory on the characterisation of the novel in a twist of genre that might be termed Gothic realism. The limitations of this analysis have also been suggested in this essay. Far more attention has been given to the influence of a domestic ideal on the feminine psyche than the ways in which domestic virtue were contested by feminists, libertarians and traditionalists in the complex political rhetoric of the mid-nineteenth century. Examination of the census materials as well as the asylum records and sources from affluent households indicate that these institutions bore the imprint of a continuing struggle between different class images, and they each carried forward their own narratives of the responsibilities of the household as well as the status of the insane. The material and emotional resources provided by the governesses' family household and personal connections, as well as her duties in policing the interior geography of the employer's domestic world, provide important clues in explaining the continuing prominence of the governess in Victorian society.

Notes

1. This essay is based on research projects generously funded by The Wellcome Trust and by the University of Exeter Research Fund. The Exminster data were collected in collaboration with my co-researchers Richard Adair and Bill Forsythe. Richard McLain and Anne Stobart assisted in gathering the Wonford data. I owe a particular debt to Robert Turner who has made an invaluable contribution to gathering and processing the asylum and census data on which much of this essay is based. Earlier versions of this paper were presented to seminars at the Universities of Bangor, Exeter,

Portsmouth, Southampton and Warwick at which contributors offered important criticisms. The ideas were discussed in detail with Helen Rogers to whom I am most grateful.

2. L. Hunt (ed.), *The New Cultural History* (Berkely: University of California Press, 1993).

3. J. Melling and B. Forsythe (eds), *Insanity, Institutions and Society* (London: Routledge, 1999).

4. R. Porter, 'Love, Sex, and Madness in Eighteenth-Century England', *Social Research*, 53, 2 (1986), 211–42: 231–2, 241–2.

5. A. Ingram (ed.), *Voices of Madness: Four Pamphlets, 1683-1796* (Stroud: Sutton; 1997), xxii, 'Everything testifies to the normal, to a desire to be restored to it, to be embraced once again by the protective certainties of the English language'.

6. E. Showalter, *The Female Malady: Women, Madness and English Culture, 1830-1980* (London: Virago, 1987), 28, 'The most significant innovation of Victorianism, however, was the domestication of insanity'. See page 52, for discussion of the preponderance of females in almost all institutions for the insane by the 1890s; J.E. Kromm, 'The Feminisation of Madness in Visual Representation', *Feminist Studies*, 20 (1994), 511–18, offers visual evidence for the Showalter thesis in relation to Shakespearean heroines and medical illustrations; *Cf.* A. Scull, *The Most Solitary of Afflictions* (New Haven: Yale University Press, 1993), 256, n.111, for emphasis on the common experience of male and female lunatics; H. Small, *Love's Madness: Medicine, the Novel and Female Insanity, 1800-1865,* (Oxford: Oxford University Press, 1996), 7, 150–6; S. Shuttleworth, *Charlotte Brontë and Victorian Psychology* (Cambridge: Cambridge University Press, 1996).

7. Showalter, *op. cit.* (note 6). Such an interpretation complies with the view that the scientific as well as literary models of the Victorian decades represented the female body as a natural economy of production and reproduction, with insanity portrayed as the result of a disorder within the bodily equilibrium. See M. Poovey, 'Speaking of the Body: Mid-Victorian Constructions of Female Desire', in M. Jacobus, E. Fox Keller and S. Shuttleworth (eds), *Body/Politics: Women and the Discourses of Science* (New York: Routledge, 1990), 29–46, for discussion of prostitution; Shuttleworth, *op. cit.*, (note 6), 72–3, 219–42; J.B. Taylor and S. Shuttleworth (eds), *Embodied Selves: An Anthology of Psychological Texts, 1830-1890* (Oxford: Oxford University Press, 1998), 184–98 and passim.

8. Shuttleworth, *op. cit.* (note 6), 219–42.

9. E.D. Ermath, *The English Novel in History, 1840-1895* (London:

Routledge, 1997), 84–5. 'This narrative continuum, then, in which consciousness, time and language mix inextricably, literally *constitutes* historical time in the same way that single-point perspective literally constitutes realistic space in Renaissance painting. ...It is the time of Newton and Kant, the time of empiricism and history'.

10. J. Swindells, *Victorian Writing and Working Women: The Other Side of Silence* (Cambridge: Polity Press, 1985), 30–3.

11. G.R. Searle, *Morality and the Market in Victorian Britain* (Oxford: Oxford University Press, 1998), 116–127, 226–7 and *passim.*

12 . Small, *op. cit.* (note 6), provides a succinct critique of the Showalter thesis.

13. S.M. Gilbert and S. Gubar, *The Madwoman in the Attic: The Woman Writer and the Nineteenth-Century Literary Imagination* (New Haven: Yale University Press, 1979), offered the seminal analysis. M. Poovey, *Uneven Developments: The Ideological Work of Gender in Mid-Victorian England* (London: Virago, 1989), 136–8, 141–3. Poovey restates the celebrated argument that when Brontë deals with the childlike dependence of women within contemporary culture, her inexpressible anger is conveyed through the form of her heroine's dreams of children and the novel itself becomes 'a hysterical text'.

14. Lady Eastlake, 'Hints on the Modern Governess System', *Fraser's Magazine,* 31 (November 1844), 571–83, in T. Broughton and R. Symes (eds), *The Governess: An Anthology* (Stroud: Sutton, 1997), 110–12. In her promotion of mutuality and social rescue, Eastlake shared some of the ideals of Ashley. Eastlake is discussed in Poovey, *ibid.,* 127–30 and quoted more fully in K. Hughes, *The Victorian Governess* (London: Hambleton Press, 1993), 163.

15. M.J. Peterson, 'The Victorian Governess: Status Incongruence in Family and Society', in M. Vicinus (ed.), *Suffer and Be Still: Women in the Victorian Age* (Bloomington: Indiana University Press, 1973), 10–14 and *passim.* P. Horn, 'The Victorian Governess', *History of Education* 18, 4, (1989), 333–44: 335–8. Horn cites the census figure of ninety-five governesses in lunatic asylums in 1851 and 136 in 1861, amongst many thousands of female inmates; Poovey, *op. cit.* (note 13), 129–30, 134–6.

16. T. Eagleton, *Myths of Power: Marxist study of the Brontës* (London: Macmillan, 1975), 10–11 provides a valuable discussion.

17. Poovey, *op. cit.* (note 13), 127–30, 144–5, notes that 750,000 domestic servants received less attention, but her main argument is that governesses encompassed the contradiction between the demand that women should rightly fulfil their maternal responsibilities and the practical necessity for many middle-class women to work unless

209

and until they found a husband. As working women, governesses were in dramatic tension with the female lunatic and the factory worker as the fundamental reference point in contemporary literature.

18. Eagleton, *op. cit.* (note 16), 75, suggests that the sexual expression of the sexual transaction between the heroine and her soul-mate is sado-masochistic in Charlotte Brontë's fiction. The more explicit and pornographic connotations of the governess role appear to be later. For the sexualisation of the domestic servant see L. Davidoff, 'Munby' in Broughton and Symes, *op. cit.* (note 14), 180, 201–4, who suggests that by the 1890s the term governess was 'freely used as part of the vocabulary of sexual obscenity' and was so closely associated with flagellation literature as to become 'virtually a synonym for "cheap and sexually available"'. Such an interpretation is open to further discussion. The domestic sphere was often preserved as a relatively unsexualised space in male-oriented pornography. See S. Marcus, *The Other Victorians: A Study of Sexuality and Pornography in Mid-Nineteenth Century England* (London: Weidenfeld and Nicolson, 1966), 128–36, for semi-realist account of *My Secret Life.*

19. A. Vickery, *The Gentleman's Daughter: Women's Lives in Georgian England* (New Haven: Yale University Press, 1998), 182, 381–2, for the case of Ellen Weedon, for example.

20. J.E. Grey, 'Introduction' to S. Fielding, *The Governess or, Little Female Academy* [1749] (Oxford: Oxford University Press, 1968), 14–17, for example. Fielding actively discussed such works as *Pamela* with her famous brother Henry Fielding.

21. L. Davidoff, 'Class and Gender in Victorian England: The Case of Hannah Cullwick and A.J. Munby', in *Worlds Between: Historical Perspectives on Gender and Class* (Cambridge: Polity Press, 1995), 104–50, particularly 134–42; see also 'Mastered for Life: Servant and Wife in Victorian and Edwardian England' in *ibid.,* 18–40.

22. Acland Papers, 1148 Madd/36/942, Eunice Mordaunt to TDA, 10 December 1850. 'When not in the drawing room May w[oul]d be with her in her bedroom or the drawing room. She w[oul]d eat with the servants & May with us, or if we did not have May Miss Hikin w[oul]d have her meals with her in the dining room. When not wanted Miss H. w[oul]d be in the housekeeper's room. As it is the good of the child we must think of not our own pleasure, it does not signify so much whether she is a pleasant companion for us, as whether she is fit for a cheerful playmate for May; – & whether she can be with her in the drawing room if wanted, not as company but

only to play with, teach, or look after her when we are too coughy or tired or busy – Of course she w[oul]d do the dressing and all. ...The great difficulty of finding exactly the person we want *temporarily*, & still more the chance & risk of what a stranger turns out, w[oul]d make me incline to Miss Hikin if she is fit in the main points'. See also 1148 Madd/36/943, letter of Eunice, 15 December 1850.

23. See for example, O. Chadwick, *Victorian Miniature* (Cambridge: Cambridge University Press, 1991), 107–10 for the sensational trial of James Rush for the murder of Isaac Jermy in Norfolk in 1848, in which a young governess was implicated.

24. Much of the frustration frequently expressed by governesses who emigrated to frontier societies such as in Australasia came with the realisation that the differences in factor endowment (an abundance of land and scarcity of capital and skilled labour) and cultural heritage meant that the status of governess work counted for less, despite the promises of the Female Middle Class Emigration Society. See P. Clarke, *The Governesses: Letters from the Colonies 1962-1882* (London: Hutchinson, 1985), 106–7 for Louisa Geoghegan's view of gentlemen and social 'mushrooms' in Victoria.

25. Eagleton, *op. cit.* (note 16), 13, 39.

26. Acland Papers, 1148 Madd/36/940, May Erskine to TDA, 28 August 1850 from Bournemouth, 'Incendiaries have taken to burning the fir woods; yesterday men were seen to set fire to it near where you saw it all black on the Poole road, in an hour it had burnt a mile deep in the wood. ...This is the third fire there has been in the woods lately'. She added somewhat laconically that the men responsible were known 'and I hope taken'.

27. The frustration of the governess in being rendered invisible in social situations provides a central theme of Anne Brontë's *Agnes Grey* as well as her sister's novels. Some of the most important governess novels of the period, such as Anne Brontë's *Agnes Grey* (1847) were also drawn from autobiographical experiences. See Charlotte Brontë's 'Biographical Notice' to *Agnes Grey* (Harmondsworth: Penguin, 1994).

28. S. Jeffreys, *The Spinster and Her Enemies: Feminism and Sexuality 1880-1930* (London: Pandora, 1985), 86, notes that by the end of the Victorian period one in three adult women were single and one in four would never marry.

29. B.L.S. Bodichon, 'Women and Work [1857]', in C.A. Lacey (ed.), *Barbara Leigh Smith Bodichon and the Langham Place Group* (London: Routledge & Kegan Paul, 1987), 36–73: 41–4 and *passim*.

30. I. Craig, 'Insanity: its Cause and Cure' [*The English Woman's Journal*,

September 1859] in *ibid.*, 305–8 and passim. The article was a commentary on the annual Report of Commissioners in Lunacy. See 312–15 and 319 for discussion of the social deprivation which fostered insanity. See also B.R. Parkes (editor of *English Woman's Journal* from 1858) 'The Market for Educated Female Labour' [originally read at the National Association for the Promotion of Social Science, October 1859], in *ibid.*, 147–8.

31. Quoted in Hughes, *op. cit.* (note 14), 165, 188–9; J.L. Hammond and B. Hammond, *Lord Shaftesbury* (London: Constable, 1923), 203–10; G.B.A.M. Finlayson, *The Seventh Earl of Shaftesbury, 1801-1885* (London: Eyre Methuen, 1981), 125–9, 242–8, for social reform and eventual move in favour of Corn Law repeal, 544 for Shaftesbury's reservations on C.O.S. policy; F.K. Prochaska, *Women and Philanthropy in Nineteenth-Century England* (Oxford: Oxford University Press, 1980), 109–10, 211–12; B. Hilton, *The Age of Atonement: The Influence of Evangelicalism on Social and Economic Thought, 1795-1865* (Oxford: Oxford University Press, 1988), 95–6, 212–15.

32. Peterson, *op. cit.* (note 15), 5–6; D. Wahrman, *Imagining the Middle Class: The Political Representation of Class in Britain, c.1780-1840* (Cambridge: Cambridge University Press, 1995), 396.

33. *Ibid.*, 399–400.

34. H. Rogers, *Women and the People* (Aldershot: Ashgate, 2000).

35. Wahrman, *op. cit.* (note 32), 400–6, for the argument that the negotiation of 'class' virtues as well as domesticity and gender had a clear political agenda. N. Elias and M. Schroter (eds), *Mozart: Portrait of a Genius* (Cambridge: Polity Press, 1993), 16, and passim discusses an analogous problem in relation to the role of the artist and patron within the rigid conventions of the aristocratic household European culture.

36. H. Bradley, *Men's Work, Women's Work: A Sociological History of the Sexual Division of Labour in Employment* (Cambridge: Polity Press, 1989), 204–09 and *passim* for a discussion of the varied working conditions of the governess. In 1851 there were more teachers than governesses and significantly more females than males employed in teaching, i.e. almost 72,000 compared to little more than 34,000 males.

37. Horn, *op. cit.* (note 15), 334, Table 1.

38. Our survey of population from the 1881 census returns for Liverpool indicates a little over 800 employed women were occupied as governesses in a population of over 800,000 whilst Glasgow reported little more than 200 in a population of more than 600,000.

This compares to approximately 1,000 governesses living in Devon, where the total population was a little over 600,000 in 1881. The low numbers in Glasgow are confirmed by the research of Dr. Eleanor Gordon on a sample of Barony households in the mid-nineteenth century. My thanks to Dr. Gordon for this information.

39. Bradley, *op. cit.* (note 36), 204–6 and passim for a discussion of the varied working conditions of the governess.

40. There were 304,217 females in 1851 (compared to 274,364 males) and 318,000 females given in 1881. In 1881 there were 94,000 women clearly indicated as unmarried and presumably qualified to marry. Since governesses were almost invariably unmarried, 572 would therefore represent 0.6% of this group, though as a proportion of employed females in their age groups they would represent a substantially higher figure.

41. The 1881 census reveals that 200 and 100 governesses respectively were residing in Newton Abbot and St Thomas on census night, with the two large cities of Devon holding noticeably fewer. The exclusivity of these census titles should not be exaggerated.

42. In 1881 the largest constituents amongst those identified as governesses in Devon were either a governess or a daughter in the household in which they resided. At least twenty-two governesses were associated with the small group of females identified as in a 'private' occupation, thirty-seven private schoolteachers, mistresses and proprietors.

43. Hughes, *op. cit.* (note 14), 22–3, 32.

44. The largest group of 'daughter' governesses in 1881 (38% of 172 in the Devon case) lived in households headed by parents of some rank and status. The majority of the 'no occupation' households appear to be retired people.

45. In contrast to what Hughes found for the earlier period there appear to have been only eight governesses living as the daughter of a farmer in Devon in 1881 and none of the sisters were living in a farming household, though three sisters-in-law are recorded.

46. In Devon in 1881 almost one half of governesses lived in houses of non-relatives with children present. Amongst the 979 governesses and former governesses in 1881, 278 were given the relationship of 'governess' to the head of household and ninety-five were said to be 'servants'. This represented two thirds of those resident. Very few governesses in 1881 were recorded as unemployed.

47. Hughes, *op. cit.* (note 14), 32, notes that the private governess was largely confined to the wealthier middle-class households but her evidence for Crediton, Devon reveals thirteen governesses who were

employed by farmers, millers and similar families, being themselves recruited locally. The 1881 census records Jane Hicles Helder living at the Earl of Devon's Powderham Castle, whilst Ellen Clare Mallett lived with Maud Heathfield at the Stoke Canon inn.

48. It was very rare for the governess or any other residential female to be identified a teacher in relation to the household head and as many residential teachers were described as governesses in such situations. Nineteen teachers were given as 'teacher' in the household and twenty as 'governess'. Only four governesses were described as 'teacher' in the household of an employer.

49. In the 24.1 employing group the situation with the household of origins was reversed in that there were twice as many male as female heads of households (forty-six versus twenty-seven in the case of a governess relation to household, and seventeen versus fifteen in households where the governess was given as a servant). In marked contrast to the governesses' household of origin, almost all the employers' households possessed residential servants ranging from one to fourteen but with an average of more than four per household, and a larger average number in households where the governess was returned as a servant. A similar pattern is evident for the census group of 1.2, which includes magistrates, and some senior officials. Amongst the 122 farmers heading households in which a governess was resident, two-thirds appear to have been employed as a teacher. A substantial majority of these householders farmed more than 100 acres and many more farmed more than 200 acres.

50. Those households with five servants or more were far more likely to have recruited a governess who was not a native of Devon, though it is noticeable that non-Devonians formed a majority in all households where residential governesses were employed. Non-English governesses were much more rarely seen in households with one or no servants.

51. Almost all of those described with the prefix or suffix 'certificated' or 'certified' in the 1881 census were teachers or schoolmistresses (a total of 111) whilst only three governesses were so described.

52. Only 218 female teachers were identifiable in the 1851 Devon census, 33% of which were aged twenty or younger.

53. There are 1,359 schoolmistresses identifiable in the 1851 census.

54. Approximately eighty governesses attracted the title of professional compared to thirteen teachers, and some of the latter were language teachers. Approximately forty-four female professors taught music or languages.

55. The 1881 census for Devon suggests that two-thirds of those

described as governess in the census were under the age of forty and less than 1% of this number was married.

56. Figures from the 1851 census show that 271, or more than 47% of all governesses were aged twenty-one to thirty and another 21% were aged thirty-one to forty. Less than 9% were older than forty.

57. There were twenty-two females identified as retired governesses in 1881, fourteen of them under sixty. Amongst the total were four heads of households all of whom were older than fifty.

58. About 5% of governesses were householders in 1881. In the Devon case there were 460 resident with non-relatives. Perhaps 175 of the total of 979 lived in relatives' households with children whilst 161 did not have any possible family pupils at that address. Here, the most common relationship to the head of household was that of governess (278 or 60% of 460) or as a servant (19% of 460). There were only nine wives in all but 224 daughters plus two stepdaughters, representing almost a quarter of the total. Much smaller numbers lived with their uncles and aunts (twenty-four). In all, forty-four governesses living as sisters to the head of the household and thirteen as sisters-in-law. About two-thirds of the governesses concerned lived with their sisters and one-third with brothers. Males headed all of the in-law households. Only seven of the sisters who headed the household were married.

59. Almost two-thirds of female teachers in 1851 were thirty or younger. Approximately half of those designated as teachers in 1881 were twenty years old or younger and a further quarter in their twenties. The proportions in a total of 1,244 teachers (former teachers, governess teachers and other ambiguous titles were excluded but not private teachers) were 632 and 350 respectively. Excluding the younger groups below twenty leaves 62.5% of teachers in their twenties, 22.3% in their thirties and 15.2% in older groups. The corresponding figures for the governess group are 60.2%, 22.7% and 17.1%. The overwhelming majority were unmarried.

60. Amongst the 1,165 variously given the title of teacher (including many private teachers), seventy-seven were married and twenty-five were widowed, representing approximately 92%, 6% and 2% of the total respectively. Somewhat surprisingly the wives included certificated teachers at publicly funded schools.

61. The two groups of schoolmistress and school mistress have been combined. In 1851 there were 1,359 in this group, of whom only a quarter were thirty or younger. About one-third of the group were married, almost all aged twenty-one or older and a large majority of wives being older than thirty. About three per cent of the group were

widows. In 1881 there were just over 1,000 female schoolmistresses in the Devon census. Relatively few schoolmistresses were younger than twenty (perhaps sixty-seven) and the largest cohort (as with the governess group) were those in the age-range twenty-one to thirty (374 of the total) but one-third of the total (334) were forty-one or older. Within the schoolmistress group approximately 189 were married and 117 were widowed.

62. Education was one of the few occupations in 1881 which revealed a substantial proportion of female heads of households employing a governess, with 176 females compared to thirteen males in this category in Devon.

63. The three towns which made up Plymouth possessed a total of 348 teachers compared to 139 governesses, whilst Exeter claimed only 127 teachers compared to eighty governesses; Newton Abbot had 202 female teachers compared to 211 governesses.

64. There were approximately 853 daughters in the Devon census for 1881, representing about 63% of all teachers, 414 of whom were pupil teachers. This latter group included a large number of females under sixteen. There were eighty-six female heads of household alongside 167 boarders and lodgers representing 6.3% and 12% of the total respectively.

65. In 1851, remarkably, the most common relationship to the head of the household amongst schoolmistresses was that of head, at 35% of the total, whilst 27% were wives of the head and 23% were daughters. Amongst the 930 women who were returned as schoolmistresses in the 1881 census a similar pattern emerges, with 318 (34%) heads of households, though with fewer wives (159 or 17%) and more daughters (287 or 31%), together with 132 boarders and lodgers and fifty-four sisters. Only a miniscule fraction of these women have 'servant' as a relationship to the head of the household.

66. J.L. Geller and M. Harris (eds), *Women of the Asylum: Voices from Behind the Walls, 1840-1945* (New York and London: Doubleday, *c.*1975). I am aware of no comparable tradition within the Voices from the asylum references here.

67. Hammond and Hammond, *op. cit.* (note 31), 204–6. The case of Mrs Turner at Acomb House had been reported in *The Times*, 28 July 1858 and taken up by *The Leeds Mercury.* Shaftesbury attacked private asylums in a Committee of the House of Commons in 1859. K. Jones, 'Law and Mental Health: Sticks or Carrots?' in G.E. Berrios and H Freeman (eds), *150 Years of British Psychiatry, 1841–1991* (London: Gaskell, 1991), 93–8: 94–5. Although much noticed by scholars, the Weldon case may have been less well

reported than others such as that of Thomas Harrison, who was illegally seized in Glasgow. See C. Cameron letter to *The Times,* 26 February 1883.

68. J. Oppenheim, *'Shattered Nerves': Doctors, Patients, and Depression in Victorian England* (Oxford: Oxford University Press, 1991).

69. *The Times,* 11 August 1883, for report on the 8,000 'private class' lunatics and 60,000 'pauper class' individuals known to the Lunacy Commission in 1883. Shaftesbury (formerly Ashley) had used the occasion of enquiries in 1859 and in 1877 to criticise physicians as well as the keepers of private madhouses. See Hammond and Hammond, *op. cit.* (note 31), 203–6; and S. Collini, *Public Moralists: Political Thought and Intellectual Life in Britain, 1850-1930* (Oxford: Oxford University Press, 1993), 287 for Dicey's *Law of the Constitution* and the wider promotion of law as central to 'the distinctive identity of the English nation'.

70. M. Anderson, '(Only) White Men Have Class: Reflections on Early 19th-Century Occupational Classification Systems', *Work and Occupations,* 21 (1994), 5–32.

71. Hughes, *op. cit.* (note 14), Table 2, 206. The figure represented 0.55% of the 25,000 females identified as governesses in 1861. Horn, *op. cit.* (note 15), 338, notes that in 1851 there were ninety-five governesses recorded in asylums which would represent about 0.45% of the 21,000 then identified.

72. *Ibid.,* 164, 'At 8s. 6d. a week, the private asylum offered cheap and just about respectable accommodation'.

73. W. Ll. Parry-Jones, *The Trade in Lunacy: A Study of Private Madhouses in England in the Eighteenth and Nineteenth Centuries* (London: Routledge & Kegan Paul, 1972), 23–4, and 55, Table 11. C. Mackenzie, *Psychiatry for the Rich: A History of Ticehurst Private Asylum, 1792-1917* (London: Routledge, 1992), Table 6.1, 170–1, for figures on governesses and others. L.D. Smith, *'Cure, Comfort and Safe Custody': Public Lunatic Asylums in Early Nineteenth Century England* (Leicester: Leicester University Press, 1999).

74. *The Times,* 11 August 1883, col. 10d, for example, noted that of the total lunatic population of 76,765, only 4,127 males and 3,796 females belonged to the 'private class'. Amongst the pauper class there were 30,355 males and 38,487 females. Many private asylums also made contracts with Poor Law unions, which placed their paupers in the care of commercial and charitable institutions, particularly when borough Guardians refused to finance the cost of their own asylums despite the provisions of the 1845 legislation.

75. The public advertisement for Wonford House provided exactly this

tempo when it sang of the opening by the Earl of Devon whilst stressing that the fees ranged according to the needs of the individual. Devon Record Office.

76. Of the twenty-two governesses with an invalidity column entry in the 1881 Devon census, four were in the County Asylum, two others blind and the disability of the others unknown. It is noticeable that even fewer of the larger host of female teachers were identified as invalids, with three of the fourteen females given as blind and the condition of the remainder unclear.

77. The forty-two female lunatics recorded as Wonford Asylum residents in 1881 included seven 'lunatics', a wife, a widow and a daughter of farmers, two tradesmen's daughters and thirty-seven for whom no occupation at all was entered.

78. Amongst 4,000 admissions, which were sampled, there were rather more than 2,000 females of whom twelve were identified as having the occupation of governess.

79. Charlotte T. entered in 1849 as a fee-paying patient, though the Order signed for Alice G. dated 28 December 1911 was filled in for a Private Patient. One of the twelve (Mary P.) examined from the sample of 4,000 admissions came from the private establishment at Plympton House and others from various other institutions.

80. Admission certificates, Susan L., Charlotte T.

81. Of the three female teachers in our 4,000 sample only one, Jessie M., was clearly identified as a teacher at school, another being a music teacher and a third a teacher of French. There was also one 'school assistant' admitted in 1892, Mary M.J.L., who may have been a pupil teacher. There were about seventeen schoolmistresses, one National Schoolmistress and two 'former' schoolmistresses, plus one wife of a schoolteacher who *may* have assisted in the classroom.

82. A search of the marital status of the Exminster schoolmistresses suggests about half were unmarried, six were widows and two or three were wives. The proportion of spinsters is similar to the census schoolmistresses, but widows were much more prominent, and wives much less prominent in the asylum than in the census population.

83. Among the schoolmistresses, two of the wives and four of the widows departed as recovered or relieved, as compared to five spinsters. Five spinsters died in Exminster, as compared to three of the seven widows even though the latter were generally older on admission.

84. Of the 312 pauper females there were perhaps seventy-one who had no occupation or whose occupation was unknown. Another sixty-four were described as servants, domestic servants, charwomen or

cooks. About fifty women admitted were or had been occupied in some form of dressmaking or needlework. Another dozen at least were in laundering. Fifty-three were described as wives or widows. There were two governesses, two music teachers, one former ladies' companion, two clerks, three nurses and one farmer on the female pauper list.

85. Marianne Albure C. was aged fifty-eight on entry and would therefore have been perhaps eighty-three on her death.

86. Rosabella J. aged thirty-two was admitted in 1889 and died in 1894, Frances Emma L. entered in 1893 and died in 1918.

87. C. Mackenzie, *op. cit.* (note 73), 97; see also J. Andrews *et al., The History of Bethlam* (London: Routledge, 1997).

88. *Ibid.,* 114 and Table 6.1, 170–1. Mackenzie found relatively few governesses in the expensive Ticehurst Asylum.

89. Nineteen females were resident at the Plympton House Asylum in 1881 and Charlotte Couderax may have been a governess, though no occupations are given in the census, whilst the four women at the private Court Hall Asylum were identified as 'imbeciles' with no occupation given. Four governesses can be seen boarding at the St Raphael's Home in Tormoham (Torquay) but the basis of their residence and the purpose of the institution remains unclear. Similarly the Ridgway Convalescent Home and the quaintly titled Delamer Servants Rest [Home] in Tormoham both included one teacher but no governesses in their number, whilst Emily White and Jane Champion were governesses and apparently convalescing at the Western Hospital for Consumption in Tormoham.

90. Wonford House records. I was assisted in this research by Ann Stobart and by Richard McLain.

91. Fewer than 300 females were entered as gentlewomen in the 1881 census of Devon and another thirty-five returned as wives of gentlemen, though a cluster of aristocratic ladies are also visible. The overwhelming majority of the gentlewomen were unmarried (sixty-one per cent) or widowed (thirty-three per cent). They were found mainly in central and southern Devon where the governesses were also predominant, with eighty-six in Newton Abbot compared to only forty-eight in Plymouth.

92. Approximately 162 gentlewomen arrived from an address in Devon, eighteen from Somerset, six from Bristol and fifteen from Cornwall out of a total of 263. It is quite possible that some of these were convalescing in Devon prior to admission, though the general point on the catchment area seems to hold.

93. Wonford House lists suggest the institution was reluctant or unable

to provide details of occupational returns for their clients in many instances. On the other hand, a comparison of public asylum and census returns indicates that the descriptions of occupations corresponded reasonably well in this period. On comparing admissions to the Devon County Asylum against census entries near the time of the 1881 census, it was found that in half of the cases (fifteen out of thirty) the entries matched exactly or were very close, with a small number of entries fairly close (four), in some (six or seven) there was an entry in one of the records but not in the other, a few could not be found, and in only one-tenth of the cases (i.e. three), there was there a clear variance in the occupations given with one of these easily understood (washerwoman in the census rather than wife of a labourer in the asylum records). This would suggest a fairly good consistency of description between very different institutions in this period.

94. Since there were five re-admissions, the age distribution could be calculated in different ways, though a sizeable majority of the women were in their middle age, aged thirty to fifty.

95. Three of the twenty-nine were married and none was widowed. See Hughes, *op. cit.* (note 14).

96. Two were aged twenty-nine to thirty, four were aged fifty-four to sixty-four, and one, forty-two.

97. Approximately 310 females were identified as suffering simply from mania or acute mania, compared to 222 suffering from melancholy or acute melancholy. Amongst governesses there were also six suffering from dementia and four from delusional insanity.

98. Ninety unmarried females died in this period compared to 135 recovered, 107 relieved and fifty-one not improved. For wives, the figures were twenty-six deaths, 106 recovered, seventy-five relieved and twenty-two not improved.

99. D. Wright, *Mental Disability in Victorian England: The Earlswood Asylum, 1847-1901* (Oxford: Oxford University Press, 2001).

100. Since Eleanor had a young daughter, Nora, aged seven months in 1881, it is conceivable that this was diagnosed as a case of puerperal insanity.

101. H. James, 'The Turn of the Screw', *Collier's Weekly* (January-April 1898); reprinted numberous times, notably in Penguin Classics (Harmondsworth: Penguin, 1985). My own interpretation is that this novella is distinct in its association with a genre of overtly supernatural literature rather than the apparent phantoms of much earlier literature.

102. Collini, *op. cit.* (note 69), 62–5. Intellectuals 'betrayed a constant

anxiety about the possibility of sinking into a state of psychological malaise or anomie, a kind of emotional entropy assumed to be the consequence of absorption in purely selfish aims'.

103. Prochaska, *op. cit.* (note 31), 109–110, 211–12; Finlayson, *op. cit.* (note 31), 544 for Shaftsbury's reservations on C.O.S. policy.

104. H. Perkin, *The Rise of Professional Society: England Since 1880* (London: Routledge, 1989), 9–13, 116–23.

105. Hilton, *op. cit.* (note 31), 95–6, 212–15; Hammond and Hammond, *op. cit.* (note 31), 203–10.

8

The Female Patient Experience in
Two Late-Nineteenth-Century Surrey Asylums

Anne Shepherd

'It is acknowledged that women are more prone to insanity than men'

Dr. Rees Philips, Medical Superintendent, Holloway Sanatorium.

This chapter will investigate how cultural perceptions of gender influenced the diagnosis, confinement and treatment of those women deemed as 'suffering' from a wide range of mental disorders during the latter years of the nineteenth century. Rather than merely illustrating the female patient experience by analysis of only one institution's population, here, two widely contrasting nineteenth-century Surrey asylums come under scrutiny. Brookwood Asylum was a large Poor Law institution, while a mere twenty miles away the middle classes were being treated at the exclusive Holloway Sanatorium. Thus, the question of class in relation to gender and incarceration can also be explored.

Introduction

The debate concerning women's relationship with psychiatric medicine during the nineteenth century was initially revived by the publication of Elaine Showalter's *The Female Malady*.[1] She argued that the predominantly male perception of insanity as a female complaint, directly resulted from the view held by much of the contemporary medical profession; namely that women's biological destiny was irrefutably linked to their mental state. This led to women's overwhelming predominance in asylum populations from 1845, though later in the private sector (1890), in all but criminal asylums and military hospitals.[2]

The assumption that nineteenth-century patriarchal society utilised psychiatric institutions simply to control difficult women rather than to cure them of genuine mental illness, quickly came under attack. In her work on women who had at one time lived in British India,[3] Waltraud Ernst questioned the appropriateness of Showalter's analysis for explaining women's experience of psychiatric disorder and incarceration. The notion that madness was primarily a female condition, Joan Busfield has argued, is based on 'stereotypical images of women as neurotic and irrational' and blames inconclusive data on the over-representation of women in asylum populations, claiming that Showalter failed to acknowledge that 'female predominance is far from monolithic'.[4]

The abundance of recent research into the social history of madness has included historical accounts of asylums and patients, such as the extensive survey of public asylums in the nineteenth century by Leonard Smith.[5] Joseph Melling, Richard Adair and Bill Forsythe have explored many aspects of the Devon County Asylum in the nineteenth century in a series of informative and fascinating publications, which pioneered new research in the social history of insanity and institutions.[6] The admission of female patients within the context of individual nineteenth-century asylums has been explored and compared to that of men, and has gone some way towards refuting allegations of social control. The evidence illustrates that disparities between male and female admissions into nineteenth-century county asylums were, in fact, comparatively small, as seen in David Wright's work on Stone, Buckinghamshire's county asylum.[7]

Charlotte MacKenzie, in her work on Ticehurst Asylum in Sussex, has drawn a picture of the upper-class psychiatric patient, illustrating that, within this private asylum, more men than women were admitted during the second half of the nineteenth century, and that the prognosis was bleak for the majority of patients.[8] She has argued that allegations of social control do not work for the private asylum, as, unlike public institutions, there was less of a class differential between the incarcerated and their keepers.[9]

While other studies have tended to centre on one institution to draw their conclusions, this contribution will focus on the experiences of female patients in two contrasting asylums located in Surrey during the latter years of the nineteenth century. These two particular institutions catered for different clienteles allowing for a fuller consideration of both gender and class; Brookwood Asylum was built to accommodate the lunatic poor of Surrey, and Holloway Sanatorium housed the middle classes.

Surrey, located in the south of England, was bordered on the north by the river Thames, and contained many picturesque towns and villages, as well as several poor parts of south London. After 1889, the new London County Council took on the administrative responsibility for several eastern parishes of the county, in addition to taking areas from Middlesex and Kent. The county was, however, predominantly rural, and so provided an ideal location for both private asylums and large Poor Law institutions that could be situated in beautiful countryside and yet easily accessed from the Metropolis.

To understand the totality of the female patient experience in the latter years of the nineteenth century, both gender and class must be taken into the equation. Whilst variations in admissions might be small, it is in the residual populations that differences become apparent. Poor women had a different psychiatric experience from that of their middle-class sisters, although there were of course some commonalities. Either way, there is little evidence to support suggestions that either of these particular institutions operated an overt agenda of social control in relation to disorderly women. That is not to say, however, that women were not expected to conform to ideas of socially acceptable behaviour, but the evidence indicates that expectations within the asylum reflected those of society outside.

State provision:
Brookwood Asylum

Brookwood Asylum was built on an elevated site of 150 acres in Knapp Hill, Woking and opened in June 1867, the year in which the Metropolitan Poor Act (30 Vic. cap. 6) was passed. Under this legislation, vast numbers of pauper lunatics were transferred from workhouses to more appropriate accommodation. Brookwood was serviced by rail from London, and the rural location offered a therapeutic dimension for the many patients sent from south London workhouses, providing separation from family and friends, which was seen by some experts as curative for the troubled mind. The issue of an asylum's location was critical. Land was cheaper in the country, and so large institutions could be built, sufficiently isolated to prevent upsetting the local population. However, asylums also needed to be accessible and transport links were important, both for delivering supplies and allowing staff and patients to easily reach recreational facilities.[10]

Described by the *Lancet* as a 'cheery hamlet of almshouses'[11] and initially able to accommodate 650 patients, the asylum expanded quickly.[12] By 1938, Brookwood was able to accommodate 1753 inmates, and was the size of a village. Indeed, to some extent, that was how the asylum functioned, as, like most other county asylums at the time, it strove for self-sufficiency and cost-effectiveness in keeping with the ethos of Poor Law institutions. The considerable farm with its dairy herd, pigs and crops allowed the Superintendent to report in 1869 that the farm's livestock had provided the asylum with 3,215 gallons of milk and 1,114 stone of pork.[13]

Private provision:
Holloway Sanatorium

Ten miles away at Virginia Water was the luxurious Holloway Sanatorium built by a bequest from the patent medicine manufacturer and philanthropist, Thomas Holloway (1800-1883). He saw the Sanatorium as filling a niche in the market, its purpose being the care and cure of the middle classes.[14] Virginia Water was only twenty miles from London, conveniently accessible by rail, and its proximity to London attested to the importance of the metropolis as a potential source of patients.

Holloway Sanatorium was opened on 15 June 1885 by the Prince and Princess of Wales and attracted much press interest, *The Builder* noting that 'the notion of erecting for such a purpose a sumptuously decorated palace is a novel idea…'.[15] The architect William Crossland had designed an outstanding neo-gothic building, standing on the elevated site of St. Ann's Heath, with a 530ft red brick and Portland stone frontage, 145ft high water tower and lavish grounds.[16] The interior was sumptuously decorated and furnished, and included an imposing dining room and recreation hall with hammerbeam roofs, theatre, billiard room and a Winter Garden.[17] Such was the opulence that its equal was deemed 'not to be found in any modern building in this country, except the House of Lords'.[18] Later, a small seaside branch operated in Hove until 1909, when larger accommodation was opened at Canford Cliffs, Bournemouth.

Horses and carriages were purchased for the patient's use, and over the years, tennis courts, a cricket pitch and Turkish baths were among the many facilities added for their entertainment and well being. Companions – initially two female and two male – were engaged to live amongst the patients to encourage normal behaviour and conversation, and were reported to be 'of the greatest use in promoting occupation and amusement'.[19] From a therapeutic perspective, the comforts and elegance available for the middle-class patients were designed to make their transition from home to institution easier. The preservation of normality by the creation of a homely but luxurious environment was believed to aid patient recovery, and, from the outset, Holloway was promoted as a different type of establishment, namely one designed to preserve middle-class propriety. 'A father will feel terrible repugnance at committing his son to a *mad-house*, whereas the notion of sending him for a time to a sanatorium seems far less dreadful...'.[20]

The intention was that deserving middle-class cases would be admitted at reduced rates supplemented by the surplus accruing from those patients able to afford higher fees.[21] The impoverished middle classes were important to the House Committee, who reported in 1886: 'The benevolent object with which the institution was founded has not been lost sight of. Several patients, including one kept gratuitously, have been maintained at low weekly rates. Indirect aid has also been given to certain patients in the shape of clothing and other extras'.[22] In January 1889, the Sanatorium was registered as a charity, and thereafter was required to accommodate at least a quarter of the patients at weekly rates of twenty-five shillings or under. These third-class patients were supplemented by the second and first-class patients, who paid between forty-two and eighty-five shillings per week.

Admissions to the two asylums: Brookwood Asylum

Brookwood was intended to relieve overcrowding at Springfield[23] and to accommodate the growing numbers of Surrey's lunatics held in unsuitable accommodation or at expensive private asylums. Upon opening, the asylum was besieged with applications from east metropolitan Surrey. In 1867, Brookwood's Committee of Visitors restricted eight metropolitan unions to a total of 280 workhouse patients, with Lambeth allotted the most – thirty-six per cent. By 15 October, five unions – Bermondsey, Lambeth, Newington, St. George's Southwark, and St. Saviours – accounted for thirty-four per cent of the new patient intake.[24] Other Guardians were not pleased; Rotherhithe complained that Brookwood's admission procedures were too slow – an accusation strongly refuted – while Newington pleaded to send more patients.

The majority of metropolitan lunatics originated from workhouses and licensed houses, and were often difficult cases despatched by workhouse masters in order to regain discipline, as frequently acknowledged by the medical superintendent in his reports. The remaining patients came from rural areas of the county. The Superintendent's 1884 *Annual Report* showed that an accountant, an architect, doctor of medicine, schoolmaster, sculptor and a surgeon's assistant had been admitted that year,[25] indicating that not all of Brookwood's patients were obvious paupers,[26] just that

Figure 8.1
Brookwood Asylum, General Patient Admissions by Sex, 1867-97.
Source: Patient Admission Registers, Surrey History Centre.

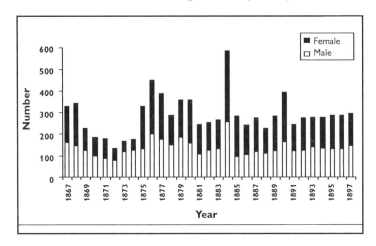

they or their families were unable or unwilling to shoulder the burden of fees for private care, which in turn could have reduced the family to pauperisation. Governesses, companions, nurses, and wives of professional men also featured in the female admissions.

During the first thirty years, 8,891 patients were admitted to Brookwood Asylum at a consistent yearly rate with the exception of 1870–72, when they fell to less than 200 per year, due to building work and alterations being carried out in the asylum. There is no significant difference between the proportions of female to male admissions to Brookwood during the first thirty years. Over this period, the average female intake stood at fifty-three per cent of the total number of patients admitted,[27] a similar figure to that of other asylums at the time. For example, at Leicestershire County Asylum, between 1860 and 1865, fifty-four per cent of the paupers admitted were women.[28] This was not unique to Britain; in his examination of South Carolina Asylum, Peter McCandless has shown that up until 1900, there was very little difference between the admission of male and female patients, and that some years, men even outnumbered the women.[29]

Relapsed cases, or readmissions to Brookwood, stood at roughly five per cent, which the Superintendent claimed was 'about one-half of the general average in English County Asylums'.[30] Neither sex was more susceptible to readmission than the other; usually relapsed cases

Figure 8.2
Brookwood Asylum, General Patient Admission by Sex 1867-97,
per cent.

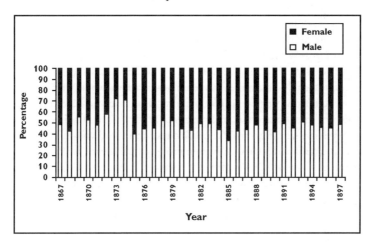

were those released at the request of friends and relatives, often against the better judgement of the medical staff. On average, they remained out of the asylum for less than a year.

Why there was no significant difference between male and female pauper admissions to Brookwood is not entirely clear. Few working-class families would have had the financial resources to pay for psychiatric treatment. Private medical care was the prerogative of the middle and upper classes and as illustrated by the many charitable applications to Holloway Sanatorium, the incidence of insanity and its treatment could cause grave financial hardship. It may be argued that the working-class woman had little time for considering her emotional or psychological problems. A mentally or physically defective woman, whatever her age, could often be maintained within the home. Her economic usefulness could continue by performing domestic duties or childcaring whilst other family members were at work. Admissions figures for Brookwood could be seen as broadly supporting this – nearly fifty per cent of female admissions were listed as having no occupation.[31] Some female occupations may have been ignored by those completing the asylum records – as previously identified in the work of Edward Higgs on the census in which he shows that working women are much under-represented in the nineteenth-century returns.[32] Occupations for female patients were wide-ranging, ballet dancers, stay makers, fur pullers and prostitutes were represented, but the majority were domestic servants. This demonstrates their vulnerability: if these women lost their jobs, then in most cases they also lost their home, thereby driving them to poverty and the workhouse.

A working-class man if unemployed, poor and perhaps ill, was arguably more of a drain on family resources. If he was married and claiming poor relief, he was also more visible to the authorities. Families may have been more likely to bring male cases to the attention of the authorities in the hope that a cure would be procured for the breadwinner – an idea explored by Charlotte MacKenzie in her work on upper-class male patients at Ticehurst. If this was true for wealthy families, then the need to restore a breadwinner to mental stability and competence was even more critical for the working-class families. The majority of men coming from the workhouse to Brookwood – some seventy-eight per cent in 1871 – were listed as having a former skill or trade, excluding those listed as labourers. Only two men out of an intake that year of eighty-six were listed as having no former occupation.

There are few differentials in the ages of the married patients admitted to Brookwood, but single men were much younger. For example, in 1871, nearly three-quarters of unmarried men admitted were aged between sixteen and thirty-five. Over one-third of single male admissions originated from workhouses and houses of correction, compared to only six per cent of married men. Most of these were noted to be dangerous or suicidal, and usually suffered from mania. Given their origin, and diagnosis, it might be deduced that many of these men were difficult to control both within society at large and in the workhouse. Insane, harmless paupers were allowed to be maintained in workhouses, however, if certified or dangerous, they could not remain there for more than two weeks. The younger male admissions to Brookwood fall into this category. Discipline was vital within workhouses and some larger unions, such as Lambeth, built special wards to cater for disruptive younger inmates. Overcrowding and misbehaviour would lead to the managerial, rather than the medical, decision to transfer these difficult cases. Professional opinion differed; some called for the removal of workhouse lunatics to the county asylum, yet others felt that for particular types of insanity the workhouse remained the most appropriate location, as patients remained within their local community.[33]

Holloway Sanatorium

Within the first six months, seventy-three certified patients plus sixteen voluntary boarders – patients without certification – were admitted. Over the first twenty years – 1885 to 1905 – a total of 2,815 certified patients and 1,258 voluntary boarders were treated. At Holloway women stayed longer and were frequently re-admitted, directly contradicting the founder's original intentions. The opening rules declared that 'no patient will be allowed to remain an inmate of the institution for a longer period than twelve months; no patient will be received whose case is considered hopeless; no patient will be allowed to enter the Sanatorium after having been discharged...'.[34]

Voluntary admissions, which accounted for thirty-one per cent of all admissions during this period, were particularly favoured by the medical staff, who believed that this procedure avoided stigma and thus promoted recovery. Voluntary boarders were frequently readmitted to Holloway, and were entitled to charitable assistance. Often patients commenced their treatment as voluntary boarders prior to certification in order to lessen the trauma of the admission, but it was generally acknowledged by the staff that they could be most demanding, behaving like hotel guests and refusing to observe hospital rules. Approximately one-third of the boarders 'drift[ed] into certifiable insanity...',[35] and the majority remained at Holloway as certified patients. Eva Margaret suffered from mania and was first bought to the Sanatorium by her mother as a voluntary boarder in 1898 at the age of twenty-one. Over the next eight years, she returned as both certified patient and boarder, eventually discharged as 'not improved' to The Coppice at Nottingham.[36] For some female voluntary patients, the Sanatorium, with its luxurious surroundings and active social life, became a safe haven and, once 'cured', many certified female patients chose to stay on as boarders. Elizabeth Ann, a 47-year-old unmarried former schoolmistress, plagued the Medical Superintendent with her declarations of love. Laundry work was found to relieve her 'erotic' disposition and she recovered, but having nowhere else to go, she chose to stay at the Sanatorium for many more years.[37]

The higher weekly fees paid by the wealthier patients supplemented those unable to pay, and so it was important that a balance be maintained between those two groups of patients. The rules and regulations for 1886 stated that no patient or boarder was to be admitted 'unless in the opinion of the House Committee, he or she has held such a respectable position in society as unfits him or her

Figure 8.3
Holloway Sanatorium, General Patient Admissions by Sex, 1885-
1905, certified patients only. Source: Holloway Admissions Registers
and Annual Reports, Surrey History Centre.

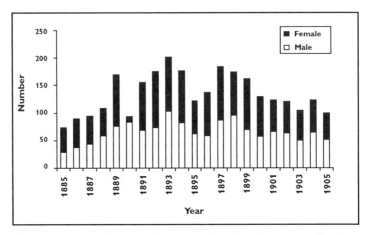

for association with paupers'.[38] Most female patients were listed as being of independent means, or described as gentlewomen. In 1893, eighty-five per cent of female admissions had no occupation and were 'of good social standing'. Those with a given occupation included a nun, a hospital matron, students and governesses. Two thirds of male patients had previous occupations, such as medical or businessmen, members of the armed forces, clergy and students.

As at Ticehurst,[39] the majority of patients, male and female, had been referred to Holloway Sanatorium by (usually male) members of their family. Unsurprisingly, reflecting the social and legal norm of nineteenth-century England, most married women were referred by their husbands, though fathers, brothers and brothers-in-law also played their part. The evidence given to the doctors by family members was regarded as a crucial contribution towards the correct assessment of the patient's insanity, and suggests a level of collaboration between lay and medical concerns. There were many different reasons why families took steps to have their relatives confined, not least, as Charlotte MacKenzie has pointed out, that the removal of a difficult family member could restore family harmony.[40]

David Wright has argued that in the public asylum families were key to the confinement process and that endeavouring to have troublesome relatives incarcerated was a calculated strategy adopted in response to the stresses induced by industrialisation.[41] At other county asylums such as Leicestershire, most inmates were despatched directly from the home to the asylum.[42] At Brookwood, roughly equal numbers originated from the workhouse as from their own home.[43] Families may well have been involved in the first step – the workhouse – but this is difficult to prove, though in 1871, Dr. Thomas N. Brushfield (Medical Superintendent, 1865-1882), commented that many older patients came in due to 'occasioning some trouble to their relatives or to the workhouse authorities' and that 'they appear to have been sent to the asylum for the mere purpose of getting them out of the way...'.[44] But this does not mean that the process was less traumatic for some poor families than for the middle classes, who arguably could afford to use the Sanatorium facilities to suit family circumstances. There is some evidence in Holloway casebooks that families placed difficult female family members there when going on holiday, or when an epileptic had more fits than they could tolerate.

Of the total number of admissions during the first twenty years, fifty-one per cent were female, although in the first eighteen months, this rose to sixty per cent.[45] That many more women than men were applying to enter the Sanatorium during the first decade caused Holloway's first Medical Superintendent, Dr. Sunderland Rees Philips (1884-1899), to observe in the that thirty to thirty-three per cent more women than men had been admitted.[46]

The majority of patients of both sexes admitted were unmarried. For example in 1890, sixty-five per cent were single of whom nearly three quarters were women. It was a phenomenon that caused Dr. Rees Philips to write in 1892, that among the single and widowed patients admitted that year; 'the female sex preponderated to the extent of forty-five and fifty-five per cent respectively'.[47] This is further verified by a sample of 1,003 certified and voluntary female patients admitted between 1885 and 1905,[48] which shows that sixty-four per cent were single (including widows). Amongst only voluntary female patients, the figure is seventy-one per cent.

According to the 1891 census, there were nearly one million more women than men in England and Wales.[49] The late-nineteenth century saw the rise of the culture of the single man; it became socially acceptable for middle-class men to delay marriage in order to establish their fortune, if indeed they married at all.[50] This was a time that saw the opening of many more men's clubs, such as the luxury Albany 'men only' accommodation in Piccadilly. It was also an era of increased prostitution. Not only were there fewer men, but also apparently fewer reasons for them to marry. Despite emerging job and education opportunities, middle-class women's perceived destiny remained marriage. As John Tosh has pointed out, for better-off families with servants there would be fewer domestic duties to occupy these unmarried women, and in lower income brackets, no option of a life long income.[51] Unmarried women may have felt marginalised, lonely, frustrated and unfulfilled, which may have in turn resulted in some psychotic behavioural patterns, or they may simply have been a burden to their families. This in turn may have impacted upon the admissions to Holloway, with the women themselves, or their relatives, choosing such a superior establishment as their refuge or prison.

The single women admitted tended to be younger, with nearly two-thirds under the age of forty-five. These were of child-bearing age, but with no legitimate and socially acceptable outlets for sexual feelings. Many women, single and married, were described as exhibiting erotic behaviour and there are many cases of married women admitted to Holloway so described, according to the evidence presented by their husbands and other (usually) male relatives.

Married women, especially those who had been married for some time, may have found their restricted lives, and attending social expectations, frustrating and unrewarding. Anxiety and depression, the mental baggage of many latter day housewives, may have contributed to the physical and psychological effects of the menopause to manifest in attention seeking behaviour or more serious types of mental disorder. Behaviour deemed inappropriate for a married woman often featured in the 'facts' recorded in the women's certificates of insanity. Typical evidence included that given by Mary Emmeline's husband, who informed the doctor that his wife's conversation was 'improper and even coarse in the presence of her children...';[52] or Ellen, whose husband testified that 'she has frequently made her escape from the house in the night and without proper clothes...', and further, 'she shows entire incapacity for managing her house and looking after herself'.[53]

Between 1885-1888, three quarters of men admitted were single (six per cent of these were widowers) and like the women, tended to be younger than their married counterparts. Whilst Charlotte Mackenzie has pointed to the model of the family prepared to spend in order to have the breadwinner cured, the high numbers of single males admitted to Holloway indicates that it may have been the income earning potential of all males that made them deemed worthy of the financial investment of treatment.

Figure 8.4
General Patient Admissions by Sex: Holloway Sanatorium 1885-1905.
Voluntary Boarders. Source: Holloway Admissions Registers and Annual
Reports, Surrey History Centre.

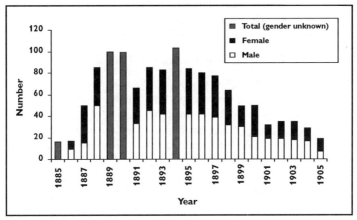

Where women clearly dominate, however, is in the numbers of residual patients calculated at the end of each year, and this is a pattern seen in both institutions. Women account for over sixty per cent of the remaining certified patients in Holloway between 1885-88, and fifty-eight per cent in 1895 – the only years for which this data is available. The majority of those remaining were unmarried or widowed.[54] This trend is repeated in the voluntary boarder sector; in 1887, women accounted for seventy per cent of the voluntary boarders admitted that year, and of those remaining at the end of the year, seventy-five per cent were female.[55] At Brookwood too, there were consistently more women left at the end of the year; from 1865 to 1896, the average was fifty-eight per cent.

This can be partially explained by the higher death rate for male patients, reflected in other registered hospitals for the insane between 1886 and 1890, including Holloway. Large numbers of men suffered from General Paralysis of the Insane (tertiary syphilis), attributed as the cause of death for three out of four men at Holloway.[56] At Brookwood, GPI was also the primary cause of death for males; for example, in 1875, forty-four men died of this disease as opposed to twenty-seven women.[57]

Poor women were also likely to have become physically fitter during their stay, as many would have enjoyed a better diet than outside, thus adding to their natural longevity. It is arguable that working-class women had less financial independence and were more likely to become impoverished if deserted and/or unable to find work, so that the very economic dependence that may have initially contributed to their incarceration, was a factor why so many remained. Their relatives may have been less likely, or able, to petition for their discharge and there would have been few employment options awaiting them upon their release, tarnished as they were by the stigma of being a discharged lunatic.

Classification of disorders and outcomes

Nearly half of Brookwood's female patients were classified as suffering from mania, as were the male patients, particularly those 'difficult' workhouse patients transferred from metropolitan Surrey. Melancholia accounted for nearly a quarter of females admitted, (similar to the men) and dementia was attributed to fifteen and twenty-one per cent respectively.

Ascertaining the causes of patient insanity was difficult. Writing in 1876, Dr. Brushfield complained bitterly that the involvement of the Relieving Officer in the clerical process led to 'defective and even perverted histories of the cases' being given to the medical officers. As a result, over two thirds of admissions in 1875 have 'not known' ascribed to their cases.[58] Nevertheless, Brushfield was confident that intemperance was the 'principle cause', particularly when it came to generating General Paralysis. He conceded that it was not always apparent on admission, but that some discharged male patients had 'admitted their disease to have been caused by the same exciting agent'. With women, he was not so sure, 'due in part perhaps to their greater reluctance to own the truth' and that 'moral causes are much more frequent among them than males'.[59] This is reflected in the annual reports, where moral causes are attributed to many more women than men.

The poor physical and mental condition of new patients was seen as the cause of Brookwood's poor recovery rates, which, for example, stood at thirty-four per cent in 1870, dropping to twenty-two per cent in 1871. Women were either discharged as recovered within less than a year, or else they became long-term patients in the asylum, as seen from the 1871 admissions when no patients were discharged as recovered after five years. This endorses findings by David Wright for Stone Asylum,[60] and also the earlier work done by Lawrence Ray, who showed that there was a fast turnover of patients within the county asylums and that this high discharge rate was neglected due to preoccupation of historians' preoccupation with the growth of institutionalisation and contemporary concerns with the accumulation of incurable cases.[61]

Figure 8.5
Brookwood Asylum. Patients remaining by Sex, (per cent) 1867-1897.
Source: Annual Reports, SHC.

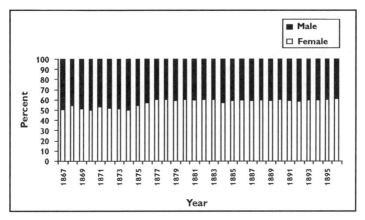

Workhouse patients were frequently received in a poor condition, and there are many instances of women who arrived excessively restrained, bruised and riddled with vermin. It was alleged that many had been retained too long by workhouse masters thus jeopardising their chances of recovery. This was not uncommon, and studies of the Devon County Asylum have revealed that patients sent from nearby Plympton workhouse were substantially less likely to recover than those sent from home.[62] Dr. Brushfield observed in 1875 that Brookwood had 'not a very favourable class of cases to deal with...' and that one in four cases were either epileptic or general paralytic. Female GPI sufferers were fewer in number, but the casebooks of both sexes reveal more typical symptoms, even though they may not have been initially recognised as such.

GPI cases invariably died shortly after admission. The *Lancet* commented that at Brookwood the disease accounted for '31.45 (per cent) of the total mortality, or 140 out of 451 deaths in all, from the opening of the asylum on June 17th, 1867, to December 31st, 1874...'.[63] It was a more problematic disease for Brookwood than for Springfield; 1875 figures show that one case in 8.5 inmates was a sufferer, as opposed to one in 22.4 in Wandsworth.[64] When in 1890 only five patients were admitted with GPI, the Medical Superintendent James Barton attributed this to the fact that only rural cases from Surrey had been admitted that year, indicating the medical association of this condition with the evils of urban life.[65]

Busfield and Showalter have both suggested that General

Paralysis was predominantly a male disorder that resulted from differences in sexual behaviour, as opposed to differential rates of diagnosis or detection.[66] Women's cases, Busfield has argued, were more likely to have been contracted from their philandering husbands than from their own promiscuity.[67] This implies that most men who contracted syphilis did so after they were married, but as John Tosh points out, it was more likely that it was promiscuous bachelorhood that made wives vulnerable, as unmarried men formed the bulk of the nineteenth-century prostitute's clientele.[68]

At Holloway, specific information on GPI may have been omitted to protect the patients and families, although this did not prevent the Superintendent commenting in 1890 that 'no less than one fourth of the gentlemen admitted during the year were found to be suffering from this fatal form of insanity, a fact which goes far to explain the higher mortality among the male than the female insane'.[69] Dr. Rees Philips believed fewer women suffered from this disease, and although women were more liable to insanity, there was also more chance of them being cured. He explained: 'The nervous organisation of the female is less stable than that of the male, and is therefore more liable to merely functional disturbance, while in the male the nervous centres, though more stable, are also more prone to serious organic lesions, such as general paralysis, from which the female is comparatively exempt'.[70] Thus the doctors at Holloway failed to make the connection when a husband and wife were simultaneously undergoing treatments for GPI.

Women at the Sanatorium suffered predominantly from the same three disorders as they did at Brookwood. Taking 1888 admissions as an example, sixty-two per cent suffered from mania, thirty-eight per cent melancholia, and twenty-four per cent from dementia. However, recovery rates were higher at the Sanatorium than at Brookwood; in 1889, they stood at nearly forty per cent for certified patients and forty-one per cent for boarders. Early admission was seen as critical to the chances of recovery and in 1890 the Superintendent proudly announced that during the previous year, twenty-four cases of acute mania had been admitted and that a hundred per cent recovery had been achieved due to their admission having been in the early stages of the disease.[71]

As at Brookwood, few female patients at Holloway were assigned a cause for their insanity, predisposing or exciting. In only relatively few cases was some form of aetiology attempted. Causes listed were wide-ranging, but a considerable number related to women's reproductive life, including confinement, childbirth, the menstrual cycle – or lack of it, and 'the change of life'. Other 'moral' causes typically associated with women were disappointment in love or family troubles. Whilst a similar proportion of men had no cause assigned, those most frequently cited were overwork and business worry, followed by self-abuse and debauchery. Domestic concerns and alcohol are given in only a handful of cases. For both sexes, other occasional reasons included sunstroke, indigestion, fright at being bitten, and excessive use of gas during a dental operation.

Eating disorders, frequently associated with suicidal tendency and conditions such as melancholia, appear frequently in Holloway casebooks, and markedly less so at Brookwood. As mentioned above, pauper patients benefited from an improved diet, and whilst some seriously disordered patients may have harboured delusions regarding food (e.g. poisoned etc.), there is considerably less evidence of self-starvation. However, food was central to the therapeutic regime of the asylum; dietary 'extras' were given to ailing patients and they were regularly weighed as part of the on-going assessment of their mental and physical health.

A different picture emerges at Holloway. Anne, a 33-year-old spinster, was regularly admitted, suffering with violent mania. She attempted to escape twice and frequently refused food, so that the attendants had no option other than to feed her three times a day with a tube. Despite her previous violent inclinations, 'she does not make the slightest resistance to the operation, walks quietly in, sits down to have it performed, opens her mouth voluntarily so that the gag is almost unnecessary'.[72] This was not usually the case; 34-year-old Emily struggled so violently at each feed that several attendants were required to hold her down during the process.[73] It has been argued that appetite disorders were viewed as having associations with masturbation and sexuality,[74] and for some late nineteenth-century clinicians, food denial was intrinsically linked to melancholia and suicidal propensity, therefore treatment was deemed imperative. Such behaviour also offended contemporary notions of recovery that centred on gaining flesh.[75] Some cases of food refusal may have taken the form of individual protests, but may not have constituted full-blown anorexia nervosa which had become a recognised clinical syndrome from 1873.

Large numbers of suicidal patients were admitted to both asylums. At Brookwood, so many patients coming from urban workhouses were described as suicidal that it is likely that such terminology was used to facilitate the discharge of difficult inmates to the county asylum. Many such cases arrived bound in straightjackets or strong dresses but did not exhibit such symptoms once under treatment. Although women were considered to be more suicidally disposed than men, Brushfield believed that all cases of melancholia were a potential risk. His primary policy of surveillance was largely successful, as there were only three recorded suicides during this period.[76]

At Holloway, some women were determined to kill themselves. In June 1886, Alice, aged forty-five and married, was admitted to Holloway with hysterical mania, allegedly caused by the onset of the menopause and the 'excitement of a noisy thoroughfare in Spain'. Just prior to her arrival, she had attempted suicide by throwing herself out of a window, thereby sustaining several scalp wounds. Once an inmate, she continued in her efforts of self-destruction. She tried to gouge out her eyes and bit her lips to the extent that she was 'now a ghastly subject with her lips swollen beyond recognition and eyes the colour of claret'. She repeatedly smashed her head against the walls and screamed continuously. Much effort was made to relieve her condition, not least for the comfort of the other patients and the staff. Hypodermic morphia, purgatives and electric therapy were all used, and she was regularly sent to the seaside branch for short visits. Emily, a 42-year-old suffered from mania and was also suicidal, the result of 'over anxiety and lactation after confinement'.[77] Various therapeutics were used to control and cure her condition, including massage, continuous baths and electricity. When particularly maniacal, she was confined to a padded room. Special attendants were assigned to such cases, and the treatments employed at Holloway, such as electric therapy,[78] indicate that the Medical Superintendents and staff were trained in the latest therapeutic techniques and approaches to potential suicide. Observation was the main weapon employed, but despite all precautions, there were two apparently unrelated suicides (one of each sex) on the same day in 1887. A subsequent inquest exonerated the Sanatorium from any blame and the event appears to have had no effect on admissions which were particularly buoyant that year.

Therapeutics in the asylums

Brookwood's rural location and considerable grounds allowed extensive outdoor employment for patients, particularly for the men, who worked in the kitchen gardens and the farm. Together with regular exercise, work was seen as curative and as providing the virtues of endeavour and self-sufficiency whilst preparing for a 'de-institutionalisation of the insane'.[79] Women were mainly employed in the kitchens, the laundry, and the sewing room to make men's clothes. They also worked in the wards, and for many years, one female patient helped the night duty nurse until the intervention of the Commissioners in Lunacy stopped the practice. As McCandless has pointed out, it should be no surprise that [moral] therapy was segregated by gender as asylums were predominantly based on a domestic ideal where men dominated and women were subordinate. Daily exercise was undertaken in the grounds, with less extensive excursions for female patients, and difficult or feeble patients restricted to the airing courts. Periodically, this activity was constrained by the asylum's building programme which caused great concern, as exercise was not only therapeutically beneficial, but tired the patients and made them more malleable.

It is difficult to gauge the extent of the medication administered to women in Brookwood – the irregular references to dosage and prescription in the case books were criticised by the Commissioners in Lunacy in 1868. There is evidence of opiates, chloral, potassium bromide and cannabis being used, but it was the avowed preference of the first two medical superintendents to prescribe moral order, fresh air and employment. They were also cheaper. Chemicals were, in the main, administered to noisy and difficult women where their behaviour disrupted the asylum routine. Sarah R., a 29-year-old widow was brought from St. Olave's workhouse and was recorded in 1872 as 'never sleeps unless chloral is given to her – this is done nightly'.[80] Treatment was suspended if it did not quickly achieve the desired results. This was seen in the case of Elizabeth K., first admitted at the age of ten in October 1867. During this and subsequent readmissions, she was subjected to a wide range of treatments – morphine, chloral, potassium bromide and cold water. Solitary confinement, eggs and brandy all failed to work. Ultimately the dietary additions and medication were withdrawn, as they were believed to be making 'her stronger to do evil'.[81]

At Holloway, despite the lack of familiarity of most patients with physical labour, some types of work were deemed valuable and so several workshops were built.[82] As a result, some men and women took part in the traditional work ascribed according to gender, although not to the same extent as at Brookwood. The emphasis at Holloway was on a moral therapy that saw entertainment and genteel occupations as being more in keeping with middle-class life than physical exertion through work. In his desire to encourage normality and socially acceptable behaviour amongst the patients, male and female companions were engaged by the Superintendent. Of suitable social origin, they lived amongst them providing companionship and social and moral guidance. By 1889, there were seven female and three male companions, all possessing musical and artistic talents.[83] Their assistance was regarded as essential for carrying out the social niceties that the Superintendent continually introduced into the patients' regime, such as in 1888, when 'a table d'hôte dinner at 6.30 with tea and music afterwards has been established for those who are well enough'. This was presided over by the Assistant Medical Officers with the specific help from the companions.[84] The sensibilities of the patients were also uppermost in the mind of the Superintendent when he reported in 1891 that 'many gentlewomen are replacing the nurses drawn from the lower classes', as he determined to surround his patients with their social familiars.[85] This continuance of 'normality' was considered essential for the confined middle-class patients. Whilst removal of the patient from family and friends was a key element of nineteenth-century psychiatry, relatives were encouraged to stay. Originally they stayed in the main building but later had cottages in the grounds. They dined with the patients and participated in amusements, often residing at the Sanatorium for some months.

Living as closely as possible to the middle-class norm that they were presumed to have enjoyed prior to admission, patients were allowed 'the utmost liberty consistent with safety...'.[86] Patients hunted, went for carriage rides, extensive walks and visited nearby towns to shop or arrange their personal affairs. They took regular excursions to places of interest, public sporting events and the London shops. Whilst such arrangements were obviously not feasible for Brookwood, both asylums believed in the therapeutic value of entertainment. Musical ability was an essential skill for all attendants, and Brookwood regularly held concerts, balls, and theatrical events alongside seasonal sports, primarily for the male patients.

Hydrotherapy was popular at Holloway, and in cases of acute mania, the continuous warm bath 'proved to be a therapeutic agent of great value'.[87] Padded rooms were included in the original construction (not so at Brookwood) and these were used for secluding the more violent and disruptive patients. Paraldehyde, sulphonal and chloral were regularly used to calm patients and induce sleep, and hypodermic morphia was also administered. Other preparations containing cannabis, strychnine, opium and cocaine also feature in the casebooks, with some of these combinations probably used to stimulate appetite. Electric therapy was used from c.1890, particularly with regard to cases of severe melancholia and suicidal tendencies in female patients where many other forms of treatment had been tried and found ineffective. The Medical Superintendent encouraged his staff to sit for professional qualifications, arranged for their training in rudimentary massage, and introduced Swedish gymnastics for both patients and staff.

Conclusion

Nineteenth-century asylum superintendents and other sections of the psychiatric profession considered women to be more prone to mental disorder but yet believed that the very weaknesses which made them so also rendered them more liable to recovery. Their illnesses were not so serious, perhaps only to be expected, given the nature of their reproductive cycles. Dr. Reece Philips frequently endorsed women's higher recovery rates, which he felt were particularly evident amongst those of the middle and upper-middle classes.[88]

Class differentials between the women admitted to these asylums were often less clear-cut than might first be supposed. Many were not seriously ill, yet others suffered from mental disorders attended by extreme symptoms. The comparatively small distinction between the numbers of men and women admitted to these two asylums, indicates that there was no overt policy of female oppression, nor is this evident in the routines and therapeutics practised by either institution. The occasional increase in female admissions can be explained by localised factors, as we have seen, in addition to being little more than a reflection of the sex variant in the population. Many similarities existed in the perception of female patients by the medical profession, and also in treatment selected for their recovery. The differences in the experiences of these women lay primarily in the extent and duration of their treatment, partially due to financial considerations, but also to some extent resulting from the attitudes of those running a Poor Law institution towards their impoverished charges.

The more significant differences lie in the residual patients – more women than men remained in the asylum, whether in the public or the private domain. Indeed, for certain groups of women, life in the asylum was preferable, though this is of course not to disregard the impact of institutionalisation amongst all patients. At Brookwood, the women, on a superior diet and freed from the rigours of extended child-bearing and dangerous employment, became healthier and lived longer. Few women were admitted suffering from GPI, the chief cause of mortality in the asylum at the time. They were also less likely to have had many relatives campaigning for their release.

At Holloway, many women chose to stay on after the successful completion of their treatment. For some female – and male – patients admitted to Holloway, the Sanatorium came to be a luxurious type of rest home that offered respite from demanding families or the scorn of the outside world. This suggests that for all women, particularly if poor or unmarried, the options for discharged female lunatics were few. As Busfield has said, it would be a mistake to assume that where there is evidence of high incidences of mental disorder in women that this is necessarily indicative of their oppression.[89] To a degree dependent on their social status, some women and their families collaborated with the medical authorities. Female incarceration was in some instances a desirable option for a variety of interested parties that cannot neatly be explained by accusations of social control.

Notes

1. E. Showalter, *The Female Malady; Women Madness and English Culture 1830-1980* (New York: Pantheon, 1985).
2. *Ibid.*, 54.
3. W. Ernst, 'European Madness and Gender in Nineteenth Century British India', *Social History of Medicine*, 9 (1996), 357–82.
4. J. Busfield, *Men, Women and Madness,* (New York: New York University Press, 1996), 14.
5. L.D. Smith, *'Cure, Comfort and Safe Custody'. Public Lunatic Asylums in Early Nineteenth-Century England* (Leicester: Leicester University Press, 1999).
6. R. Adair, J. Melling and B. Forsythe, 'Migration, Family Structure and Pauper Lunacy in Victorian England; Admissions to the Devon County Pauper Lunatic Asylum, 1845-1900', *Continuity and Change*, 12 (1997), 373–401; B. Forsythe, J. Melling and R. Adair, 'The New Poor Law and the County Pauper Lunatic Asylum', *Social History of Medicine*, 9 (1996), 335–55; J. Melling and B. Forsythe (eds), *Insanity, Institutions and Society, 1800-1914* (London: Routledge, 1999).
7. D. Wright, 'The Discharge of Pauper Lunatics from County Asylums in mid-Victorian England. The Case of Buckinghamshire' in Melling and Forsythe (eds), *Insanity, Institutions and Society, op. cit.* (note 6), 93–112.
8. C. MacKenzie, 'Social Factors in the Admission, Discharge, and Continuing Stay of Patients at Ticehurst Asylum, 1845-1917', in

W.F. Bynum, R. Porter and M. Shepherd (eds), *The Anatomy of Madness, Volume II, Institutions and Society* (London: Tavistock, 1985), 147–74; MacKenzie, *Psychiatry for the Rich; A History of Ticehurst Private Asylum*, (London: Routledge, 1982).

9. MacKenzie, 'Social Factors', *op. cit.* (note 8), 159.

10. C. Philo, 'Fit Localities for an Asylum: The Historical Geography of the Nineteenth-Century Mad-Business in England as Viewed Through the Pages of the Asylum Journal', *Journal of Historical Geography*, 13 (1987), 398–415: 411.

11. 'Report on Brookwood Asylum', *Lancet* (4 Dec. 1875), ii, 817–20.

12. Intermittent building programmes occurred from 1874, and 50 acres of additional farmland were purchased in 1880.

13. Brookwood Asylum, Report of the Medical Superintendent for the Year 1869, 26, contained in the Third Annual Report of the Committee of Visitors of the Surrey County Lunatic Asylum, presented to the Court of Quarter Session, 5 April 1870. Wellcome Library for the History of Medicine.

14. Thomas Holloway died before the completion of his two philanthropic projects, the other being Royal Holloway College.

15. *The Builder*, 7 January 1882.

16. A. Harrison-Barbet, *Thomas Holloway, Victorian Philanthropist* (Egham: Royal Holloway, 1994), 46.

17. J. Taylor, *Hospital and Asylum Architecture in England 1840-1914. Building for Healthcare* (London: Mansell, 1991).

18. *The Builder, op. cit.* (note 15).

19. The Superintendent's First Annual Report for 1886, 10.

20. *The Builder, op. cit.* (note 15).

21. Minutes of the Annual and Ordinary Meetings of the General Committee for Holloway Sanatorium, Surrey History Centre (henceforth SHC) Ac 2620/1/1, February 1887, 3–4.

22. Minutes of the Annual and Ordinary Meetings of the General Committee, 15 November 1887. SHC Ac 2620/1/1.

23. Springfield, Wandsworth, was Surrey's first county asylum.

24. Report for the Quarter Sessions, 15 October 1867, in Brookwood Minutes of the Committee of Visitors 1867-68. SHC, Ac 1523/1/9/1.

25. Brookwood, Report of the Medical Superintendent for 1884, (henceforth RMS).

26. R. Adair, B. Forsythe, and J. Melling, 'A Danger to the Public?: Disposing of Pauper Lunatics in Late-Victorian and Edwardian England Plympton St. Mary Union and the Devon County Asylum, 1867-1914', *Medical History*, 42 (1998), 1–25: 25.

27. Brookwood Admission Registers, SHC Ac 1523/3/21/1-15.

28. P. Bartlett, *The Poor Law of Lunacy* (Leicester: Leicester University Press, 1999), 153.

29. P. McCandless, 'A Female Malady? Women at the South Carolina Lunatic Asylum, 1828-1915', *Journal of the History of Medicine and Allied Sciences*, 54 (1999), 543–71: 554.

30. Brookwood, RMS for 1878, SHC Ac 1523/1/1/1, 27.

31. These include those women listed as 'wife of' or 'widow of'.

32. E. Higgs, *Making Sense of the Census: The Manuscript Returns for England and Wales 1801-1900* (London: HMSO, 1989).

33. For a comprehensive discussion of the Poor Law in relation to lunacy, see Bartlett, *op. cit.* (note 28).

34. Anonymous article, probably by George Godwin, *The Builder*, 7 January 1882.

35. Holloway, RMS for 1891, 59.

36. Holloway, Female Case Books, SHC Ac 3473/3/1, 6, 7, & 29.

37. *Ibid.*, SHC Ac 3473/3/1, no. 96.

38. *Regulations for the Holloway Sanatorium, Hospital for the Insane, St. Ann's Heath, Virginia Water, 1886*, SHC Ac 2620.

39. MacKenzie, *op. cit.* (note 8), 159.

40. *Ibid.*

41. David Wright, 'Getting out of the Asylum: Understanding the Confinement of the Insane in the Nineteenth Century', *Social History of Medicine*, 10 (1997), 137–55.

42. Bartlett, *op. cit.* (note 28), 156.

43. For example, in 1878, 45 per cent came from home and 42 per cent form the workhouse, and by 1897, 49 and 43 per cent respectively.

44. Brookwood, ARMS 1871, 17.

45. Holloway Sanatorium, Annual Reports 1886-1906, Minutes of the Annual and Ordinary Meetings of the General Committee for Holloway Sanatorium, SHC Ac 2620/1/1.

46. Holloway, RMS for 1892, 72, SHC Ac 2620/1/1. Female admissions periodically slowed down due to the lack of available beds and applications were duly refused.

47. Holloway, RMS, *ibid.*

48. Holloway, Alphabetical Register of Female Patients, SHC Ac 3473/3/37.

49. 14,949,624 women as opposed to 14,052,901 men.

50. John Tosh, *A Man's Place. Masculinity and the Middle Class Home in Victorian England* (London: Yale University Press, 1999), 130.

51. *Ibid.*, 152–3.

52. Holloway, Female casebook, SHC Ac 3473/3/, no. 3.

53. *Ibid.*, no. 26.
54. Voluntary boarders are not included in these figures.
55. Holloway, RMS, 1887, 18.
56. Holloway, RMS 1891, 60.
57. Brookwood, RMS 1875, 18.
58. Brookwood, RMS 1875, 20.
59. Brookwood, RMS 1875, 21.
60. David Wright, 'The Discharge of Pauper Lunatics', *op. cit.* (note 7), 100–103.
61. L.J. Ray, 'Models of Madness in Victorian Asylum Practice', *Archives of European Sociology*, xxii (1981), 229–64. Ray used selected data from Surrey and Lancaster asylums.
62. Adair, Forsythe, and Melling, 'A Danger to the Public?', *op. cit.* (note 26), 12.
63. 'Report on Brookwood Asylum', *Lancet* (4 Dec. 1875), ii, 227.
64. *Ibid.*, 229.
65. Brookwood, RMS for 1890, in Surrey County Council Reports 1891, SHC, 9.
66. Busfield, *op. cit.* (note 4), 19; Showalter, *op. cit.* (note 1), 111.
67. Busfield, *op. cit.* (note 4), 19.
68. Tosh, *op. cit.* (note 50), 130–1.
69. Holloway, RMS 1891, 59.
70. *Ibid.*, 60.
71. Holloway, RMS 1890, 48.
72. Holloway, Female Case Book, SHC Ac 3473/3/1, case no. 83.
73. *Ibid.*, case no. 147.
74. J. Ussher, *Women's Madness: Mysogyny or Mental Illness?* (New York: Harvester Wheatsheaf, 1991), 78.
75. J.J. Brumberg, *Fasting Girls. The Emergence of Anorexia Nervosa as a Modern Disease* (Cambridge, Mass., Harvard University Press, 1998) 141–53.
76. For a fuller discussion on suicide and the county asylums, see A. Shepherd and D. Wright, 'Madness, Suicide and the Victorian Asylum: Attempted Self-Murder in the Age of Non-Restraint', *Medical History*, 46 (2002), 175–96.
77. Holloway Sanatorium, Female Case Book, SHC Ac 3473/3/1, case no. 204.
78. The effects of electric therapy are described in Holloway Sanatorium female casebooks from 1890.
79. M. Finnane, 'Asylums, Families and the State', *History Workshop Journal*, 20 (1985), 134–48: 142.
80. Brookwood Female Case Book, SHC Ac 1523/2/21/3.

81. *Ibid.*, 1, 3.
82. Holloway, RMS 1891, 62.
83. Holloway, RMS 1889, 28.
84. Holloway, RMS1888, 26.
85. Holloway, RMS 1890, 61.
86. *Rules for Admission to Holloway Sanatorium*, 1886, SHC Ac 2620.
87. Holloway, RMS 1890, 48.
88. Holloway, RMS 1891, 73.
89. Busfield, *op. cit.* (note 4), 236.

9

A Class Apart?
Admissions to the Dundee Royal Lunatic Asylum
1890-1910[1]

Lorraine Walsh

Our perceptions of 'class' and what it meant to be a pauper or a private patient require redefinition before we can draw any firm conclusions on the importance of class to the patient experience in the nineteenth-century Scottish asylum. This chapter argues that a range of influences within the asylum, including financial concerns and a striving for respectability, led to the reconceptualisation of the private patient in this period, thus negating any direct translation of rich and poor into private and pauper. Such an interpretation challenges Scull's suggestion that divisions between private and pauper asylum patients was an accurate reflection of class divisions within Victorian society.

Introduction

Ladies and Gentlemen requiring the benefit of the Institution can be accommodated with commodious apartments in Gowrie House, the recently erected Private Asylum, apart from the other Patients, with a servant if required.[2]

Insanity, and its possible causes, was clearly identifiable with class issues for many nineteenth-century medical, and often lay, men. Many of these connections were made in order to illustrate what they saw as sharp differences between the susceptibility of the upper and lower classes to mental illness both in general and in its variant forms. For some nineteenth-century commentators, moral causes of insanity 'naturally affected the rich and educated differently to the poor and uneducated';[3] consequently, this difference was seen to extend to their respective forms of treatment. Isaac Ray, in his observations on several European asylums,[4] was of the opinion that patients from the 'educated and affluent' classes needed much greater attention than those from a 'poor and laboring [sic]' background,[5] while physicians, such as Esquirol, believed that the influence and authority which they exercised over poorer patients, further augmented by the social standing of the physician in relation to the patient, could provide almost instantaneous cures.[6] In Scotland, the apparent susceptibility of society's wealthier members to mental illness was highlighted by W.A.F. Browne who went on to implement his ideas on the benefits of class segregation at the Crichton Royal,[7] an asylum not far from the Scottish border that was well patronised by the English gentry. As Donnelly has argued, for contemporaries it appeared that '[t]o a significant degree the rich and poor [were seen to have] suffered different insanities'.[8]

The idea that the treatment and handling of the institutionalised insane was centred on a decidedly class-based system has been advanced in the work of, among others, Andrew Scull. For Scull, the social structure of the nineteenth-century asylum was an accurate reflection of the class-based society outwith the gates.[9] Jonathan Andrews, in a recent study of the historical value and utility of patient case notes, has highlighted the fact that the patient experience revealed by such records was 'prejudiced in favour of the wealthy, educated, articulate or extrovert patient' with the result that these patients 'tended to be regarded as more interesting and to receive more attention' than the other less 'interesting' cases.[10] While Andrews does not specifically discuss class issues, the implication is that it was the 'better' class of private patients, those individuals who were more likely to be wealthy, educated and articulate, that were seen as the subject of greater interest, and perhaps value, to asylum physicians. The largely undifferentiated mass of pauper patients, by virtue of their status, having apparently little to offer.

This chapter aims to demonstrate that it is our perceptions of 'class' and what it meant to be a pauper or a private patient that require redefinition before we can draw any firm conclusions on the importance of class to the patient experience. The direct translation of what is perceived to have been the accepted societal roles of wealthy and poor individuals into the asylum experience of private and pauper patients, has the potential to result in the oversimplification of a complex situation that was influenced by factors other than class interests or concerns. Rather than simply employing the somewhat complicated and indeterminate concept of 'class', other factors can usefully be brought into the equation. 'Status', as differentiated from 'class' by Weber, may prove helpful, although the usage of the terminology is still far from fixed in time and place. However, Geoffrey Best's suggestion that respectability, rather than class, was the 'sharpest of all lines of social division',[11] is perhaps a more useful concept to employ within the context of the asylum, where the attainment of respectability and socially acceptable behaviour was an essential tenet of moral therapy. Respectability – particularly in the case of the poor – was the key to acceptance, or at least tolerance, within wider society, being a necessary prerequisite for the receipt of parish relief and charitable monies in general. The overwhelming predominance of the middle classes – for whom respectability was a credo – in the management of the Scottish charitable asylums also makes for its central importance within such institutions.

An examination of the experience of the pauper and private patients within the asylum after they have been stripped of their 'class' or society-based realities and affiliations, such as home and family, workplace, and associations, is crucial to an understanding of the relevance of class to the asylum environment.[12] In what ways, if any, was this background articulated within the asylum setting? And to what extent did the category of 'asylum patient' override and perhaps replace these previously given aspects of an individual's social standing? This chapter will examine the impetus behind the separation of classes within one Scottish institution, the Dundee Royal Lunatic Asylum, in addition to evaluating the effect of a class-based system on patient diagnosis and the likelihood of recovery and discharge from the institution. The patient experience in the Dundee Royal as a mixed class institution from 1890-1903 will be considered, in addition to the patient experience within the asylum as a solely private institution from 1903 – and the creation of the new District Pauper Lunatic Asylum – up to 1910 and the eve of the Lunacy (Scotland) Bill (1911). The experience of this Scottish institution should shed light on the wider asylum experience, and the implications of class-based analysis within the context of institutional provision generally.

Divide and rule?

Unlike their English counterparts, Scottish asylums, largely as a result of their charitable basis, had a history of maintaining both pauper and private patients. By the end of the nineteenth century that policy had begun to change. This change was partly the result of external influences and the creation of new bodies, such as the District Boards of Lunacy which became responsible for the maintenance of pauper lunatics, but was also a response to changes from within the asylum itself. Opened as a charitable institution in 1820, Dundee Royal Lunatic Asylum had by 1883 moved outwith Dundee to Westgreen, a country area on the outskirts of the city. Although the Dundee Royal remained an asylum for the reception of both pauper and private patients throughout the period 1890-1903, a physical separation of these two groups of patients had begun by the mid-1890s. The opening of Gray House in 1895, for the reception of solely private patients, was the first time that completely separate accommodation had been provided by the asylum for its private clientele. Previously all classes of patient had been accommodated within the one institution, albeit in separate parts of the building. However, by adopting this new policy of providing completely separate private accommodation the Dundee Royal was following a distinctive trend of the period. The 'lavishly constructed' Craig House was opened for private patients of the Edinburgh Royal Asylum in 1894,[13] and the building of Carnegie House, planned for the reception of 'private patients at the higher rates', was under way at Montrose Royal Asylum by 1895.[14] The creation of District Boards of Lunacy in Scotland, charged with responsibility for the maintenance of pauper lunatics, added further impetus to this class separation. However, Dundee's activity predated this development by several years. How can this 'trend' be explained?

Jonathan Andrews, in a discussion of the Glasgow Royal Asylum, notes that the movement at the end of the nineteenth century to reduce the numbers of pauper patients within the Glasgow Royal Asylum was an attempt by the directors and medical officers to improve the status of the institution, and to create further accommodation for the increasing numbers of potential patients from the middle classes. By 1897 no pauper patients remained in the Glasgow Royal.[15] The asylum had some measure of success in raising its profile and as a result began attracting patients from as far afield as India, South Africa and Australia.[16] The Dundee Royal was as eager to accommodate more patients from the 'intermediate' middle classes as was the Glasgow Royal, but Dundee was also reluctant to be rid of its coterie of pauper lunatics. Financial considerations lay at the root of this concern. Although the Dundee Royal had always accepted both pauper and private admissions the number of pauper patients had always exceeded the number of private cases. This situation had led to the development of a vicious circle where the asylum's attempts to create an atmosphere conducive to the attraction of increased numbers of private patients were hampered by the large numbers of paupers resident within the institution. Yet at the same time the lack of private patients' fees, and thus income, resulted in a continuing need to maintain large numbers of paupers, whose fees were paid by the Parochial Boards, in order to maintain a reasonably secure financial basis for the institution.

Accommodation was a problem encountered by the majority, if not all, of the Scottish and English asylums due to the apparently ever-growing numbers of 'pauper lunatics'. In England this situation led to the establishment of a 'national network' of pauper asylums in the wake of the 1845 Asylums Act, followed by a further spate of building activity to accommodate the intermediate class of patient.[17] In Scotland the relatively delayed programme of new building, and then solely for the accommodation of private patients, was to do little to solve the more general problem of overcrowding. This was a situation readily acknowledged by the Commissioners in Lunacy when they noted, in 1897, that the directors of the Dundee Royal were planning to erect a separate building for the use of the 'intermediate class' of private patients (this new building was the planned Gowrie House which was to replace the rented accommodation provided by Gray House). The number of this class of patient resident in the asylum was comparatively small, being only fifty-nine out of a resident population of almost 500,[18] and the planned new building was to accommodate only sixty patients. The Commissioners commented that, 'It will be evident that the removal of fifty private patients of the intermediate class who are resident in the main building to the new asylum... will not set free the accommodation necessary to meet the future requirements'.[19]

Nonetheless, the Commissioners clearly supported the principle of the development of separate accommodation for private patients and were full of praise for the existing separate private accommodation at Dundee provided by the rented Gray House. Secluded and far removed from the public road the Commissioners considered the arrangements to be in accordance with 'the modes of life usual in a well-appointed country mansion'.[20] The Dundee Royal physician, Dr. Rorie, was also eager to praise the separate accommodation, commenting in 1899 that,

> Gray House... continues to prove a valuable adjunct in the treatment of the private patients, and to afford a quiet and homelike place of residence for such as do not require the rigid supervision of an Institution. Several ladies have recently left it recovered, who, I feel sure, would not have done so had they been placed in less favourable surroundings.[21]

Indeed, several case book entries refer to the improvement to be found in patients who were moved into the separate private accommodation. Rorie failed to express, however, any corresponding view that the pauper patients, housed in the main asylum building, might also have benefited from such a rarified atmosphere. Despite this, Dr. Rorie was at pains not to appear overly biased towards the private patients, and he emphasised the benefits to the pauper patients – as evidenced in their 'freedom from irritability and excitement' – of the relief from overcrowding in the main asylum due to the movement of patients to Gray House.[22] It is debatable, however, whether the removal of such a small number of patients would have impacted in any great way on the patients in the main asylum, particularly as those private patients paying the lowest rate of board were still resident in the main building and would presumably have occupied the best quarters of the house.

The separation of patients in this way was more than an attempt to separate physically the different 'classes' of patient. In effect the directors were trying to create in Gray House something more akin to a convalescent home, 'its arrangements... entirely free from features of an asylum character',[23] something which is at odds with the asylum's claims to be moving more in the direction of a medical facility. In 1892 it had been noted in the annual report that 'every year this asylum... is becoming more and more an hospital for the treatment of mental and other allied nervous diseases, and less and less a place for the mere detention of patients'.[24] Although this was a view which continued to be echoed in subsequent years it is far from clear that this was actually the case. Indeed the number of deaths was often as high as the number of 'cures' per annum.[25] However, by providing separate accommodation for private patients in a smaller and less institutional facility, the Scottish asylums were following the example of English private asylums which had always been small-scale, home-like and intimate.[26]

A further, and ultimately central, reason for the development of the new building for the accommodation of private patients appears to have been the acute awareness on the part of the asylum directors of the changes planned for the asylum system in Scotland. Concern over the prospect of further interference, as they saw it, regarding the dispatch of local pauper lunatics led the directors of the institution to resolve to 'appeal to the Secretary for Scotland against the order and regulations erecting the Parish of Dundee into a separate Lunacy District'. The Dundee Royal along with several other Scottish asylums had a long history of rebuffing governmental legislative attempts to take control over what were essentially charitable, independent institutions.[27] However, this appeal was to come to nothing and the Dundee District Board of Lunacy, with its acquired responsibility for pauper lunatics, was established in 1899. As a direct result it became necessary that the Dundee Royal broaden its appeal to potential private patients from both the middle and upper classes.

This development was important on two fronts. Firstly, in that the asylum required a *raison d'etre* and therefore had to repackage itself as a private institution, and secondly, patient numbers had to be sufficient to maintain the economic viability of the asylum. The construction of Gowrie House, a completely separate building for the accommodation of private patients, meant that the Dundee Royal Asylum could literally stand alone as a private institution. Therefore the decision to shape the new accommodation as a separate building, rather than as a new wing to the existing asylum as had previously been the case with building expansion throughout the history of the institution, had been as much a tactical decision with regard to the future of the asylum as a move towards the separation of patients for reasons of status or class.

Class versus classification

The classification of patient admissions in terms of social status was a difficulty for the nineteenth-century asylum administrators and remains a problem for historians today. While it has been argued that such classification in relation to social class had become part of the 'normal arrangements in both private and public asylums by the latter part of the eighteenth century'[28] many Scottish asylums, such as the Edinburgh Royal [29] as well as Dundee, made little attempt to classify their patients in this way. Patients arriving at the Dundee Royal Asylum were subdivided and classified according to their ability to pay a specified level of board. As the board might be paid by someone other than the patient themselves, such as a relative, patron or employer, such classification was not in itself indicative of the patient's social status. Further than this, there appears to have been little, if any, concern at the Dundee Royal to differentiate in any way amongst pauper and private patients in terms of administration. Admissions were simply listed in the annual report by occupation, the only differentiation being one of gender rather than class. Entries for both pauper and private admissions were also mixed indiscriminately in the case books,[30] which again were more likely to be separated by gender than by class.[31] Therefore, in order to ascertain the social status of patients entering the mixed-class asylum, a judgement has to be made using the available information, which in the case of the Dundee Royal Asylum comprises occupational details provided by annual reports, and patient histories recorded in the case notes. The aim here is not to attempt to establish any detailed analysis of patient admissions in relation to occupational groupings, but rather to ascertain the relationship between social status and patient categorisation (either private or pauper) and to demonstrate the difficulties inherent in ascribing both social status and potential asylum status as either a pauper or private patient to particular occupational categories.

Classes are commonly established through such economic indicators as occupation and an individual's relationship to the modes of production, however, such a system of categorisation can be misleading.[32] Elizabeth McK., a housekeeper, was admitted to the Dundee Royal as a private patient in 1891.[33] A comparison with two other housekeepers, Margaret H. or S. and Jessie R. or L., who entered the asylum as *pauper* patients in 1903,[34] indicates that, in the asylum setting, an automatic assignation of a specific class to the occupation of housekeeper would be incorrect. Similarly, while significant numbers of domestic servants entered the asylum as pauper patients, nonetheless several servants were also classified as private patients in 1907, 1908 and 1910. The breadth of occupational groupings relating to the nineteenth-century working and middle classes makes it almost impossible to construct a system of commensurability between occupation and status with any measure of success or accuracy.[35]

Once resident in the asylum, an individual's status was not immune to change. For those patients whose care was reliant on family finances the possibilities of such a change in status were manifest. Removed from the marketplace, such individuals became reliant on existing rather than prospective funds for their continued maintenance. A prolonged period of residence could quickly eat into available capital resulting in rapidly changing fortunes. Helen W. was originally admitted to the Dundee Royal Asylum as a private patient in 1891, however, after ten years in the asylum her funds were failing and she was reduced to the status of pauper patient, chargeable to Inverkeithing Parish in Fife. As a result she was transferred to Fife and Kinross District Asylum as a pauper lunatic.[36] Furthermore, the fact that the financial responsibility for many of the patients was borne by individuals other than the patients themselves nullifies any indicator of asylum classification that relies on personal status or occupation. Essentially, entry to the Dundee Royal Asylum as a pauper or private patient was related less to an individual's social position and more to the funds available for their maintenance within the institution. Factors such as the relationship of the patient with his family, community and possible patrons, in terms of available financial support, are crucial to the equation.

There is little doubt, however, that different levels of care did exist for the designated 'classes' or groups of patient within the asylum itself. But again this was essentially a financial consideration rather than the response of the asylum to the sensitivities of the class system. The fact that 'Suitable dinners were served to the different classes of patients'[37] was simply the result of the provision of care at a level commensurate to the amount of money paid by individuals for board, rather than a response to any perceived needs or requirements indicated by the status of the patients. In some asylums the different levels of accommodation were linked to the state of mind of the patient rather than to any consideration of their social class, although as Anne Digby notes in her discussion of this practice at the York Retreat, it would seem that this extent of social mixing may only have taken place in exceptional cases rather than on a regular basis. This was again a purely financial decision, taken in order to avoid the objections of the relatives of the higher class of patients. The high level of income generated by this class of patient was too important to the financial well being of the asylums for it to be placed in jeopardy.[38] Such exceptions did occur at the Dundee Royal, but rather than demonstrating any classification of patients on a medical basis, this was an example of the need for patients to conform to standards set by the asylum.[39] Individuals who did not conform could easily find themselves ejected from their private quarters if they did not comply with those standards. Elizabeth M. was admitted as a private patient in 1894. After four years she was moved into Gray House, only to be removed two years later, 'having become dangerous', not being returned to the separate private accommodation again until after several years had elapsed.[40] Respectable behaviour, rather than social status, proved the deciding factor. Cases such as this indicate further that there was no automatic admission to, or retention of patients in, the private accommodation but that patients had first to conform. The advertised image of Gray House was one of a calm and quiet convalescent home and any such disruptive patients, regardless of their social class or status, were not to be tolerated.

Such striving for respectability was extended to the wholesale incorporation of the Protestant work ethic within the asylum, and increasingly the private patients were expected to be usefully employed within the institution. Helen M. was admitted to the asylum as a private patient in 1890. She was only eighteen years old and had previously been a resident in the Larbert Institution for Imbecile Children since the age of eight. Helen initially occupied herself with a little sewing but by 1897 she was 'assisting' in the private wards. This increased level of activity was recorded in conjunction with the comment that her level of intelligence also appeared to be increasing.[41] Eliza K. was also admitted to the institution in 1890 as a private patient but by 1897 she too was recorded as assisting with the housework.[42] Pauper and private patients did on occasion also work together. Marjory K., a former sack machiner from Dundee, worked in the asylum laundry before being transferred to the lunatic wards of the Dundee East Poorhouse.[43] Elizabeth McK. a former housekeeper from a Perthshire farm, entered the asylum as a private patient, yet in the same year as Marjory K., Elizabeth could be found 'working industriously' in the laundry regardless of her status as a private patient.[44]

It was anticipated that all the private patients in Gowrie House should be employed in some capacity. The annual report of 1908 noted that, 'Practically all the patients who can work are induced to do something useful, and the record of employment shows that 40 of them, 17 Gentlemen and 23 Ladies, were employed',[45] while the following year it was noted that 'Useful employment, *chiefly of a household and domestic nature*' [author's emphasis] was found for 20 Gentlemen and 28 Ladies'. The putting to work of private patients who might previously have spent their days occupying themselves with parterre and needle, backgammon or bowls, or perhaps with music 'in an hour of langour and ennui'[46] suggests that the desire to demonstrate to the public that the patients were being usefully employed, and could thus prove themselves to be worthy and respectable citizens, now overrode the traditional occupations and pastimes associated with the image of the private patient.[47] More importantly, however, this situation was also the result of the increasing number of middle-class individuals who were entering the asylum as private patients on the lower and often subsidised rates of board, and who were thus contributing to the reconceptualisation of the private patient.

For the asylum directors themselves, private patients constituted those 'persons the expense of whose maintenance [is] defrayed by their relatives and friends'.[48] There was thus no direct correlation of social standing with the status of private patient. Indeed, the majority of 'private' patients were in fact financially supported, at least in part, by the asylum itself, with very few individuals paying the highest rates of board. The 1905 Report of the Commissioners in Lunacy commended the Dundee Royal for the 'extent to which the Directors provide[d] for patients of limited means at low and unremunerative rates of board'. The Commissioners went on to bestow their 'warmest recognition' on the 'important service... rendered to the community by contributing towards the care and treatment of persons of this *class* in the excellent accommodation of this asylum'.[49] In reality, the extent of this 'enlightened benevolence' meant that of the sixty-seven patients resident in the asylum when visited by the Commissioners, fifty-one individuals were paying between £25 and £40 per annum, fifteen of whom were paying the lowest rate of £25.[50] The levels of board for private patients at this time ranged from £25–£180 per annum.[51] This situation continued throughout this period with the total sum expended by the asylum in subsidising their private patients, from June 1908 to June 1909, amounting to slightly more than half of the monies raised by the institution from the patients' board as a whole.[52] It would therefore be wrong to assume that all patients admitted to the private accommodation at the Dundee Royal were from a similar background, or that a great many of them were treated in a *markedly* different manner from those classified as 'pauper' patients.[53] Indeed, patients could and did move between the two categories of patient, entirely on the basis of financial, rather than class-based, considerations. It could even be argued that there was as great a class distinction in Gowrie House as had ever existed in the mixed class asylum.

From 1905 to 1910 the former occupations of the patients admitted to Gowrie House were overwhelmingly what would be considered middle class, and on occasion working class, in nature, thus exceeding the class-based limitations of the acknowledgement that Gowrie House had been 'designed and built as an establishment for private patients belonging to the middle and upper classes'. Shop assistants, grocers, dressmakers, merchants, servants, housekeepers and teachers, all swelled the ranks of the private patients in Gowrie House. The realities of the patient experience in the Dundee Royal, which included the availability of a heavily subsidised rate of board plus the need for the asylum to fill its beds in order to retain viability, meant that the patient profile in the Dundee Royal as a private institution was overwhelmingly – and for the directors disappointingly – middle class. While some female patients of 'no occupation' were admitted whose background was possibly more genteel in character, the very high ratio of subsidised to non-subsidised patients demonstrates that the majority of the patients resident in Gowrie House did not match what has been accepted as the profile of the private patient.

Such a situation within the asylum goes some way in challenging Andrew Scull's suggestion that 'the division between the pauper and the private lunatic reflected accurately the basic class division of Victorian society'.[54] Many subdivisions of the class system existed within the arbitrary terms of working class, middle class and upper class, and correspondingly there was a similar spread of social status within what was called the pauper and private class of patients. While this situation has, perhaps, always been demonstrable through the various levels of board charged to the patients, the wide discrepancy of social status which existed within the categories of pauper and private patients and the way in which, for the Dundee Royal at least, the private asylum was less an exclusive institution and more a re-creation of the old mixed class asylum on a smaller scale, has been less widely acknowledged.

Arrivals and departures

Social status, as interpreted within the wider community, could and did affect the entry of patients into the asylum. Individuals were regularly admitted to the Dundee Royal from a wide variety of institutions including other asylums, prisons, both the ordinary and lunatic wards of the poorhouses, the Dundee Royal Infirmary, and charitable institutions such as The Home (a small charity for 'fallen women'). Ultimately the Scottish asylum found itself, by the second half of the nineteenth century, as just one player in the system of mixed care that England had experienced from a much earlier date.[55] The comparatively late development of poorhouse provision in Scotland, combined with the relative lack of private madhouse accommodation, had created something of a monopoly of care of the insane by the chartered asylums throughout the first half of the nineteenth century. A recent study by Richard Adair, Bill Forsythe and Jo Melling notes that, for England, 'the Victorian Poor Law, and more particularly the Union workhouse, was an important filtering stage in the assessment of those who might be identified as pauper lunatics'.[56] For Adair *et al.* 'the pauper lunatic was "made" by the Poor Law machinery at local level'.[57] In Scotland, that position was filled by the aforementioned referral network of official organisations, such as the poorhouse - the Dundee Inspector of Poor acting as the petitioner in numerous cases of pauper admissions to the asylum - and the town's charitable organisations.

This network of charities and referral systems could prove of benefit to the less advantaged patients. Such an individual on arriving at the Dundee Royal from another institution or charitable organisation would have had a reasonable chance of bringing a medical history with them, in that they would have been under observation and may have been able to provide some background details on first admission, or those details may have been sought out by the police office or the poorhouse officials. The situation could be quite different with middle- or upper-class patients. In 1904 the asylum medical report complained that, 'a great many of the patients are brought to the asylum unaccompanied by a relative or friend, and even when friends do come they are extremely reticent in giving information'.[58] On the other hand, some of the more 'outrageous' of the impoverished patients entered the asylum with a full report of their colourful history. William M., a married man from Dundee, entered the asylum as a pauper lunatic in October 1890. Admitted under a Sheriff's warrant as a 'dangerous lunatic', a newspaper clipping appended to the patient's case notes further described the activities which had led to his detention by the police, including his 'habit of going about the house cursing and swearing, and brandishing a knife, and also running out to the street in his night shirt'. The final straw had been an alleged assault upon his wife and daughter.[59]

Patients from more salubrious or sheltered backgrounds, whose distress was not so public and indeed often purposefully concealed, were often less fortunate in terms of the recognition of, and acting upon, their mental condition. Although Elizabeth M. had been regarded as insane for two years, she had continued to act as housekeeper in her brother's home – despite that fact that she did not 'engage in any work'- before her eventual admission to the asylum as a private patient.[60] Andrew T., a young man from a middle-class background, presented himself with his parents at the Dundee Asylum in an attempt to gain entrance as a voluntary patient. To do so was only possible with the sanction of the Lunacy Board, which necessarily involved some slight delay, therefore immediate admission was not possible. However, the young man took the matter into his own hands and the next day attempted to take his own life. After being admitted to the Dundee Royal Infirmary with wounds to the throat he was eventually transferred and admitted to the asylum.[61]

Generally, the physical condition of the patients upon admission appears not to have differed greatly across the range of social classes. The condition of those classified as private admissions in 1903-4 were considered to be 'very poor', while 'in the large amount of eighty per cent the disease was looked upon as unfavourable or incurable'.[62] As far as the Dundee Royal was concerned it was 'the termination of the third year' of residence which could 'for all practical purposes be regarded as the period which separates the curable from the incurable forms of mental disease'. Any further treatment could then be expected to ameliorate rather than cure symptoms.[63] There appears to have been little discrimination between the pauper and private patients with regard to long-term care. Both groups of patients were seen as bringing in regular income to the institution. The death of a 91-year-old patient in 1891 marked the end of a period of sixty years continuous residence in the asylum. The annual report for that year described how the patient's 'recollection of the events connected with his admission... remained unclouded to the last hours of his life', without any apparent awareness of the potentially sinister image conjured up by this statement.[64]

While some diagnoses appeared to have become unfashionable by the turn of the nineteenth century, others were coming into favour. 'Religious excitement' was in steady decline as a recognised causative agent over this period, at least at the Dundee Royal, although this state of affairs was perhaps not unconnected with the fact that the asylum was at this time in the process of attempting to raise funds for a chapel building. Intemperance, on the other hand, was a rising star, claimed as second only to heredity as a causative agent of insanity. 'Drink' was described as the 'plague spot in our social life'.[65] Although alcoholism was recognised as a factor in the admission of private patients to the asylum, the identification of the problem of intemperance continued to be associated with, and described in terms of, a working-class problem. Other alleged causes of mental illness, such as sexual intemperance and drug abuse, were also discreetly referred to in consideration of the private patients. Irritation in cases where patients were deemed responsible for their own mental breakdown, whether private or pauper, was not always successfully concealed within the annual reports. In the medical section of the 1909 annual report it was noted that forty-two per cent of admissions to Gowrie House were the result of 'selfish indulgences in excesses of various kinds', and it was considered that 'if these cases had avoided these indulgences and obeyed the ordinary laws of hygiene and health they would not have required the help of a mental Hospital'. The physician does not go as far as to reveal the nature of these activities in the body of the report but an examination of the medical tables indicates that the cases involved alcohol, drugs and the transmission of venereal disease. Nonetheless, the preservation of the image of the private asylum as a place of comfort, seclusion and restfulness could not be compromised by the inclusion of drunken or lecherous madmen – or women. It was easier to use the example of the working classes to discuss such medical matters in the annual report, which was after all in the public domain, and therefore to avoid compromising the position of the 'better' sort of private patient which the asylum desperately wanted to attract.[66]

A central difference in the class-based patient experience in terms of admission and release from the Dundee Royal Asylum appears to have lain in the ability of the wealthier patients to leave the institution, although not recovered, and to be settled elsewhere. Those patients with adequate funds could be removed from the institution and perhaps boarded with friends in the country, while those of impoverished means and thus reliant on the parish could expect to languish in the asylum or be transferred to the lunatic wards of the poorhouse, or to another asylum. Pauper patients were occasionally boarded-out under the auspices of the parish. [67] Harriet Sturdy argues that the 'economical nature' of the system of boarding-out would have given encouragement to the continually financially straitened asylums to remove patients from the institutions to other forms of care wherever possible.[68] This was certainly the case with some of the other Scottish asylums, such as the Edinburgh Royal, but was not a practice favoured at Dundee. This may have been due to the increasing concern to portray the medical nature of the institution, boarding-out taking the form of a palliative rather than curative option. Dr. Rorie had also considered that the majority of the insane were too dangerous to the local community to be boarded-out with any safety; a view obviously not shared by everyone. Nonetheless, the reason why the Dundee Royal Asylum strove to maintain pauper patients within the institution was as much a financial concern as a medical or safety issue, and those who did find themselves, like Margaret H. or S., being boarded-out in places such as Muirhead (a country district adjacent to Dundee) had previously been removed from the asylum by the Parish Council.[69]

Conclusion

The Dundee Royal had always been an institution for the reception of both pauper and private patients and it was with a good deal of reluctance and not some little resistance that the asylum lost its decision-making powers over pauper patients and became a private institution. The decision to convert the asylum into an institution for the sole reception of private patients was a response to changes in the wider Scottish system of asylum care and management, and was taken purely in the hope of maintaining the asylum as a viable institution. However, the separation of the 'classes' made little difference to the private clientele which the asylum attracted. The new private patients admitted between 1904 and 1910 were drawn predominantly from the ranks of the middle, and even the working, classes. The mismatch of traditionally conceived roles of wealthy and poor, and private and pauper, as witnessed at the Dundee Royal, suggests the need for a reappraisal of our ideas on the role played by class in the construction of the asylum patient.

Ultimately the separation of patients by 'class' at the Dundee Royal Lunatic Asylum was as much a practical and financial decision – reflecting the status of the asylum and Dundee itself within the wider context of the Scottish system of institutional care for the mentally ill – as the result of a change in attitude towards the treatment and care of patients based upon their social status. While routes in and out of the asylum remained divided along class lines, and insanity continued generally to be articulated in class-based terms – the most obvious example being the use of working-class 'weaknesses' such as alcoholism to illustrate supposed causative agents of mental illness which in reality affected a broad spectrum of individuals – this did not always make for a system which repressed the poor and favoured the wealthy. What could appear as the over-bearing machinery behind the 'creation' of the pauper lunatic could instead be viewed as the early stages of a social service network, highlighting cases of mental illness and channelling them towards appropriate care systems. For the more affluent amongst the mentally ill, the need for secrecy often obscured the need for help. Thus there was no Foucault-inspired 'great confinement' of the poor and impoverished in the Scottish asylums, but rather inclusion on the terms of a shared mental instability plus the ability – either personal or sponsored – to afford the cost of maintenance within the institution.

The Dundee Royal remained very much in the second-rank of the Scottish lunatic asylums, in the shadow of much grander institutions at Glasgow, Edinburgh and Dumfries, and as a result attracted the business of the solid middle classes or the respectable working classes, while the more affluent sought solace in more salubrious surroundings. Nevertheless, the Dundee Royal continued to aspire to the 'better class' of patient. As far as the asylum directors were concerned, however, that 'better class' of patient was to be measured solely in terms of their monetary value. Class or social status meant little once the patient entered the gates of the institution. The patient was labelled and classified according to the standards set by the asylum and that classification was based purely on the spending power of that individual or of their relatives or friends. It was a system that could see domestic servants classed as 'ladies' and shop assistants as 'gentlemen'. Thus the image of the 'private' and the 'pauper' asylum patient has to be reconsidered for at least this Scottish asylum – and no doubt for others too. The direct translation of rich and poor into private and pauper is an over-simplistic and unrealistic method of approaching the role which class had to play in the Scottish asylum, faced as it was with myriad other concerns, including financial viability, competition for patients and the future development of the asylum system.

Notes

1. I would like to thank Rab Houston, Marjorie Levine-Clark and the anonymous referees, for their comments on an earlier draft of this chapter.
2. Dundee University Archives (DUA), THB 7/4/9, Dundee Royal Lunatic Asylum (DRLA) *Annual Report* (*AR*) (1904), my emphasis.
3. G.M. Burrows, *Commentaries on Insanity* (1828), in V. Skultans (ed), *Madness and Morals. Ideas on Insanity in the Nineteenth Century* (London: Routledge & Kegan Paul, 1975), 38.
4. I. Ray, 'Observations on the Principal Hospitals for the Insane in Great Britain, France and Germany', *American Journal of Insanity*, II (1846), 387–8, in G. Grob, *Mental Institutions in America. Social Policy to 1875* (London: Collier MacMillan, 1973), 227.
5. *Ibid.*
6. J. Goldstein, *Console and Classify. The French Psychiatric Profession in the Nineteenth Century* (Cambridge: Cambridge University Press, 1990), 132–3.
7. L.D. Smith, '"Levelled to the Same Common Standard"? Social Class in the Lunatic Asylum, 1780-1860', in O. Ashton, R. Fyson & S. Roberts (eds), *The Duty of Discontent. Essays for Dorothy Thompson* (London: Mansell, 1995), 142–66: 145, 155. (However, Browne may well have been talking more about asylum-based classification rather than social class).
8. M. Donnelly, *Managing the Mind* (London: Tavistock, 1983), 123. See also, for eighteenth-century constructions of mental illness, R.A. Houston, *Madness and Society in Eighteenth-Century Scotland* (Oxford: Oxford University Press, 2000).

9. A. Scull, *The Most Solitary of Afflictions. Madness and Society in Britain 1700-1900* (London: Yale University Press, 1993), 354–5.

10. J. Andrews, 'Case Notes, Case Histories, and the Patient's Experience of Insanity at Gartnavel Royal Asylum, Glasgow, in the Nineteenth Century', *Social History of Medicine*, 11 (1998), 255–81: 266.

11. G. Best in T. Koditschek, *Class Formation and Urban-Industrial Society (Bradford, 1750-1850)* (Cambridge: Cambridge University Press, 1990), introduction. See also for a coherent discussion of the various approaches, and the inherent difficulties, involved in any discussion of 'class'.

12. See J. Bourke, *Working-Class Cultures in Britain, 1890-1960* (London: Routledge, 1994) for a further discussion of these ideas in relation to the working classes.

13. A.W. Beveridge, 'Madness in Victorian Edinburgh: A Study of Patients Admitted to the Royal Edinburgh Asylum under Thomas Clouston, 1873-1908. Part I', *History of Psychiatry*, 6 (1995), 21–54: 26.

14. A. Presley, *A Sunnyside Chronicle. A History of Sunnyside Royal Hospital* (Dundee: Tayside Health Board, 1981), 19–20.

15. J. Andrews, 'The Patient Population', in J. Andrews & I. Smith (eds), *'Let There be Light Again'. A History of Gartnavel Royal Hospital from its Beginnings to the Present Day* (Glasgow: Gartnavel Royal Hospital, 1993), 106.

16. *Ibid.*, 108.

17. Smith, *op.cit.* (note 7),144, 147.

18. The number of patients resident in the Asylum at the date of the annual report of 1897 was 472 plus one 'absent by escape'.

19. DUA, AccM/370/130, DRLA *AR* (1898), extract from the Report of the Commissioners in Lunacy (1898).

20. DUA, THB 7/4/8, *AR* (1896), extract from the Report of the Commissioners in Lunacy (1895).

21. DUA, AccM/370/130, DRLA *AR* (1899).

22. DUA, AccM/370/130, DRLA *AR* (1900).

23. DUA, AccM/370/130, DRLA *AR* (1897), extract from the Report of the Commissioners in Lunacy (1896).

24. DUA, THB 7/4/6, DRLA *AR* (1892).

25. For example, over the period of the annual report 1899-1900 forty-six of the admissions in that period 'recovered' while forty-one died, DUA, AccM/370/130, DRLA *AR* (1900). Figures for following years are similar.

26. Scull, *op. cit.* (note 9), 293.

27. See L. Walsh, '"The Property of the Whole Community": Charity

and Insanity in Urban Scotland. The Dundee Royal Lunatic Asylum 1820-1850', in J. Melling and B. Forsythe (eds), *Insanity, Institutions and Society 1800-1914. A Social History of Madness in Comparative Perspective* (London: Routledge, 1999), 180–99.

28. Smith, *op. cit.* (note 7), 150–1.

29. Beveridge, *op. cit.* (note 13), note 30.

30. The only distinction appears to have been applied with respect to attaching a photograph of the patient to their case notes. The majority of photographs appear to have been of pauper patients.

31. For an example of a mixed gender case book see for the year 1890 and for gender-specific case books see for the year 1902.

32. For further discussion of these difficulties see S. Edgell, *Class* (London: Routledge, 1997), 33–6.

33. DUA, AccM/370/94, DRLA case book (1890-), 673.

34. DUA, AccM/370/100, DRLA female case book (1902-).

35. The fact that the institutionalised automatically also become 'unemployed' raises further interesting questions in relation to the application of a theoretical construct based upon the identification of class or status in relation to the modes of production.

36. DUA, AccM/370/94, DRLA case book (1890-), 349–351.

37. Excerpt from the Dundee Combination Board Report (1888) in DUA, THB 7/4/3, DRLA *AR* (1889).

38. A. Digby, *Madness, Morality and Medicine. A Study of the York Retreat, 1796-1914* (Cambridge: Cambridge University Press, 1985), 182–3.

39. L.D. Smith has identified a similar regard for social order and respectability in the post-1808 asylums established in England, *op. cit.* (note 7), 152.

40. DUA, AccM/370/100, DRLA female case book (1902-).

41. DUA, AccM/370/94, DRLA case book (1890-) 25–26.

42. *Ibid.*, 189–91.

43. *Ibid.*, 369–71.

44. *Ibid.*, 673–6.

45. DUA, AccM/370/134, DRLA *AR* (1908).

46. Dundee Local Studies Library, Lamb Collection 434 (20), DRLA *AR* (1836).

47. The Dundee Royal does not fit with the more generally accepted argument that menial work was not required of the 'first-class' patients, see Smith, *op. cit.* (note 7), 158. It is only by encouraging greater investigation of asylum practice at the local level that these generalisations can be tested – and no doubt challenged. For a comparison with the early years of asylumdom see R.A. Houston,

'Institutional Care for the Insane and Idiots in Scotland Before 1820: Part 1', *History of Psychiatry*, 12 (2001), 3–32.

48. DUA, AccM/370/130, DRLA *AR* (1897).

49. DUA, THB 7/4/10, DRLA *AR* (1906), my emphasis.

50. Extract from the Report of the Commissioners in Lunacy (1905) quoted in the DRLA *AR* (1906), *op. cit.* (note 49).

51. In order to put these figures into perspective, the Dundee Social Union reported in 1905 that less than ten per cent of the male textile workers in Dundee earned more than £1 per week – a figure not attained by any women working in the jute industry. The wages of flax and jute spinners hovered around seven to ten shillings per week between 1880-1900, R. Rodger, 'Employment, Wages and Poverty in the Scottish Cities', in R.J. Morris and R. Rodger (eds), *The Victorian City. A Reader in British Urban History 1820-1914* (London: Longman, 1993), 73–113: 97. Pauper rates stood at around twelve shillings per week in the late 1890s.

52. The reason why some patients and not others were subsidised by the Asylum are not immediately obvious, and further work is required in this area. While some funds did exist for the maintenance of individuals within the Asylum, such as Grieve's and Riddoch's mortifications, these sources of financial support were established in the early years of the Asylum for pauper patients.

53. This is not to imply, however, that private and pauper patients were treated alike in all respects. It is clear from the level of accommodation and meals provided, for example, that differences did exist. However, those differences were dependent on the level of board paid for the maintenance of the patient, and not the social status of the individual, as has previously been implied by the use of the terms 'private' and 'pauper'.

54. Scull, *op. cit.* (note 9), 354–5.

55. L.D. Smith, 'The County Asylum in the Mixed Economy of Care, 1808-1845', in Melling and Forsythe, *op. cit.* (note 27), 33–47.

56. R. Adair, B. Forsythe and J. Melling, 'A Danger to the Public? Disposing of Pauper Lunatics in late-Victorian and Edwardian England: Plympton St. Mary Union and the Devon County Asylum, 1867-1914', *Medical History*, 42 (1998), 1–25: 3.

57. *Ibid.*

58. DUA, THB 7/4/9 DRLA *AR* (1904).

59. DUA, AccM/370/94, DRLA case book (1890-), 229–32.

60. DUA, AccM/370/100, DRLA female case book (1902-).

61. DUA, AccM/370/94, DRLA case book (1890-), 285–8.

62. DUA, THB 7/4/9 DRLA *AR* (1904).

63. DUA, THB 7/4/7 DRLA *AR* (1890).

64. DUA, THB 7/4/5 DRLA *AR* (1891).

65. DUA, THB 7/4/9 DRLA *AR* (1904). The temperance cause was strong in Dundee. Edwin Scrymgeour, founder of the Prohibition Party of Great Britain, defeated Winston Churchill in Dundee in the 1922 general election.

66. 'Drink' was, however, listed as an exciting cause of insanity for six out of the fourteen private patients admitted in 1905-6.

67. Harriet Sturdy has noted, in her study of the system of boarding-out in Scotland, that the practice was never a major feature of DRLA policy, although by the turn of the nineteenth century Dundee City parish was sending 'considerable numbers' to board in Fifeshire, 'Boarding-out the Insane, 1857-1913: A Study of the Scottish System' (unpublished PhD thesis, Glasgow, 1996), 113: footnote 66. For further discussion of 'boarding-out' from a Scottish perspective see R.A. Houston, '"Not Simple Boarding": Care of the Mentally Incapacitated in Scotland During the Long Eighteenth Century' and H. Sturdy and W. Parry-Jones, 'Boarding-out Insane Patients: The Significance of the Scottish System 1857-1913', in P. Bartlett and D. Wright (eds), *Outside the Walls of the Asylum. The History of Care in the Community 1750-2000* (London: Athlone Press, 1999), 19–44, 86–114.

68. Sturdy, *op. cit.* (note 67), 86.

69. DUA, AccM/370/100, DRLA female case book (1902-).

10

'A Menace to the Good of Society':
Class, Fertility, and the Feeble-Minded
in Edwardian England

Mark Jackson

During debates on the Feeble-Minded Persons (Control) Bill in
1912, Josiah Wedgwood expressed concerns that legislative
provisions to compulsorily detain the feeble-minded would be
used primarily to restrict the liberty of women and the working
classes. Wedgwood's objections to legislation proved futile. In
1913, the Mental Deficiency Act invested local authorities with
the powers to confine mental defectives in certain circumstances.
In spite of contemporary efforts to expose the class and gender
assumptions evident in the legislation, historians have paid
relatively scant attention to the impact of class and gender (or
the interaction between the two) on debates about mental
deficiency. The aim of this chapter is to redress this imbalance by
unravelling the complex interplay of class and gender in framing
Edwardian understandings of feeble-mindedness. Focusing on a
particular set of exchanges that took place in Manchester in
1911, this chapter highlights and analyses crucial incongruities in
the logic of Edwardian reformers and exposes the conflict
between the rhetoric and practice of pioneers of segregation.

Introduction

During parliamentary debates on the Feeble-Minded Persons
(Control) Bill introduced by Gershom Stewart in 1912, Josiah
Wedgwood, Liberal M.P. for Newcastle-under-Lyme and a staunch
supporter of individual liberty, voiced a number of concerns about
proposed measures to compulsorily detain the feeble-minded. First,
although he recognised the value of homes for the feeble-minded, he
insisted that such institutions should be voluntary, and dismissed
compulsory detention as the product of expediency rather than
justice. Secondly, he exposed the Bill's failure to define feeble-

mindedness sufficiently precisely, and warned against the dangers of bestowing increased powers of certification on medical specialists. Thirdly, and perhaps most importantly, he challenged what he regarded as the class and gender bias inherent in the Bill. Convinced that such legislation would be used primarily to restrict the liberty of women and the working classes, Wedgwood claimed that the 'spirit at the back of the Bill is not the spirit of charity, not the spirit of love of mankind. It is the spirit of the horrible Eugenic Society which is setting out to breed up the working classes as though they were cattle'.[1] Although Wedgwood's objections to compulsory detention were supported by Frederick Banbury and others, a government Bill was successfully passed in 1913. The Mental Deficiency Act invested local authorities with the powers to confine mental defectives if they were found without visible means of support, had been convicted of a criminal offence, were detained in an asylum, prison, industrial school or inebriate reformatory, or if, in the case of women, they were in receipt of poor relief when pregnant with, or while giving birth to, an illegitimate child.[2]

In spite of Wedgwood's exuberant efforts to expose the covert class assumptions inherent in Edwardian policies for controlling mental defectives, and in spite of a growing body of historical literature addressing the relationship between class and insanity (largely in the context of the Poor Law),[3] until recently historians have paid relatively scant attention to the impact of class concerns on debates about mental deficiency. The works of Donald Mackenzie, Geoffrey Searle, David Barker, Gillian Sutherland, Greta Jones, and Gareth Stedman Jones have certainly provided extensive insights into the class composition of eugenists, Fabian socialists, and other political and professional groups involved in establishing segregatory policies for the feeble-minded.[4] However, these studies have generally failed to unravel the classist assumptions inherent in contemporary rhetoric or to link that rhetoric clearly to institutional practices adopted in the early-twentieth century. More recently, Mathew Thomson and, to a lesser extent, Tim Stainton have explored the manner in which the elaboration of novel segregatory policies for the feeble-minded interacted not only with 'anxieties about regulating the boundaries of responsible citizenship', but also more broadly with the process of 'adjusting to democracy'.[5] In this context, Thomson is probably right to suggest that since the notion that mental defectives were 'fundamentally different from normal responsible citizens' was 'often held most firmly by members of the "respectable" working class, the segregation of mental defectives cannot be dismissed as a simple "class issue"'.[6] However, this assessment underestimates the extent to which the scientific rhetoric that legitimated segregatory policies in the early-twentieth century was indeed suffused with assumptions about both class differences and feeble-mindedness.

It is also striking that historians have focused far less on class than on gender (and very little on the interaction between the two) in their accounts of the emergence of novel welfare provisions for mental defectives in late-Victorian and Edwardian England. Recently, for example, Pamela Cox has constructively explored the manner in which the relationship between crime and mental status was reconfigured in the context of mentally deficient and delinquent young women, Jan Walmsley has examined the impact of the 1913 Mental Deficiency Act on women, and Lucia Zedner has explored the relationship between feeble-minded women and crime.[7] A recent issue of the *British Journal of Learning Disabilities* focused primarily on the interplay between gender, policy, and practice within the history of learning disabilities, but afforded little attention to class issues.[8] This omission is grave, since, as Simon Szreter, Richard Solloway and others have shown, late-Victorian and Edwardian concerns about gender were closely linked to those about class, most notably in the context of debates about differential class fertility rates.[9] More particularly, as I have suggested elsewhere, it is also probable that in an increasingly class conscious society,[10] contemporary understandings of feeble-minded women were more strongly shaped by middle-class concerns about the uncontrolled sexuality and criminality of the lower classes, than by issues of gender alone.[11]

The aim of this chapter is to begin redressing this imbalance in the history of mental deficiency by unravelling the complex interplay of class and gender concerns in framing Edwardian understandings of feeble-mindedness. In part, I want to highlight and analyse crucial incongruities in the logic of Edwardian reformers that betray contemporary class anxieties. At the same time, I want to indicate points of conflict between the rhetoric and practice of those pioneers of segregation. The bulk of the chapter will focus on a particular debate about the class distribution of feeble-mindedness that took place following a presentation by Dr Alfred Tredgold at a conference on the 'care of the feeble-minded' organised by the Manchester and Salford Sanitary Association in 1911.[12] Of course, a closely focused local study of this nature can make generalisations about Edwardian England difficult. But, for a number of reasons, both Alfred Tredgold and Manchester offer instructive insights into contemporary

273

understandings of, and approaches to, the problem of the feeble-minded.

Dr Alfred Tredgold (1870-1952) was nationally and internationally acclaimed for his work with the feeble-minded. A Licentiate of the Royal College of Physicians and a Member of the Royal College of Surgeons, Tredgold had been the resident physician at the Northumberland County Asylum, a research scholar in insanity and neuropathology for London County Council, and assistant at the Claybury Pathological Laboratory. He had given evidence to the Royal Commission on the Care and Control of the Feeble-Minded, acted as consulting physician to the National Association for Promoting the Welfare of the Feeble-Minded and to the Littleton Home for Defective Children, and was the author of numerous articles on the problems apparently linked to feeble-mindedness.[13] His major work, *Mental Deficiency (Amentia)*, first published in 1908 and dedicated 'to all those persons of sound mind who are interested in the welfare of their less fortunate fellow-creatures', provided contemporaries with a detailed account of the incidence, aetiology, pathology, symptoms, and treatment of mental deficiency.[14] Published in eight editions before his death in 1952, *Mental Deficiency* established Tredgold's reputation as an expert in the field.

Manchester was no less illustrious in the fight to combat the problem of the feeble-minded. The Manchester and Salford Sanitary Association conference was held at the crest of a wave of public and political pressure on the government to enact legislation enforcing the segregation of the feeble-minded. The movement to manage the feeble-minded more effectively had gathered momentum in the closing decades of the previous century. The combined experiences of teachers, workhouse officials, prison medical officers, and asylum superintendents had convinced a number of professional groups that children who were unable to benefit from ordinary elementary education and adults who were unable to provide for themselves constituted a menace to social stability and a threat to the strength of the nation. Such convictions were in part sustained by prominent professional preoccupations with the psychiatric, anthropological, and imperial ramifications of hereditarian theories of degeneration that were sweeping through Europe in the late-nineteenth century.[15] Believing that feeble-mindedness was the root cause of a wide range of social problems (crime, poverty, promiscuity, illegitimacy, alcoholism, epilepsy and insanity), English reformers began to advocate the establishment of discrete institutional provisions for the feeble-minded. Special schools and colonies, they argued, would not only remove a substantial proportion of the criminal and pauper classes both from the streets and from other institutions but would also prevent the feeble-minded from transmitting their hereditary taint to future generations.[16]

In the first decade of the twentieth century, Manchester arguably constituted the political fulcrum of this process of pathologising and segregating the feeble-minded. Driven by the pioneering zeal of its secretary, Mary Dendy (1855-1933), the Lancashire and Cheshire Society for the Permanent Care of the Feeble-Minded (founded in Manchester by Dendy in 1898) had taken advantage of permissive legislation of 1899 and opened the Sandlebridge Boarding Schools and Colony for the feeble-minded in 1902. Supported by funds from local education authorities, the Board of Education, Poor Law Unions, and private donations, the Colony rapidly expanded. Dendy's energetic advocacy of her policy of permanent, life-long segregation on local, national, and international stages swiftly secured Sandlebridge a persistently high profile in the professional, political, and public eye.[17] Fortified by the findings of the Royal Commission on the Care and Control of the Feeble-Minded, Mary Dendy and her compatriots in Manchester acquired a reputation as pace-setters in the race to eradicate the problem of the feeble-minded.[18]

In the light of Manchester's pre-eminence in the field, it is not surprising that the Sanitary Association managed to attract Alfred Tredgold and a host of local dignitaries to its conference, which was also well attended by local physicians, medical officers of health, poor law guardians, teachers, penitentiary workers, and philanthropists. While this mix clearly reflected the broad range of professional groups that were drawn towards eugenic measures to control the feeble-minded, it is important to note that many of the doctors involved in the debate were prominent not only in the generation and legitimation of local initiatives but also in the mobilisation of national resources for controlling a supposedly proliferating population of feeble-minded children and adults. Analysis of Tredgold's paper and the subsequent debate about the class distribution of feeble-mindedness can therefore illuminate more than parochial political interest. It can also shed light on broader national concerns about class, fertility, and the feeble-minded.

Class, fertility and the feeble-minded

Both in his presentation to the Manchester and Salford Sanitary Association in 1911 and in a variety of other publications around that time, Alfred Tredgold insisted that the feeble-minded could be identified by virtue of a particular constellation of mental, physical, and behavioural characteristics. Mentally, the feeble-minded were marked by a lack of 'vital quality' stemming from an 'imperfect development of the cells of the brain'. As a result, while they might be 'capable of earning a living under favourable conditions', the feeble-minded were 'incapable of competing on equal terms with their normal fellows, or of managing themselves and their affairs with ordinary prudence'. This incapacity to function successfully (or, in the case of children, to benefit from ordinary elementary education) inevitably led to their inability to remain in employment and to their dependence on the State.[19] As Tredgold had asserted in his textbook, first published in 1908, such mental weaknesses were often accompanied by the physical stigmata of degeneration, or what Tredgold referred to as 'anomalies of anatomical development and physiological function'. Derived from the same 'inherent defects of the germinal plasm' that Tredgold believed to be the cause of mental weaknesses, anatomical anomalies of the ear, skull, palate, and so on, along with evidence of various physiological dysfuntions, could be used for diagnostic purposes.[20]

In addition to mental and physical peculiarities, the feeble-minded exhibited particular behavioural characteristics. 'For the feeble-minded are not merely defective in intellect', Tredgold insisted in 1911, 'many of them are obstinate, passionate, and devoid of self-control; others are weak-willed and amenable to any suggestion; whilst a considerable proportion have definite criminal tendencies'. It was these attributes, together with their propensity for 'waywardness, fickleness, and bad temper' and their tendency to vagrancy, that defined the feeble-minded as a 'menace to the good of society'.[21] Critically, Tredgold was adamant that this pattern of mental, physical, and behavioural abnormalities constituted a distinct pathological condition, and that the feeble-minded differed qualitatively from the normal population: 'the first point that I desire to insist upon is that feeble-mindedness is not the lowest grade of the normal, but that it is a definite abnormality – that it is, in fact, a disease'. Although he acknowledged that appropriate training in the right environment might enable the feeble-minded to be partially self-supporting, Tredgold maintained that feeble-mindedness, like more severe types of mental deficiency, was incurable. 'In short,' he informed his audience in Manchester, 'the feeble-minded and the normal are separated by an impassable gulf, and the essential feature of this condition is its permanence and incurability'.[22]

Tredgold was also keen to refute the view that feeble-mindedness was 'the immediate product of bad housing, improper feeding, and other errors of the environment'. Arguing that there was no essential difference between idiocy and feeble-mindedness, he asserted that both were caused by 'morbid inheritance' rather than a poor environment:

> The causation of mental defect has now been investigated with very considerable thoroughness, and there is not the slightest doubt that, in the great majority of cases, it is not due to disease or accident incident upon the individual, and not to a faulty environment, but to an inherent incapacity of the brain cells to develop, to something wrong with the seed and not with the soil in which it is grown. My own conclusion is that ninety per cent of all cases are the result of heredity.[23]

The significance of this aetiological understanding of mental deficiency was that, in the eyes of Tredgold and many of his contemporaries, the feeble-minded could transmit the defect inherent in their 'germ plasm' to their offspring, thereby spreading deficiency to succeeding generations. In a passage that captures the desolate tones of much contemporary rhetoric, Tredgold was quick to emphasise the dangers involved in the hereditary transmission of feeble-mindedness and an array of attendant degenerate conditions to a supposedly normal, healthy population:

> The feeble-minded, the insane and the epileptic have been allowed to mate to such an extent with healthy stocks that, although the full fruition of the morbid processes may have been thereby delayed, the vigour and competence of many families has been undermined, and the aggregate capacity of the nation has been seriously reduced. The taint is, in fact, slowly contaminating the whole mass of the population.[24]

Tredgold supported his belief in the hereditary nature of feeble-mindedness in two ways. In the first instance, he cited findings from family studies, in which he had 'noticed that the blood relations of the feeble-minded, whilst not, it may be, actually suffering from mental defect or certifiable insanity, were decidedly abnormal. They were lacking in mental and moral fibre, and the want of this inevitably caused them, throughout the whole of life, to follow the line of least resistance; the consequence being that a very large number were alcoholics, prostitutes, criminals, paupers, or chronic unemployed'.[25] From a classificatory perspective, Tredgold's views on this were evidently inconsistent (a point that, as I shall show later, James Niven fixed on in the ensuing discussion). Tredgold's assertion that the presence of abnormalities not amounting to mental defect in the families of the feeble-minded (or, as he suggested elsewhere, that the birth of 'mentally dull and backward' children to mentally deficient women)[26] proved the inheritance of feeble-mindedness is incompatible with his insistence that feeble-mindedness constituted a disease aetiologically and pathologically distinct from mere backwardness and abnormality.

Tredgold's second argument in support of his contention that feeble-mindedness was inherited related to his understanding of the class distribution of the condition. Refuting beliefs that 'slum life' was a prevalent cause of feeble-mindedness, Tredgold claimed:

> ...that mental defect is just as common amongst the rich and well-to-do as amongst the dwellers of the slums, that idiocy and imbecility are even commoner in the depths of the country than they are in the towns, whilst I am sure that most of you will have noticed that, speaking generally, the street urchin, even in the densely populated and squalid regions of the city of Manchester, is by no means less sharp than his cousin of the country side. I admit that personal ill-health may *retard* mental (and physical) development, but it rarely produces that permanent arrest which is the essence of mental defect.[27]

Tredgold's denial of a relationship between class and feeble-mindedness, a theme that he had first tentatively elaborated in his book of 1908,[28] stands in stark contrast to the explicit classist assumptions that permeated the text of Tredgold's presentation in Manchester. His characterisation of the feeble-minded and their families as alcoholics, prostitutes, criminals, and paupers who were devoid of self-control and, in the case of women, promiscuous and overly fertile, resonated with two specific sets of contemporary concerns about the threat of the lower social classes that peaked around the turn of the century, namely anxieties about the 'social residuum' and about differential class fertility rates.

In the first instance, Tredgold's language is clearly reminiscent of that used to describe the social residuum in the late nineteenth century. As Gareth Stedman Jones has eloquently argued, in the last decades of the nineteenth century the emerging professional middle classes became increasingly anxious about the political threat posed by an expanding body of casual labourers. Although the surveys of Booth and Rowntree helped to allay fears about the political threats posed by lower-class workers, the residuum (including both the semi-criminal and the shiftless casual earners) clearly remained a social problem. The failure of sanitary reforms, slum clearance, or the closer organisation of charity to eradicate the social threat of the casual poor was rationalised as the product of the biological weakness of that 'class' of the population. Social-imperialist links between unemployment, poverty, ill-health, and imperial decline, and the efforts of advocates of the new economic liberalism to draw clearer boundaries between the respectable working class and the residuum, facilitated the emergence of more coercive and interventionist policies aimed at what were often referred to as the dangerous or predatory classes.[29] Thus, Alfred Marshall and Samuel Barnett advocated 'labour colonies' for the casual poor.[30]

The continuity and overlap between Tredgold's construction of the feeble-minded and late-nineteenth-century accounts of the residuum is evident. Tredgold's depiction of the shiftlessness, waywardness, and fickleness of the feeble-minded, of their inability to remain in employment, and of their tendency to drift into crime, poverty, and prostitution (exemplified by case histories in his text of 1908)[31] neatly parallels earlier portrayals of the social residuum. Significantly, Tredgold's conflation of mental defectives with the poor and criminal classes was echoed elsewhere. For some years, Mary Dendy had been attempting to justify permanent custodial care for the feeble-minded by outlining the inevitable (indeed biological) links between feeble-mindedness, pauperism, and crime, links that she made explicit in a paper presented to the Economic Section of a British Association conference in 1901.[32] Crucially, such links between poverty, crime, and mental deficiency came to particular fruition in the creation of the category of the 'moral imbecile'.[33]

Significantly, parallels between the feeble-minded and the social residuum also extended to the elaboration and implementation of particular policies. The farm colonies advocated by Mary Dendy, Alfred Tredgold and many others in the first decade or so of this century reproduced Marshall's and Barnett's earlier schemes for labour colonies directed at solving the problems of housing and unemployment. In both contemporary rhetoric and practice, then, the feeble-minded were identified as a distinct class of people co-extensive with the lower and criminal classes. In some senses, the feeble-minded had merely replaced the social residuum as the focus of middle-class paranoia about the threats that racial degeneration posed to the maintenance of law and order and the survival of Britain's imperial power.

Tredgold's image of the feeble-minded also drew on, and resonated with, contemporary concerns about differential class fertility in a manner which exemplifies the complex interplay between notions of class, gender, and deficiency in this period. As a number of excellent historical studies have made clear, late-nineteenth and early-twentieth-century anxieties about declining national birth rates were dominated by concerns about the greater fertility of the lower classes and the consequent threat to national efficiency.[34] In this way, as Richard Soloway has suggested, 'the population question quickly became inseparable from the question of class'.[35] Significantly, many of the assumptions about lower-class sexual behaviour and fertility were reproduced in discussions of the feeble-minded, particularly in relation to feeble-minded women.

There were several strands to contemporary concerns about the fertility of the feeble-minded. First, feeble-minded women were understood to demonstrate what Tredgold referred to in 1908 as 'pronounced erotic tendencies' and to be 'utterly lacking in any sense of shame, modesty, or even ordinary decency'.[36] Mary Dendy was more forceful. 'Certainly there is one evil with which the feeble-minded cannot be charged', she commented ironically in 1910, 'they are not responsible for the decreasing birth rate. It is as though, when the higher faculties have dwindled, the lower, or merely animal, predominate in an unusual degree'.[37]

Secondly, feeble-minded women supposedly possessed insufficient will-power to resist male sexual advances. According to Tredgold, 'even the best-behaved, and those of good parentage brought up amid every refinement, are often so facile that it is utterly unsafe for them to be at large without protection'.[38] It was in this context that segregation of the sexes within institutions was regarded as serving the dual purpose of keeping pauper, criminal, and prostitute classes off the streets and preventing them from propagating.

Thirdly, the unrestrained sexuality of the feeble-minded resulted in the birth of large numbers of both legitimate and illegitimate children. Many contemporaries estimated that the families of the feeble-minded were substantially larger than those of the normal population.[39] Given the apparently hereditary nature of the condition, the majority of these children were expected to be feeble-minded or degenerate in some way. The imagined social consequences of this process were immense. Not only were the feeble-minded thought to be filling workhouses, gaols, and asylums to overflowing but they also posed a distinct threat to the future of the nation. As Tredgold warned his audience in 1911, in tones reminiscent of alarmist rhetoric about both differential fertility rates and the social residuum:

> ...very few of the children of these feeble-minded mothers are up to the normal standard of mental vigour, most of them are defective and must inevitably lead a parasitic existence at the expense of society. When we remember that thousands of such children are born each year, we begin to get a glimpse of the manner in which feeble-mindedness is permeating the country and swamping the mental and moral vigour of the community.[40]

Finally, Tredgold and his contemporaries highlighted the extent to which modern life (and particularly certain welfare measures) had exacerbated the problem of the feeble-minded by facilitating their survival. In earlier times, the higher mortality rates of the lower classes and the unfit had partially compensated for their greater fertility. However, the increased availability of charitable and state relief for those unable to care for themselves or their families guaranteed their survival. 'We so interfere with his life', wrote Mary Dendy in 1910, 'as to make it possible for the trouble to be handed on, when if we had let him alone he would have died from the natural hardships of his condition. In fact, for generations past we have chosen to play the part of Providence to our weaklings; sometimes a benevolent Providence, but almost invariably a foolish one'.[41] Such sentiments, strongly reminiscent of earlier concerns (voiced particularly by the Charity Organisation Society) that indiscriminate charity discouraged the social residuum from seeking regular work,[42] were used by Dendy to demand a more rational, scientific approach to the problem of the feeble-minded.

Significantly, in addition to alluding indirectly through his language to the equivalence of the feeble-minded and the lower classes, Tredgold made a more direct link between the two in his address in 1911.

> Consider for a moment the birth-rate. As you are well aware, this has been steadily declining since the year 1876, and it is now the lowest on record. If the decline affected equally every class in the community, the general character of the nation would, of course, remain the same, and our only concern would be with the numerical diminution. But the decline is far from general throughout all

classes, it is practically confined to the best elements. It is the steady, persevering, industrious, progressive, and capable members (whatever may be their social status) who are having fewer children; whilst the insane, the feeble-minded, the paupers, the criminals, and the whole parasitic class of the country are continuing to propagate with unabated and unrestricted vigour.[43]

Tredgold's attempt to dissociate capability, productivity, and respectability from social status is as unconvincing as his general claim that there was no differential distribution of feeble-mindedness according to class. Tredgold's language, his imagery, his case histories, the implicit links that he established between the feeble-minded, the social residuum, and the fertility of the lower classes, as well as the nature of his proposed solutions, betray the extent to which the problem of the feeble-minded was a problem of class. Indeed, Tredgold's adoption of class metaphors was central both to his classification of the feeble-minded as a distinctly pathological class in society and to his successful mobilisation of support for segregatory policies in the form of special classes and colonies. Institutional provisions for the feeble-minded would save the State the enormous expense of supporting the parasitic pauper and criminal classes, and prevent the social and political threat of an expanding residuum of semi-vicious, highly fertile, casual labourers. At the same time, such forceful condemnations of the biological and behavioural attributes of the lower classes served to consolidate the position of middle-class professionals as the guardians of national morality and the agents of national regeneration. In constructing an 'impassable gulf' between the normal and the pathological, Tredgold was clearly delineating the boundary between the middle and the lower classes. In this way, the early-twentieth-century fabrication of the feeble mind was not merely a product of class relations. It was intimately bound up with the processes of class formation.[44]

Conflict and consensus on class

In the discussion that followed Tredgold's paper to the Manchester and Salford Sanitary Association conference in 1911, two central questions dominated proceedings: the relative impact of heredity and environment in the aetiology of feeble-mindedness; and the class distribution of the condition. Given Tredgold's assertion that the absence of a class distribution demonstrated the hereditary nature of feeble-mindedness, these two issues were clearly closely linked. Analysis of the debates demonstrates that these questions were also tied up both with the vexing problem of the accurate identification and classification of the feeble-minded and with the construction of class identities.

The discussion was started in a critical tone by Dr Charles Melland (1872-1953), honorary physician to the Northern Hospital for Children in Manchester and author of an extensive survey into feeble-mindedness and epilepsy in the Manchester region.[45] Melland agreed with Tredgold that the inheritance of feeble-mindedness had been 'conclusively demonstrated', and he dismissed the role of environment by suggesting that any child that benefited from changing the environment or from education could not be 'truly feeble-minded but rather mentally backward'.[46] However, Melland was undecided about the benefits to be gained from compulsory segregation, largely because of the impracticalities of segregating whole families of degenerates. His arguments are significant, since they highlight the extent to which eugenic policies for controlling the feeble-minded remained contested in this period.

> There is finally the question of eugenics. That is a very big question. As I said before, if it were only a matter of segregating the comparatively small number of feeble-minded persons and preventing them having any children, and so stamping out the whole process in one or two generations, it would be very simple, but when one comes to consider the collaterals, how many are there of us who have not got some degenerate, a nervously degenerate person, in our own families? I am inclined to think that if one carries the eugenic process to its logical conclusion, there are very few families you could inquire into where there was not some bar to marriage, where there was not some slight reason for thinking that the children might show some defect, and where, if one were to carry it to its logical conclusion, one would forbid the question of marriage. Although one is extremely impressed with the theory underlying the process of eugenics, of course, one sees it applied so much in breeding in agricultural processes, yet one is not quite convinced that it can be applied in the same way to the human species.[47]

Melland's scepticism was also evident in his rejection of Tredgold's opinion that feeble-mindedness was as common in better class areas as it was in the slums. 'My experience', he asserted, 'has led me to the conclusion that feeble-mindedness is somewhat more frequent among the slum dwellers than among the better classes'. This distribution, he argued, did not prove that 'bad surroundings are the cause of feeble-mindedness' but that 'feeble-minded persons, and those who are likely to have feeble-minded children, naturally tend to sink down into the poorer neighbourhoods.[48]

Melland's focus on the question of class was immediately picked up both by Dr Joshua Cox (1857-1927), honorary physician to the Lancashire and Cheshire Society for the Permanent Care of the Feeble-Minded,[49] and by Mary Dendy. Cox agreed with Tredgold that there was 'a large amount of feeble-mindedness among the children of the middle and upper classes' and that the 'poor have no monopoly of the affliction'. However, he noted that middle-class parents were more reluctant to admit their children to Sandlebridge.[50] Mary Dendy also supported Tredgold, insisting that 'it was not in the schools in the slum districts that we found the worst cases. We found more cases in the rather better class schools'. Arguing that the same state of affairs existed in Australia, New Zealand, and Canada, Dendy asserted that any identifiable geographical distribution was not attributable to class but to inbreeding:

> In Essex, which is a county somewhat separated in its traditions and ways from other people, feebleness of mind and idiocy obtain to an enormous extent. In the Isle of Wight it is something appalling. In the remote valleys of Switzerland it is exceedingly bad. Sir Clifford Allbutt says that in the remoter dales of Yorkshire it is exceedingly bad. It is always where there is much inbreeding.[51]

In rejecting any influence of class on the geographical distribution of feeble-mindedness and in emphasising the role of inbreeding, Dendy was reiterating a dominant belief in heredity as the major cause of feeble-mindedness. While Dr James Niven (1851-1925), Medical Officer of Health for Manchester and a member of the Eugenics Education Society,[52] accepted that heredity might be the major aetiological factor, and while he had elsewhere acknowledged the value of Mary Dendy's work at Sandlebridge,[53] he strongly challenged the opinions of Tredgold, Dendy, and the others on the issue of class distribution.

> It seems to me a most extraordinary thing if you do not have more feeble-mindedness among children in the slums. Otherwise what is the disadvantage of feeble-mindedness? If feeble-minded people rise to all sorts of positions, if they can get good houses and estates and so on, if they can occupy good positions in society, it seems to me that feeble-mindedness is no very great disadvantage. Speaking from

my own personal knowledge, I do not know of any feeble-minded children amongst those who are better off.[54]

More particularly, Niven was concerned that the absence of a class distribution was incompatible with heredity as the major causative factor.

> DR. NIVEN: The argument is these people become prostitutes and sink into the lowest ranks of society.
> MISS DENDY: They do.
> DR. NIVEN: The moment the support is withdrawn they must sink downwards. Where is this perpetual fountain of feeble-mindness among the better classes? If you have this inheritance then those people who have made rank and position must have been feeble-minded people. It was, therefore, no disadvantage in making rank and position.[55]

Faced with Niven's criticism of both their logic and their experience, Dendy and Tredgold adopted various strategies. First, Dendy modified her argument to allow some form of class bias in the prevalence of the condition. Demonstrating her determination to defend the middle classes as the guardians of mental and physical vigour, she argued that 'the children of the very rich, the enormously rich, the children of the so-called upper-ten, and the children of the very poor are the worst'.[56] Dendy's retrenchment was immediately supported by Dr Henry Hutton, a physician at the Children's Hospital and a lecturer in children's diseases at the Victoria University in Manchester: 'I should say definitely that the number that occur among the poor is out of proportion to that occurring in the middle classes and the well-to-do; and that among the upper classes, the very highest classes, the proportion does increase again'.[57]

Tredgold was more dismissive of Niven's argument. Admitting that 'it is very difficult to define our classes', he agreed with Mary Dendy that 'feeble-mindedness and degeneracy is certainly just as pronounced in the Upper Ten as it is in the masses'. However, he continued to insist that it was 'not a condition which is monopolised by any social stratum'.[58] More imperiously, he then disputed Niven's understanding of the principles:

> DR. MELLAND: Dr. Niven's point was that their forbears, who must necessarily also have been feeble-minded, have got themselves into that position.
> DR. TREDGOLD: Whoever made that remark evidently utterly

fails to appreciate what heredity is. No one contends that the immediate antecedent of the person who is feeble-minded is also necessarily feeble-minded. It is not so at all.[59]

However, Tredgold's dismissal of Niven's argument was as unconvincing as his attempt to dissociate class from feeble-mindedness. According to Tredgold's own evidence, the close blood relations of the feeble-minded *were* generally either feeble-minded or 'alcoholics, prostitutes, criminals, paupers or chronic unemployed', that is socially abnormal in some way.[60] Significantly, Tredgold and others were quite prepared to use such evidence to support a diagnosis of feeble-mindedness in individual cases and to classify the feeble-minded as inherently pathological and socially problematic.

In Manchester in 1911, Niven's strident voice of dissent was largely isolated. S.T. Lord, a member of the Rochdale Education Committee, did suggest the need for 'a more accurate discrimination between backward children and those who are actually feeble-minded'. And J. Schofield, a poor law guardian, decried what he referred to as 'excessive condemnation of the working classes or the lower classes of society'.[61] Nevertheless both speakers (and the other participants) generally accepted Tredgold's and Dendy's construction of feeble-mindedness as an inherited pathological condition that was no more common in the lower classes than in the higher classes. In doing so, they effectively dismissed the claims of educationalists that the environment constituted a major factor in the aetiology, and indeed treatment, of feeble-mindedness. More particularly, in the present context, they also tacitly condoned prevailing prejudices about both the lower classes and the feeble-minded, and about the links between them.

The consequences of this consensus were immense both locally and nationally. Participants at the conference and members of the Manchester and Salford Sanitary Association drafted a resolution stressing the need for urgent legislation on the lines of the recommendations of the Royal Commission on the Care and Control of the Feeble-Minded. The signed resolution was presented to government by a deputation from the Association later that year.[62] Two years later, after further extensive campaigning on the part of Mary Dendy, Alfred Tredgold, Ellen Pinsent, members of the Eugenics Education Society and the National Association for Promoting the Welfare of the Feeble-Minded, and many others, the eventual passage of the 1913 Mental Deficiency Act and the 1914 Elementary Education (Defective and Epileptic Children) Act compelled local authorities to provide special schools and classes for defective children and to build separate institutional facilities for feeble-minded adults.[63] By emphasising the power of local authorities to institutionalise defectives who had been found guilty of a criminal offence or who were in a prison, reformatory, or criminal lunatic asylum and defective women who were in receipt of poor relief at the time of giving birth to an illegitimate child, the 1913 Act effectively crystallised a set of manifestly classist assumptions about the cause of a wide range of social problems. Significantly, the Lancashire and Cheshire Society for the Permanent Care of the Feeble-Minded, to which many of the speakers at the Manchester conference generously donated their services and financial support, claimed some credit for the Bill's successful passage through Parliament. From the proud perspective of members of the Society, the Mental Deficiency Act was sure to be 'recognised as the greatest measure of social reform that has, as yet, been given to the nation'.[64]

Conclusion

Although more research is needed to elucidate the precise implementation of the Mental Deficiency Act at both local and national levels, there is some evidence to suggest that Josiah Wedgwood's fears that the Act would be used preferentially to incarcerate women and the lower classes were justified. According to Jan Walmsley, in her study of Bedfordshire, the impact of gender on admissions is evident in two ways: first, more women than men were admitted in the years immediately after the Act; and secondly, records from such admissions suggest 'that the sexual behaviour of girls and young women was a major determinant of their fate in a period when facilities designed to deal with people under the 1913 Act were at a premium and when local authorities were specifically instructed to deal only with urgent cases'.[65] However, local examples of this nature need to be treated carefully. At Sandlebridge prior to 1913, and contrary to the dominant trend established in the last decade of the nineteenth century, the admission of boys and men had routinely outnumbered the admission of girls and women, a pattern that reflected Mary Dendy's beliefs that feeble-mindedness was more prevalent in men than women and that criminal men posed as many social problems as promiscuous women.[66] While the passage of the 1913 Act may have shifted the balance towards the admission of women, Mathew Thomson has pointed out that statistics from the Registrar General's Office demonstrate that 'there were more men than women in mental deficiency institutions' in the 1940s and

1950s. However, Thomson also notes that 'female defectives were being kept in institutions longer than men'.[67]

There is also some limited evidence to support Wedgwood's fears about class. Although Mary Dendy had strongly denied any clear class distribution of feeble-mindedness at the Manchester conference in 1911, Sandlebridge itself clearly catered predominantly for feeble-minded children of the poor. Of the first 284 children admitted to Sandlebridge, only five were private admissions; the remainder were paid for by Poor Law Unions and Local Education Committees.[68] This trend appears to have continued at a national level after the 1913 Act. According to Thomson, for example, by the 1940s the 'institutionalization of male defectives was proportionately most likely among families in the lowest social groups, especially in feeble-minded cases'. A similar, although less marked, class distribution was evident in the female admissions.[69]

Of course, this institutional bias against women and the lower classes was not new. Preoccupation with lower-class and female defectives had dominated discussions well before legislation in 1913. Medical journals in the 1890s and 1900s had regularly published letters and editorials bemoaning the lack of institutional provisions for pauper imbeciles and the feeble-minded.[70] And late-nineteenth-century concerns about immorality, illegitimacy, and differential class fertility ensured that the majority of early initiatives in this field, such as the homes established by the Metropolitan Association for Befriending Young Servants in the 1890s, had focused almost exclusively on providing suitable institutions and training for women.

For contemporaries discussing the need for greater regulation of defectives in the early-twentieth century, these biases were in some senses simply the product of harsh social and economic realities. According to Mary Dendy, for example, the traditional tendency to focus on feeble-minded women was merely a product of the fact that 'at every crisis of her career the woman is more likely to come under notice than the man',[71] a point that was also being made by American reformers during this period.[72] In a similar vein, Dr Henry Ashby (1846-1908), honorary physician to the Manchester Hospital for Sick Children and a consulting physician to the Sandlebridge Colony, pointed out in his evidence to the Royal Commission on the Care and Control of the Feeble-Minded that in 'the poorer classes the child of fifteen or sixteen has to earn its living; in the richer class provision can be made for life; they are protected; they no longer come upon the parish, or have temptations that the others have; they are looked after'.[73]

However, it is also clear that the institutional segregation of female and lower-class defectives served distinct ideological purposes in the late-nineteenth and early-twentieth centuries. Permanent segregation not only served as a means of effectively limiting the propagation of degenerates by restricting their sexual behaviour, but also crucially established a convenient physical and ideological distance between the 'fit' and the 'unfit', between the healthy middle classes, on the one hand, and the polluted and contaminated residuum, on the other. In this context, the conflation of the feeble-minded with the supposedly promiscuous, criminal, and degenerate lower classes by Alfred Tredgold, Mary Dendy, and other Edwardian reformers constituted not only a crucial strategy for mobilising support for new institutional policies but also a potent tool in the elaboration and regulation of class boundaries. In a society preoccupied and divided by class relations and immersed in the problems of defining citizenship and 'adjusting to democracy',[74] compulsory segregation of the feeble-minded operated as a conspicuous reminder of the moral superiority, professional expertise, and political authority of the middle classes.

Acknowledgements

I am, as always, indebted to the Wellcome Trust for providing the financial support for the research on which this chapter is based. The ideas presented here were first explored in a seminar at Oxford Brookes University and I am grateful for the constructive comments made by participants on that occasion. I am also particularly grateful to Jonathan Andrews and Anne Digby for their support and comments.

Notes

1. *Parliamentary Debates*, (1913), 38, cols. 1467-77.
2. *Mental Deficiency Act*, 1913, 3 and 4 Geo. 5, c.28. For further discussion of debates and the terms of the Act, see: M. Thomson, *The Problem of Mental Deficiency: Eugenics, Democracy, and Social Policy in Britain, c. 1870-1959* (Oxford: Clarendon Press, 1998); Mark Jackson, *The Borderland of Imbecility: Medicine, Society and the Fabrication of the Feeble Mind in Late Victorian and Edwardian England* (Manchester: Manchester University Press, 2000).
3. See, for example, other chapters in this volume, as well as: P. Bartlett, *The Poor Law of Lunacy: The Administration of Pauper Lunatics in Mid-Nineteenth Century England* (London: Leicester

University Press, 1999); J. Melling and B. Forsythe (eds), *Insanity, Institutions and Society* (London: Routledge, 1999); L.D. Smith, '"Levelled to the Same Common Standard?": Social Class in the Lunatic Asylum, 1780-1860', in O. Ashton, R. Fyson and S. Roberts (eds), *The Duty of Discontent: Essays for Dorothy Thompson* (London: Mansell, 1995), 142–66.

4. See, for example: D. Mackenzie, 'Eugenics in Britain', *Social Studies of Science*, 6 (1976), 499–532; D. Mackenzie, review of G.R. Searle, *Eugenics and Politics in Britain, 1900-1914*, in *British Journal for the History of Science*, xl (1978), 89–91; D. Mackenzie, 'Karl Pearson and the Professional Middle Class', *Annals of Science*, 36 (1979), 125–43; G. R. Searle, *Eugenics and Politics in Britain, 1900-1914* (Leyden: Noordhoff International Publishing, 1976); Searle, 'Eugenics and Class', in C. Webster (ed.), *Biology, Medicine and Society 1840–1940* (Cambridge: Past and Present Publications, 1981), 217–42; Searle, 'Eugenics and Politics in Britain in the 1930s', *Annals of Science*, 36 (1979), 159–69; D. Barker, 'How to Curb the Fertility of the Unfit: The Feeble Minded in Edwardian Britain', *Oxford Review of Education*, 9 (1985), 197–211; D. Barker, 'The Biology of Stupidity: Genetics, Eugenics and Mental Deficiency in the Inter-War Years', *British Journal for the History of Science*, 22 (1989), 347–75; G. Sutherland, *Ability, Merit and Measurement: Mental Testing and English Education 1880-1940*, (Oxford: Clarendon Press, 1984); G. Jones, *Social Hygiene in Twentieth-century Britain*, (Beckenham: Croom Helm, 1986); G. Stedman Jones, *Outcast London: A Study in the Relationship between Classes in Victorian Society*, (Oxford: Clarendon Press, 1971); P.M.H. Mazumdar, 'The Eugenists and the Residuum: The Problem of the Urban Poor', *Bulletin of the History of Medicine*, 54 (1980), 204–15.

5. Thomson, *op. cit.* (note 2), 35, 6; T. Stainton, 'Equal Citizens? The Discourse of Liberty and Rights in the History of Learning Disabilities', in L. Brigham, D. Atkinson, M. Jackson, S. Rolph and J. Walmsley (eds), *Crossing Boundaries: Change and Continuity in the History of Learning Disability* (Kidderminster: BILD Publications, 2000), 87–102.

6. Thomson, *op. cit.* (note 2), 76.

7. P. Cox, 'Girls, Deficiency and Delinquency', in D. Wright and A. Digby (eds), *From Idiocy to Mental Deficiency: Historical Perspectives on People with Learning Disabilities* (London: Routledge, 1996), 184–206; Jan Walmsley, 'Uncovering Community Care: Evidence in a County Record Office', in D. Atkinson, M. Jackson, and J. Walmsley (eds), *Forgotten Lives: Exploring the History of Learning*

Disability (Kidderminster: BILD Publications, 1997), 95–106; J.
Walmsley, 'Women and the Mental Deficiency Act of 1913:
Citizenship, Sexuality and Regulation', *British Journal of Learning
Disabilities*, 28 (2000), 65–70; L. Zedner, *Women, Crime, and
Custody in Victorian England* (Oxford: Clarendon Press, 1991).

8. M. Jackson (ed.), *British Journal of Learning Disabilities*, Special
    Issue, 28 (2000).

9. S. Szreter, *Fertility, Class and Gender in Britain 1860-1940*
    (Cambridge: Cambridge University Press, 1996); R.A. Soloway,
    Birth Control and the Population Question in England, 1877-1930
    (Chapel Hill: University of North Carolina Press, 1982).

10. H. Perkin, *The Rise of Professional Society: England Since 1880*
    (London: Routledge, 1989).

11. Jackson, *op. cit.* (note 2), 148.

12. The proceedings were published as Manchester and Salford Sanitary
    Association, *Proceedings at a Conference on the Care of the Feeble-
    minded* (London: Sherratt and Hughes, 1911).

13. See, for example: A.F. Tredgold, 'The Feeble-Minded – a Social
    Danger', *Eugenics Review*, I (1909-10), 97–104; A.F. Tredgold, 'The
    Feeble-Minded', *Contemporary Review*, xcvii (1910), 717–27.

14. A.F. Tredgold, *Mental Deficiency (Amentia)*, (London: Bailliére,
    Tindall and Cox, 1908).

15. D. Pick, *Faces of Degeneration: A European Disorder, c.1848-c.1918*
    (Cambridge: Cambridge University Press, 1989); I. Dowbiggin,
    'Degeneration and Hereditarianism in French Mental Medicine
    1840-90: Psychiatric Theory as Ideological Adaptation', in W.F.
    Bynum, R. Porter and M. Shepherd (eds), *The Anatomy of Madness:
    Essays in the History of Psychiatry Vol. I.* (London: Tavistock
    Publications, 1985), 188–232.

16. For an overview of these developments, see: Jackson, *op. cit.* (note 2);
    M. Jackson, 'Institutional Provisions for the Feeble-Minded in
    Edwardian England: Sandlebridge and the Scientific Morality of
    Permanent Care', in D. Wright and A. Digby (eds), *From Idiocy to
    Mental Deficiency: Historical Perspectives on People with Learning
    Disabilities* (London: Routledge, 1996), 161–83.

17. On Dendy's life and work, see: Jackson, *op. cit.* (note 2), 53–88; H.
    McLachlan, *Records of a Family 1800-1933*, (Manchester:
    Manchester University Press, 1935), 135–84. Her publications
    included: M. Dendy, *The Importance of Permanence in the Care of the
    Feeble-Minded*, (pamphlet, n.d, originally published in 1899 in the
    Educational Review); M. Dendy, *Feebleness of Mind, Pauperism and
    Crime* (Glasgow: Glasgow Provisional Committee for the Permanent

Care of the Feeble-Minded, 1901); M. Dendy, *Feeble-Minded Children*, (Manchester, 1902); M. Dendy, 'The Feeble-Minded and Crime', *Lancet* (24 May 1902), 1460–3; M. Dendy, *The Problem of the Feeble-Minded* (Manchester, 1910); M. Dendy, 'The Feeble-Minded', *The Medical Magazine*, xx (1911), 686–98; M. Dendy, 'Feeble-Minded Children', *The Journal of State Medicine*, xxii (July 1914), 412–18.

18. Jackson, *op. cit.* (note 2), 53–88.
19. Tredgold, 'The Problem of the Feeble-Minded', in Manchester and Salford Sanitary Association, *op. cit.* (note 12), 7.
20. Tredgold, *op. cit.* (note 14), 78–97, 148.
21. Tredgold, *op. cit.* (note 19), 7. On the relationship between feeble-mindedness, pauperism and vagrancy, see Tredgold, *op. cit.* (note 14), 281–92.
22. Tredgold, *op. cit.* (note 19), 6.
23. *Ibid.*, 16.
24. *Ibid.*, 17.
25. *Ibid.*, 16.
26. Tredgold, *op. cit.* (note 14), 290–1.
27. Tredgold, *op. cit.* (note 19), 15–16
28. Tredgold, *op. cit.* (note 14), 128, 'The labouring classes have no monopoly of morbid heredity, and, although I am unable to give any actual figures, my general impression is that mental defect is just as prevalent amongst the upper as the lower classes of this country'.
29. H. Ellis, *The Task of Social Hygiene* (London: Constable and Co., 1912), 38.
30. Stedman Jones, *op. cit.* (note 4), 303–4.
31. Tredgold, *op. cit.* (note 14), 147–58
32. Dendy, *Feebleness of Mind, Pauperism and Crime, op. cit.* (note 17).
33. Jackson, *op. cit.* (note 2), 140–2. See also Stephen Watson, 'Malingerers, the "Weakminded" Criminal and the "Moral Imbecile": How the English Prison Medical Officer Became an Expert in Mental Deficiency, 1880-1930', in Michael Clark and Catherine Crawford (eds), *Legal Medicine in History* (Cambridge: Cambridge University Press, 1994), 223–41.
34. P. Fryer, *The Birth Controllers* (London: Secker and Warburg, 1965); Soloway, *op. cit.* (note 9); Szreter, *op. cit.* (note 9).
35. Soloway, *op. cit.* (note 9), 48.
36. Tredgold, *op. cit.* (note 14), 290
37. Dendy, *The Problem, op. cit.* (note 10), 7.
38. Tredgold, *op. cit.* (note 14), 290.
39. See, for example, *Report of the Royal Commission on the Care and*

Control of the Feeble-Minded, Vol. 8 (Cd 4202, London, 1908), 198–202.

40. Tredgold, *op. cit.* (note 19), 10.
41. Dendy, *The Problem, op. cit.* (note 10), 21.
42. Stedman Jones, *op. cit.* (note 4).
43. Tredgold, *op. cit.* (note 19), 18–19.
44. For a discussion of a similar process in the North American context, see Nicole Hahn Rafter, *Creating Born Criminals* (Champaign: University of Illinois Press, 1997).
45. W. Brockbank, *Honorary Medical Staff of the M.R.I., 1830-1948* (Manchester: Manchester University Press, 1965), 180–1.
46. Manchester and Salford Sanitary Association, *op. cit.* (note 12), 22. Such circularity in the criteria used to classify the feeble-minded prompted S.T. Lord, a medical member of the Rochdale Education Committee, later in the discussion to demand 'a more accurate discrimination between backward children and those who are actually feeble-minded' – *ibid.*, 35.
47. *Ibid.*, 24.
48. *Ibid.*, 23–4.
49. W.J. Elwood and A. Félicité Tuxford (eds), *Some Manchester Doctors* (Manchester: Manchester University Press, 1984), 195.
50. Manchester and Salford Sanitary Association, *op. cit.* (note 12), 24–5.
51. *Ibid.*, 26-7.
52. 'Obituary', *British Medical Journal*, (10 October 1925), 673-4; 'Obituary', *Lancet*, (10 October 1925), 783. A comprehensive collection of Niven's published papers is in the Manchester Collection, John Rylands Library, University of Manchester.
53. J. Niven, *Poverty and Disease* (London, 1909), 41.
54. Manchester and Salford Sanitary Association, *op. cit.* (note 12), 31.
55. *Ibid.*, 31.
56. *Ibid.*, 31.
57. *Ibid.*, 33.
58. *Ibid.*, 39.
59. *Ibid.*, 39–40.
60. Tredgold, *op. cit.* (note 19), 16.
61. Manchester and Salford Sanitary Association, *op. cit.* (note 12), 35, 38.
62. See Manchester and Salford Association Minute Book, in the Local Studies Library, Central Library, Manchester, M126/1/1/2, 70-89.
63. *Mental Deficiency Act*, 1913, 3 & 4 Geo. 5, c. 28; *Elementary Education (Defective and Epileptic Children) Act*, 1914, 4 and 5 Geo.

5, c. 45.

64. *Annual Report of the Lancashire and Cheshire Society for the Permanent Care of the Feeble-Minded* (1913), 12–13.

65. Walmsley, 'Women', *op. cit.* (note 7).

66. Jackson, *op. cit.* (note 2).

67. Thomson, *op. cit.* (note 2), 247–8.

68. Jackson, *op. cit.* (note 2).

69. Thomson, *op. cit.* (note 2), 248.

70. See, for example: *British Medical Journal*, (23 July 1892), 203; *British Medical Journal*, (10 February 1894), 318; *British Medical Journal*, (17 November 1894), 1127; *British Medical Journal*, (24 November 1894), 1026; *British Medical Journal*, (9 February 1895), 328; *British Medical Journal*, (14 December 1895), 1513–14.

71. Dendy, *The Problem*, *op. cit.* (note 10), 21.

72. W.E. Fernald, *The History of the Treatment of the Feeble-Minded* (Boston: Geo. H. Ellis, 1893).

73. *Royal Commission on the Care and Control of the Feeble-Minded*, Vol. 1 (London, 1908), 586. Significantly, Ashby himself believed feeble-mindedness to be more common in the 'lowest social grade' – *ibid.*, 580.

74. See: Thomson, *op. cit.* (note 2); Perkin, *op. cit.* (note 10).

11

Class and Gender in Twentieth-Century British Psychiatry: Shell-Shock and Psychopathic Disorder

Joan Busfield

This chapter explores the ways in which class and gender permeated psychiatric practice in twentieth-century Britain. It first outlines the historical context and changing character of psychiatric ideas and practice, dividing the century into four main periods – Custodialism under attack, 1890-1929; Integration and Medical Innovation, 1930-1953; Community Care and Public Sector Expansion, 1954-1973; and Privatisation and Commercialisation, 1974 to the Present. The chapter then uses the prism of two psychiatric categories – shell-shock and psychopathic disorder to examine in some detail the ways in which class and gender are embedded in psychiatric work.

Introduction

The aim of this chapter is to explore the ways in which class and gender permeated psychiatric practice in twentieth-century Britain. To facilitate this exploration I use the prism of two psychiatric categories with different trajectories – shell-shock and psychopathic disorder. I have chosen to focus on two disorders more commonly identified in men than women since, precisely because of this, they highlight issues of class and gender in twentieth-century British psychiatry particularly effectively.[1]

I want to begin however by outlining the very marked changes in psychiatric ideas and practice over the twentieth century, pointing to some of the class and gender dimensions of that practice. This provides the historical context for the subsequent examination of shell-shock and psychopathic disorder. The analysis I present draws on a range of documentary sources – legal and policy documents from the relevant periods, epidemiological studies of the class and gender distribution of mental disorder, a range of clinical literature, mostly psychiatric, and some secondary sources. The quality of the data, including the attention to class and gender, varies. The reports of the Lunacy Commissioners through to 1913 are particularly useful since they are relatively comprehensive; the tables routinely distinguish between male and female inmates and some data are provided on inmates by occupation. Subsequent official statistics on mental health services have often not provided a gender breakdown of service users, and almost no data on social class.[2] However, in the post-war period there have been some systematic epidemiological studies of the distribution of mental disorder based either on community surveys or on treated cases. Initially the focus was on class, as in Hollingshead and Redlich's classic US study *Social Class and Mental Illness*.[3] In the late 1960s and early 1970s, with second-wave feminism, attention shifted to gender, and more recently there has been some epidemiological work on ethnicity.[4] However, these studies vary in the spectrum of disorders they cover and are relatively infrequent; it is necessary therefore to make inferences from the data across time and place. Such inferences always need to be treated with caution but can be justified where specific findings have been well replicated.

Narratives of twentieth-century British psychiatry

The trajectory of psychiatric work in Britain over the twentieth century can be portrayed in a number of different ways. First and most obviously, it can be portrayed as a shift from mental health services dominated by the asylum as the locus for the care and treatment of madness to one in which services are more dispersed across the community. The idea of a linear trajectory from the asylum to the community highlights an important change over the century that can be seen across a number of Western countries, including the U.S., though there are notable differences in timing. However, the description not only offers a linear model of change that does not fit the uneven character of developments in service provision, it also ignores other significant changes, most obviously consideration of the character of provision within the community, and the changes that have occurred in the boundaries of mental disorder.[5] A common alternative is to focus on the role of professional groups in the mental health sphere and to portray developments in the twentieth century as a part of the 'medicalisation', 'psychiatrisation' or 'psychologisation' of everyday life.[6] Here the focus is on the expansion of professional power and the spread of professional ideas into new territories, the term psychologisation emphasising that it is not just doctors or psychiatrists who have been involved but a whole range of new 'psy' professions.[7]

Though this second narrative highlights the changing power of professionals, like the first it suggests a simple, linear model of change; it also ignores changes in service arrangements and the content of mental health work. There is a need, therefore, for a more complex characterisation of changes in twentieth-century psychiatry. I have suggested elsewhere that it is useful to divide the history of psychiatry in twentieth-century Britain, which I treat as the long twentieth century covering the years 1890 to the present, into four periods.[8] These are: Custodialism under Attack, 1890-1929; Integration and Medical Innovation, 1930-1953; Community Care and Public Sector Expansion, 1954-1973; and Privatisation and Commercialisation, 1974 to the present.[9] Whilst the periods are largely, though not exclusively, bounded by major legislation, a key focus of my analysis is on the different 'welfare regimes' – to use Esping-Andersen's term – of the relevant period.[10]

(a) Custodialism under Attack, 1890-1929

The beginning of the first period in British twentieth-century psychiatric history is marked by the passage of the 1890 Lunacy Act, which was the culmination of nineteenth-century concerns to protect the individual from the threat of wrongful detention by tightening the formal procedures of certification for those admitted to an asylum. In many respects the Act reflected the philosophies and policies, which Esping-Andersen sees as typifying liberal welfare regimes, that had found expression in nineteenth-century poor-law arrangements, arrangements which continued to operate throughout the period.[11] Concern for the liberty of the subject, clearly embodied in the Lunacy Act, was one of these values. So, too, was the belief that individuals should look after their own needs, and that public welfare should be a last resort available only to those in extreme need without any alternative means of support – the philosophy underpinning the 1834 Poor Law Amendment Act. In the case of those considered mad, as for others in severe need, the formal processes of pauperisation with the attendant stigma, were a prerequisite of public assistance. And to ensure that only the needy received help, those given support were to be no better off than those in work, a principle reinforced by a commitment to provide assistance primarily in institutions. If well-regulated, such institutions could, it was argued, serve as places of reform, and in the case of mental diseases be potentially therapeutic – a belief reinforced by philanthropic ideals that lunatics benefited from retreat from the pressures of the world. However in practice the desire to keep public asylum costs to a minimum led to large-scale, highly regimented, custodial institutions, providing little in the way of active therapy and serving to confine lunatics, some on a relatively long-term basis.[12]

A degree of class stratification occurred within the publicly-funded asylums. Though most inmates were pauper patients (in part because severe mental disorder was more commonly identified at the bottom of the class structure but also because pauperisation was a condition of public assistance), some private patients were admitted and were provided with special facilities – more space and privacy, better food and so forth.[13] More important, however, was the stratification between different types of institution. Alongside the public asylums were the smaller and far less numerous voluntary asylums run on a charitable basis for the 'deserving poor' and those in middling circumstances, as well as the private madhouses for the more affluent. The asylum system was consequently highly stratified in terms of social class, with different provision for different social groups – a class stratification cross-cut by gender. Though the numbers of men and women detained did not differ markedly, asylums and madhouses segregated them spatially and treated them differently. Gender divisions were especially marked in the large-scale public asylums where there were male and female wings and where the more amenable pauper patients (but not private patients) were put to work, and a clear gender division of labour operated. Female inmates engaged in domestic work; male inmates were employed on the farms and gardens of the asylum estates and in heavy work indoors.[14]

However, although the custodial asylums were still dominant in this period, their ascendancy was being challenged on a number of fronts. In the first place, strong criticisms of the asylum system had been voiced throughout the second half of the nineteenth century and these criticisms continued and were strengthened following the 1890 Lunacy Act, which reflected legal rather than medical concerns. Critics, many of whom were doctors working outside the public asylums, argued that asylums should be transformed from custodial institutions into proper hospitals. One strategy, they argued, was to introduce voluntary admission so that treatment could be provided before illness had become intractable.

A second, related challenge came from the competition from services provided outside the asylums. Whilst asylums had provided the foundation of the emergent specialism of psychiatry, other doctors, particularly those specialising in neurology, offered help to those with mental troubles (often less severe) in their consulting rooms and in voluntary and private hospitals. These doctors, whose activities had grown in the second half of the nineteenth century, used a range of therapeutic techniques such as rest cures, hypnosis, hydrotherapy, electrical treatment and various drugs, competing with asylum psychiatrists to treat the more affluent patients.[15] They called for asylums to become proper hospitals and for the development of publicly-funded outpatient services and special units for voluntary patients away from the asylums. This was the context in which the interest in psychoanalytic accounts of psychiatric disorder increased – an interest that shell-shock helped to foster (see below). Psychoanalytic accounts challenged biological, particularly hereditarian, explanations of mental disorder that had become increasingly prominent in the final decades of the nineteenth century, and had helped to sustain the asylum system and the belief in the need for long-term, custodial care. Psychoanalysis, in contrast, offered a more optimistic model of mental disorder and an alternative model of treatment that did not necessarily require inpatient care, so strengthening the demand for more outpatient services and helping to undermine the asylum system.

Third, the liberal welfare regime in which public provision was a matter of last resort was increasingly challenged, most notably by the introduction of more expansionary schemes of state welfare founded on principles of insurance in which employment, not extreme poverty, was the basis of entitlement. Legislation between 1906 and 1914 introduced compulsory state health and unemployment insurance for certain categories of workers, as well as pension provision. Such schemes constituted the first stages of a corporatist welfare state.[16] Whilst state insurance was introduced in Britain alongside the existing poor-law provision and did not entirely supplant it, the minimalist poor-law philosophy was increasingly undermined. In 1929 the Local Government Act that marks the end of this period, abandoned poor-law terminology altogether, though not all poor-law principles and practices.

(b) Integration and Medical Innovation, 1930-1953

The Report of the 1924–6 Royal Commission on Lunacy and Mental Disorder affirmed the central importance of viewing mental disorder as a form of illness to be treated as far as possible like other illnesses, and advocated a largely medical approach. In an oft-quoted passage the Report asserted:

It has become increasingly evident to us that there is no clear line of demarcation between mental illness and physical illness. The distinction as commonly drawn is based on a difference in symptoms. In ordinary parlance a disease is described as mental if its symptoms manifest themselves predominantly in derangement of conduct, and as physical if its symptoms manifest themselves predominantly in derangement of bodily function. The classification is manifestly imperfect. A mental illness may have physical concomitants; probably it always has, though they may be difficult of detection. A physical illness on the other hand may have, and probably always has, mental concomitants. And there are many cases in which it is a question whether the physical or mental symptoms predominate.[17]

The implications were clear: mental illness should be assimilated to physical illness; detention should give place to treatment and there should be a greater role for the medical profession.

The 1930 Mental Treatment Act, which marks the beginning of this second period, gave legal expression to the Commission's main recommendations. It replaced the language of asylums with that of mental hospitals, pauper patients with 'rate-aided' patients, and lunacy with 'persons of unsound mind'. It also gave powers to local authorities to fund outpatient clinics and permitted voluntary admission, accepting the Commission's view that certification was a major barrier to the early treatment considered fundamental to successful preventive medicine. Because of its expansionary implications, the Act represented a major move away from the last resort philosophy that had governed the nineteenth-century public asylums.

A more active therapeutic regime followed these legislative changes, particularly in the second half of the decade.[18] From the mid-1930s a range of sleep and shock treatments were introduced in mental hospitals to treat those with acute mental health problems, including insulin coma therapy, Cardiazol-induced convulsions and electro-convulsive therapy (ECT), with ECT soon becoming dominant as it was cheaper, simpler and safer than the chemically-induced coma or convulsion therapies. New efforts were also made to rehabilitate long-stay inmates with the development of habit training programmes and of open-door policies in some institutions, efforts that were strengthened by rehabilitative programmes for soldiers developed in the Second World War. In addition, the new psychiatric outpatient clinics, usually attached to general rather than mental hospitals, offered various forms of psychotherapy, as did the growing number of child guidance clinics, as well as private psychoanalysts and psychotherapists in their consulting rooms.[19]

In some respects class and gender stratification continued unchanged during this period. However, voluntary admission was accepted much more quickly for private than for pauper patients (in 1936, sixty per cent of private admissions to public asylums were voluntary, compared with only thirty-two per cent of rate-aided admissions).[20] In contrast in this period gender differences in the use of voluntary admission were small. However, women were more likely than men to be treated by some of the new physical treatments, such as ECT.[21]

(c) Community Care and Public Sector Expansion, 1954-1973

I have identified the third period in British twentieth-century psychiatric history as starting in 1954, a year in which the number of residents in psychiatric hospitals reached its peak before beginning to decline. It was also the year in which a new Royal Commission on the Law Relating to Mental Illness and Mental Deficiency in England and Wales started work – the Commission that recommended a policy of community care in its 1957 Report. And finally, it was the year in which new chemically-synthesised psychotropic drugs began to be used in psychiatric hospitals. All three events were crucial to the introduction of community care – a policy in which services outside the asylum were first envisaged as supplementing, and then as replacing the old asylums. Viewed as a supplement to mental hospital care, the policy does not look very new since the Mental Treatment Act had introduced the possibility of publicly-funded outpatient clinics, and private psychiatric work based on the consulting room was already expanding. The novelty for England and Wales (but not Scotland) came in the initial focus on community care for those with long-term mental health problems – care which was to be provided by the public sector in the form of training provision, residential homes and professional support.[22] These patients, who would typically have already spent a period in a mental hospital, were now to be relocated where possible into the community. Consequently community care was initially quite narrowly defined as a form of public sector after care or continuing care for long-stay patients, though the term came to embrace the full range of services, both public and private, provided outside the mental hospital for a wide range of patients – with acute problems, chronic problems, and less severe mental disorders.

The introduction of the new chemically-synthesised drugs was crucial in three respects. First, the drugs helped to legitimise the policy of community care by making professionals and the lay public believe that the 'florid' symptoms of mental disorder could be kept under control even when patients were in the community.[23] Second, the new drugs, like the physical treatments such as ECT before them, helped to legitimate a bio-medical approach to mental illness, although in this period understandings of mental disorder and approaches to treatment were diverse and eclectic.[24] Third, the drugs, particularly the minor tranquillisers and anti-depressants, introduced from the early 1960s onwards, expanded the range of individuals seeking medical help for mental health problems, usually from general practitioners rather than specialists.

The expansion of medical work in relation to the more common mental disorders was undoubtedly facilitated in Britain by the establishment of the National Health Service, which greatly improved access to medical services for the whole population, and by the decision to include mental health services in the NHS. The NHS, which began operating in 1948, represented the clearest move in Britain towards a social democratic welfare regime characterised by universal provision of services above minimum standards.[25] Its establishment led to important changes in the clients receiving help for mental health problems. Before this the treatment of less severe disorders mainly took place in the private sector and was largely restricted to the more affluent, who by the 1940s received various forms of psychotherapy or the somewhat limited range of drugs available. The NHS did not provide easy access to psychotherapy because GPs lacked the necessary training and treatment was time-consuming and relatively expensive. But the new tranquillisers were cheaper and could be prescribed by GPs, and soon became readily available to all social groups.

The expansion in those seeking help for less severe psychological problems had important implications in relation both to class and gender. First, it arguably somewhat reduced, though it did not eradicate, class divisions in relation to individuals receiving treatment for these disorders, which like the more severe mental disorders, tended to be more common in the working than the middle or upper classes.[26] However, though access to GP services was improved, there continued to be differences in the type of treatment received, with a bias towards physical treatments for working-class patients and some form of psychotherapy for those of higher status.[27] In contrast, however, there is evidence that improved access and the wider use of psychotropic medication for the less severe disorders increased gender divisions in relation to mental health problems. Women were identified as having disorders such as anxiety and depression far more than men, and so were more frequently prescribed the new psychotropic drugs by their GPs.[28] There were also changes in the degree of gender segregation in mental hospitals and psychiatric units in this period, with mixed wards and shared activities becoming the new orthodoxy – changes not strongly contested until the 1990s.[29]

A further key feature of the period was the increasing proliferation of mental health practitioners. A few social workers were employed in British mental hospitals prior to the second world war and following the war their numbers increased rapidly. Clinical psychologists were first employed in Britain in the 1950s and then, as with social workers, their numbers quickly expanded.[30] From the 1960s, the work of psychiatric nurses began to diversify with new 'outreach' nurses working in the community (to become community psychiatric nurses), and some psychotherapists were employed in the public sector. Whilst psychiatric nurses, whether working in hospitals or in the community, tended to accept psychiatric models of disorder notwithstanding their own professionalising endeavours, clinical psychologists were more successful in developing their own distinctive approaches – first behaviour therapy and then cognitive behaviour therapy.[31] This expansion of the 'psy' professions brought more women into the mental health care labour force as well as increasing proportions from ethnic minority groups.[32]

(d) Privatisation and Commercialisation, 1974 to the Present

The fourth period in the twentieth-century history of psychiatry in Britain is characterised by the growing use of the private sector in mental health services and growing commercialisation. These changes to some extent represent a retreat from the universalising models of a social democratic welfare regime and a return to liberal models more characteristic of the nineteenth century. The period was initiated by a fiscal crisis following the major rise in oil prices in the early 1970s, which led to increasing government concern about public expenditure.[33] The proportion of GDP taken up by public expenditure had been steadily increasing over the post-war years, but with the particular combination of economic stagnation and rapid inflation – stagflation – brought about by the economic conditions of the first half of the 1970s, there was a new concern about the levels it had reached.[34] Consequently the Labour Government sought to curtail expenditure, policy documents of the period referring to the ways in which the lack of finances would slow down the implementation of community care.[35] The restriction of resources to the NHS, which continued throughout the 1980s and 1990s, had a profound effect on the levels of service that could be provided in the face of demographic changes and medical innovations, and helped to encourage the growth of private provision. In addition, the new right ideology of the 1979 Conservative Government, with its explicit hostility to the public sector and support for private provision – the hallmark of a liberal welfare regime – led to models of health care, including community care, in which the private sector was to have a greater role.

Precisely what was meant by the private sector in the context of community care varied. In some contexts, it clearly meant the support provided by family and friends (and charitable groups) – care invaluable where available, but all too often inadequate in the case of difficult, awkward and dependent individuals. In other contexts it meant the greater involvement of private companies in the provision of services for the mentally ill. Government support for the private sector was both direct and indirect. On the one hand, explicit policy initiatives were designed to support the expansion of private health care, including mental health care, and to introduce a more entrepreneurial culture into the NHS. On the other hand, and just as importantly, the general sympathy to the market from governments encouraged those working in the private sector to be more dynamic and innovative.

One example of explicit support was the significant changes to consultants' NHS contracts by the government in 1980. These made it easier for NHS consultants to work in the private sector.[36] There were also some tax concessions on private medical insurance. The 1981 Budget marginally raised the threshold for tax relief on private insurance to earnings of less than £8,500 – a modest but nonetheless symbolic gesture.[37] Then in 1989, the government introduced tax relief on private medical insurance for the over-60s, an important change since a high proportion of those with private medical insurance in Britain are covered by company schemes, which usually do not continue on retirement.[38] Government commitment to the market and to private sector values and practices was also directly applied to the NHS. Business style managers (later termed chief executives) were introduced following the 1983 Griffiths Report, there was a new emphasis on efficiency and value for money, including requirements for the competitive tendering of cleaning and catering services, and then in 1991 an internal market was created.

The dual conditions of a lack of investment in the NHS and an emphasis on the market also provided indirect support to private-sector bodies, encouraging them to become more commercially minded.[39] In 1978, BUPA (the British United Providential Association), a major figure in the private insurance market and a non-profit making organisation, which already ran private nursing homes on a providential basis, set up BUPA Hospitals as a for-profit organisation. With the advent of the Conservative Government in 1979 these activities expanded, for instance, with new publicity campaigns for private medical insurance and hospitals.[40] Less noted was the clear government support for the pharmaceutical industry and the psychotropic drugs they increasingly provided – support in which the medical profession had a strong interest as its near monopoly over prescribing is an important source of medical power.

The rapid increase in the use of psychotropic (and other) drugs in the second half of the century clearly has some disadvantages for government because of the high cost of the drugs bill to the NHS. At various times governments have sought, usually rather ineffectually, to reduce the cost, for instance by requiring the substitution of generic for branded drugs.[41] In addition, because of the scandals associated with some drugs (thalidomide is the most obvious example) governments have imposed licensing requirements on the sale of new drugs. And more recently the Labour Government has sought to assess, through the new National Institute for Clinical Excellence (NICE), the effectiveness and value for money of new medical treatments, including new drugs, as the basis for regulating their use in the NHS. Yet at the same time governments have a very direct interest in sustaining and supporting the pharmaceutical industry and in not circumscribing its activities to any great extent. This is because the industry is a very significant part of the British economy, contributing to the country's GDP and directly employing a large number of people. Consequently there are major tensions between the regulatory role of government and its desire to have a flourishing pharmaceutical industry, tensions that the industry tries to exploit by emphasising its value to the economy and by protesting against what it sees as unnecessary restrictions.[42] However, notwithstanding efforts at regulation, over the period since 1974 the importance of the industry to medical work has increased enormously. This is especially true for psychiatry where medication has become the standard form of treatment for an expanding range of psychiatric problems.

The growth of the private sector during the era of Conservative governments, which has largely continued since Labour came to power in 1997, has had important implications in relation both to class and gender. First, public provision for those with acute and long-term mental health problems has been cut back, and specialist public services have increasingly focused on those with severe mental health problems, particularly those considered dangerous – a group where those from the lower social classes, men and ethnic minorities tend to be over-represented. These changes are reflected in an absolute and proportionate increase in compulsory admission, which had reached low levels in the 1970s and 1980s.[43] And with this increase came a shift in the gender distribution in the use of compulsion, with proportionately more men than women now admitted under a legal section.[44] Second, the increasing reliance on psychotropic drugs to treat the more common mental disorders has had particular implications for women, since they are still more likely than men to be identified as having disorders such as anxiety and depression and therefore to end up using some form of psychotropic medication.

The case of shell-shock

Shell-shock, the psychological disorder identified amongst troops in France in the First World War, provides an interesting case study of the class and gender dimensions of psychiatric practice. The term was first coined in 1915 by Charles Myers, a medically qualified psychologist, appointed to the Royal Army Medical Corps to arrange the dispatch of soldiers suffering from mental and nervous disorders from France to England. He used the term to describe three cases of nervous disorder in soldiers who had been at the frontline.[45] Their symptoms involved partial paralysis, loss of memory and disturbances of vision, speech, taste and smell – symptoms rather similar to those of hysteria. Initially he believed the symptoms were associated with being under the direct line of fire, the term shell-shock reflecting this presumed aetiology. The term rapidly embedded itself in lay consciousness continuing in common use long after most doctors, including Myers, had argued that the causation was psychological, involving the build up of exhaustion and fear over a period of time, and did not result from the physical effects of exploding shells.[46] Doctors preferred to talk of war neuroses but the concept never had the same popular appeal.

Class was crucial to the new category of shell-shock in two major ways. First, there was a tendency to differentiate two class-related types of war neurosis. On the one hand, there was the hysterical form Myers first described in which bodily symptoms of paralysis, loss of sight, deafness, etc were dominant, which was held to be more common amongst privates and non-commissioned officers.[47] Hysteria was a disorder that had been especially linked with women and its association with men in this context was arguably particularly stigmatising. On the other hand, there was a form more psychological in its symptoms, closer to anxiety states and neurasthenia, held to be more common amongst commissioned officers. Neurasthenia, a very poorly defined category of disorder first delineated in the US in the second half of the nineteenth century, had initially been associated with upper-class men and was viewed as a disease of civilisation.[48] It was therefore a more appropriate psychological disorder for officers.[49]

The second way in which class featured in discussions of shell-shock was in the debates surrounding its aetiology and treatment. The character and causes, as well as the treatment, of shell-shock were highly contested amongst clinicians and between clinicians and military men. As far as many members of the military establishment were concerned, shell-shock posed a major threat to the maintenance of fighting strength, since the military could ill-afford the loss of significant numbers from the front, particularly for any length of time. What the military leaders (and this included the French and German as well as the British) wanted above all was for such men to be returned promptly to the frontline. Not surprisingly, many argued that men who claimed to be suffering shell-shock lacked courage and were suffering from 'funk' or were malingering, and those who deserted were liable to be court-martialled, and some were peremptorily shot. Others argued that the soldiers who broke down were mad and should be certified and placed in asylums. In either case the blame was often placed on hereditary predispositions, some military men arguing that 'the soldiers who become affected by shock were weaklings or were descended from mentally afflicted or nervous parents', thereby reflecting a psychiatric Darwinism – the prevailing orthodoxy.[50]

Yet it was difficult for the military establishment to sustain such views in face of the fact that officers as well as privates broke down. Indeed, allowing for the far higher numbers of privates than officers, the data suggested that *rates* of breakdown were actually higher amongst officers.[51] To claim that these officers were all weaklings was highly problematic given their class origins. Indeed, the doctors who had experience of dealing with shell-shocked soldiers increasingly argued that anyone could break down given the severity of the conditions: 'It would be a gross misrepresentation of the facts to label all the soldiers who suffer from mental troubles as weaklings' since even 'the strongest man when exposed to sufficiently intense and frequent stimuli may become subject to mental derangement'.[52] Whilst 'neuropathic tendencies' would increase the likelihood of a breakdown, they were not a prerequisite.[53]

As this discussion also brings out, gender was as important as class in the contests surrounding the framing of shell-shock. Shell-shock was a problem not just because it posed an immediate threat to military strength, but also because it posed a threat to the notions of manliness so central to military endeavour. The acceptance of shell-shock as a mental disorder in a context where manliness was at a premium is of considerable interest. It required an acceptance that fighting men, one of the key embodiments of masculinity, could suffer from nervous disorder. Yet nervous disorder, to a far greater extent than madness or lunacy, was a gendered concept. In the nineteenth century nerves or nervous disorders had come to be particularly associated with women, since they were considered more emotional and less rational than men.[54] In this context the idea that shell-shock was a form of nervous disorder constituted a strong challenge to gendered expectations. Its acceptance can be only explained because the alternatives were even more problematic. I have already argued that the class characteristics of many of the men who broke down militated against the widespread acceptance that breakdown was simply a matter of cowardice in men who lacked moral strength. Military discharge or even summary death, whilst they would help to affirm values of courage and discipline, were also unthinkable in the face of the large numbers who broke down.[55] Equally the class composition of sufferers posed a problem for the idea that all who broke down suffered from lunacy and should be sent to asylums – an approach that was also problematic because it would mean the loss of too many soldiers from the frontline. Moreover the denial of agency, usually more problematic in relation to male behaviour, had the advantage in this case that the issue of possible resistance to fighting was not brought centre stage. A war neurosis, difficult though it was for military men to accept, was a marginally preferable alternative, particularly if it could be associated with a rapid return of soldiers to the front. Here disposal and treatment were crucial. A policy of treating soldiers close to the frontline where possible, and of providing assertive treatment and then sending them back very quickly to the front, helped military men to accept the reality of psychological breakdown, even though it posed dangers of giving legitimacy to the exemption of the faint-hearted from frontline duties.

Although the term shell-shock was quickly rejected by psychiatrists, to be replaced by war neurosis, and then in the 1970s following the Vietnam war, by the concept of post-traumatic shock disorder, it played an important role in psychiatric history by encouraging greater familiarity with psychodynamic ideas and helping to bring them to wider popular attention. This had important consequences for psychiatry. On the one hand, these ideas formally marked out a broader terrain of mental disorder than lunacy had done, and led to a particular focus on the psycho-neuroses and to services for those with neurotic complaints. They therefore enhanced the shift towards services outside the asylum already visible in the second half of the nineteenth century. On the other hand, they provided accounts of mental disorder which, unlike late-nineteenth century ideas concerning neurasthenia and hysteria, concentrated on the psychological realm and, following Freud, frequently, though less so in the case of shell-shock, focused on familial relationships in early childhood. The impact of these changes were not however the same for men and for women.

For men who broke down during the war and afterwards, the acceptance of shell-shock was significant: it provided a response which had the advantage to them and their families that it eschewed the harshness and cruelty of the court-martial (summary or otherwise), did not involve the stigma of cowardliness or malingering, and did not call their underlying sanity into question, or challenge their family heredity.[56] It also brought more men, particularly working-class men, into contact with the mental health services. Moreover, it provided a legitimate, even heroic explanation of their disorder. Their illness was the result of doing their duty in war. Yet at the same time shell-shock still called their masculinity into question, whether the diagnosis was neurasthenia or hysteria. Both disorders, but especially hysteria, were associated in people's minds with some failure or weakness of will – a perception that may help to account for the reluctance of many who suffered from shell-shock to talk about their problems. In the words of Oppenheim 'The Great War may have demonstrated beyond doubt that psychological agents can, by themselves, utterly disrupt the body's functions, but the lesson did nothing to mitigate the certainty that nervous breakdown unmanned men'.[57] Men were still strongly deterred by prevailing conceptions of masculinity from seeing themselves as mentally disturbed and were required to find other ways of expressing their feelings. Similarly the doctors whom they encountered were more likely to look for alternative conceptions of their problems (many people in primary care contexts still present a physical problem as their primary complaint, mentioning a mental problem only secondarily).[58] Arguably, however, whilst mental breakdown continued to be defined as unmanly, the acceptance of shell-shock did help to bring about some changes in conceptions of masculinity. It was one indicator of the sacrifice that men had had to make in the war, a sacrifice more commonly involving the loss of life and limb, that to some extent challenged certain components of Victorian notions of masculinity, including the idealisation of war and of military values.

For women, the consequences were rather different, though they relate to the same two areas: the expansion of mental health services and the spread of psychodynamic ideas. In the first place, shell-shock by encouraging the development of specialist units in general hospitals for the treatment of nervous disorders, and of publicly-funded outpatient clinics, as well as the spread of psychodynamic ideas, helped to ensure that more and more women ended up as patients with some nervous complaint. This was because of the way in which femininity, particularly middle and upper-class femininity, still emphasised the vulnerability, lack of self-control and emotional expressiveness of women, even though some of the harsher features of nineteenth-century assumptions about women's biological inferiority had been modified.[59] Under the influence of Freud such women increasingly received diagnoses of anxiety neurosis, phobias or obsessions, and the term neurasthenia gradually fell into disuse as did that of hysteria.

The aetiological accounts of mental disorder that Freud and others provided were also of particular relevance to women. In many respects they were an improvement on the pessimistic, anti-therapeutic focus on heredity that had characterised thinking about mental disorder. Freud's emphasis on the inner world was of profound significance and provided a way of thinking about underlying psychological dynamics that had considerable value, especially in understanding the psycho-neuroses. At the same time it played on women's greater tendency to focus on the inner world rather than external pressures in seeking to account for their mental disorder, a difference evidenced in the contrasting narratives men and women offer for their use of psychotropic medication.[60] In particular the Freudian focus on fantasy, especially in relation to sexual abuse, helped to ensure that the reality of women's social situations was too often ignored.[61] It was not until the 1970s and 1980s that feminism began to bring the reality of sexual and physical violence against women to public attention, including the sexual abuse of patients by doctors and therapists. And, notwithstanding some false claims of abuse, it would be hard to overestimate the importance of sexual abuse in understanding mental disorder amongst women. It is ironic however, that the greater awareness of this abuse still largely produces only a palliative response in terms of the prescription of drugs, and that the sexual abuse of women by men is all too rarely viewed as reflecting any psychological pathology in men.

Psychopathic disorder

Psychopathic disorder is arguably more a legal than a psychiatric category. I use the term here because of its ongoing legal significance in British psychiatry. Official psychiatric classifications instead use the term anti-social conduct disorder or dissocial personality disorder. The International Classification of Diseases describes the latter as 'usually coming to attention because of a gross disparity between behaviour and prevailing social norms' and as characterised by:

(a)   callous unconcern for the feelings of others;

(b)   gross and persistent attitude of irresponsibility and disregard for social norms, rules and obligations;

(c)   incapacity to maintain enduring relationships, though having no difficulty in establishing them;

(d)   very low tolerance to frustration and a low threshold for discharge of aggression, including violence;

(e)   incapacity to experience guilt and to profit from experience, particularly punishment;

(f)   marked proneness to blame others, or to offer plausible rationalisations, for the behaviour that brought the patient into conflict with society.[62]

As this description indicates, the disorder is constructed around behaviour and personality rather than thought, emotions and feelings, the usual referents of the term mental disorder. The starting point of this disorder is unacceptable conduct and the links with criminal behaviour are strong. In particular the labels tend to be especially applied to those who enter the mental health services via the courts. Such disorders consequently stand on the boundary between wrongdoing and mental sickness and there are major, ongoing debates over whether they should be regarded as 'mental' disorders and whether they can be distinguished from antisocial behaviour more generally.[63] Should the conduct in question be viewed as acts of an individual who is attributed agency and responsibility (and so might lead to punishment) or as the product of mental sickness where agency should, at least in this respect, be denied.

Like shell-shock, psychopathic or dissocial personality disorder is more commonly identified in men than women, and like shell-shock its acceptance into the framework of mental disorders has been highly contested, contests that similarly focus around issues of agency and the denial of responsibility. However it differs markedly from shell-shock in that it is not deemed a neurosis – a disorder involving emotional and psychological conflict. In that respect it does not fracture gender expectations to the same extent. Psychopathic disorder also differs from shell-shock in its class linkages. Unlike shell-shock there is no claim of class-related *types* of psychopathic disorder. Rather the disorder is specifically linked to those of the lower class – a relation that arises because of the focus on antisocial conduct and the link with criminality and the criminal justice system.[64] Those in the working class are far more likely than middle-class individuals to be apprehended for some criminal offence, though the reasons for this association are hotly contested.[65] Related to this is the fact that the working-class individuals are more likely to enter mental health services via the courts.[66]

Present day concepts of antisocial conduct disorder and dissocial personality disorder have their precursors in the nineteenth-century concepts of moral insanity and moral defect. Moral diseases of the mind were first described in Germany by Grohmann in 1818. In Britain, J.C. Prichard introduced the term moral insanity in 1833, describing it in his 1835 *Treatise on Insanity* as characterised by:

> morbid perversion of the natural feelings, affections, inclinations, temper, habits, moral dispositions and natural impulses, without any remarkable disorder or defect of the intellect or knowing or reasoning faculties and particularly without any insane illusion or hallucination.[67]

We can see here a mixed and apparently rather ad hoc list of emotions and behaviours. Two features differentiated moral insanity from other forms of insanity. First, as the extract makes clear, the condition did not necessarily involve any disorder of the intellectual faculties or reason – usually regarded as the defining feature of insanity. Second, and related to this, underpinning the emotions and behaviours was some perversion of the 'moral and active principles of the mind' so that 'the power of self-government is lost or greatly impaired'.[68] The disorder was one of will, agency or responsibility rather than of reasoning. In practice the category of moral insanity was primarily used 'to describe criminal activity and vicious, immoral, or anti-social behaviour' and its class connotations were strong.[69] As Michael Donnelly puts it: the category was 'effectively constructed as a generalisation (and exaggeration) of attributes which polite society recognised widely among sections of the labouring classes'.[70] The concept also in practice had gender connotations and was more likely to be applied to men than women. Men were more likely to be engage in criminal activities and to be judged unable to distinguish right from wrong. When applied to women it was for rather different behaviours. Women who had illegitimate children or were seen as sexually profligate (a judgement more often made of women than men) were liable to be identified as morally insane.

By the end of the nineteenth century the terms moral defective and moral imbecile had largely replaced moral insanity in Britain, and the term psychopath had also begun to be used.[71] The 1904-8 Royal Commission listed moral imbeciles as one of nine classes of mental 'defect' (used here as a generic term referring to all types of mental disorder) defining them as 'persons who from an early age display some mental defect coupled with strong vicious or criminal propensities'.[72] The focus in this description on vicious or criminal propensities indicates a formal shift in emphasis from the concept of moral insanity. There the focus had been on immorality rather more generally defined. Here it was on particular forms of immorality – the vicious and the criminal – arguably a narrowing of the concept that had arisen from the de facto use of the earlier term, a narrowing that in practice made the links with class and gender even stronger.

The focus in the description of moral imbeciles on early onset, and the use of the term propensities indicates that, like other mental disorders, the condition was generally viewed as a product of heredity, frequently visible from childhood, with the term imbeciles suggesting there was no clear separation from 'feeble-mindedness'. It was also considered difficult to treat, though appropriate training in childhood might have some impact. Such views persisted during the first half of the century, although psychoanalytic theorists began to suggest that early-childhood experiences could be crucial to the aetiology of what was now usually called psychopathic disorder.[73]

There were also some efforts, following rehabilitative work with soldiers in the Second World War, to use therapeutic communities for the treatment of individuals with psychopathic personalities.[74]

The term psychopathic disorder was given new significance in British psychiatry in the 1959 Mental Health Act where it was distinguished from other types of mental disorder and given special status in relation to compulsory powers of admission for treatment (as opposed to admission for observation or in an emergency). These treatment powers could only be used for psychopathic patients who were under twenty-one. Psychopathic disorder was defined in the Act as 'a persistent disorder or disability of mind (whether or not including subnormality of intelligence) which results in abnormally aggressive or seriously irresponsible conduct on the part of the patient, and requires or is susceptible to medical treatment'.[75] This definition was qualified by an explicit statement applicable to all types of mental disorder listed in section four of the Act that 'Nothing in this section shall be construed as implying that a person may be dealt with under this Act as suffering from mental disorder, or from any form of mental disorder described in this section, by reason only of promiscuity or other immoral conduct'.[76] Promiscuity or immorality alone could not be the grounds for the use of compulsory powers. This was a significant qualification that reflected the move from the old concept of moral insanity and affirmed the links with men and criminality.

The case for restricting the use of compulsory powers for admission for treatment of patients with psychopathic disorder was based on three intertwining ideas: that where possible individuals with the disorder should be dealt with in mental hospitals rather than the criminal justice system; that psychopathic disorder was difficult to treat (it did not appear to be amenable to the physical treatments introduced in the later-1930s and 1940s); and that there were few mental health facilities available for its treatment (therapeutic communities were small in scale and limited in number). The Royal Commission that preceded the Act set out the case for the special legal status: 'The circumstances in which the use of compulsion is justifiable [within the psychiatric system] are however more limited in relation to psychopathic patients than in relation to mentally ill or severely subnormal patients'.[77] This was because, although compulsion might be necessary for the protection of the public, the Commission considered that: 'it is quite essential that no patient should be compelled to enter hospital unless the hospital can provide care, training or treatment suited to his needs' which was not usually the case with psychopathic disorder.[78] The implication was that if treatment facilities were not available (and few were) and an offence had been committed, the individual should continue to be dealt with through the criminal justice system

Despite ongoing problems with the concept, clearly set out in the 1975 Butler *Report of the Committee on Mentally Abnormal Offenders*, the 1983 Mental Health Act retained the concept and specifically focused on treatability.[79] Compulsory admission for treatment depended on a judgement 'that such treatment is likely to alleviate or prevent a deterioration of his condition' thereby reaffirming the legal situation in relation to compulsory powers within the mental health system. [80] However the Act added sexual deviancy and dependence on alcohol or drugs to promiscuity and immoral conduct as conditions that could not in themselves be the basis of compulsory powers.[81] It also indicated that the disorder had to be of a nature of degree that made hospital treatment appropriate.

During the 1990s there were increasing concerns about the risks posed by psychiatric patients in the community, partly as a result of the very significant reductions in the numbers of psychiatric beds in the 1990s. These concerns were undoubtedly heightened by incidents such as the murder of Jonathan Zito in 1992. As a result some argued that the special legal status of psychopathic disorder was an anomaly, contending that it prevented the compulsory detention in a psychiatric bed of some of those most liable to be dangerous who could have entered the psychiatric system from the criminal justice system. It should be possible to detain such patients, even if they could not be treated. However, the Government's proposed solution of legislative change to permit longer-term detention in psychiatric facilities of those with psychopathic disorder, even if there is no prospect of benefit from treatment, raises three major problems. First, there is a lack of suitable facilities for the management of this group of patients. The 1975 Butler Report had called for the provision of regional secure units but few have been established. Second, there is the human rights issue of using compulsion on the basis of *predictions* of dangerousness rather than actual offences (an issue that applies to the compulsory detention of schizophrenic patients deemed dangerous as much as to those judged psychopathic and is compounded by the fact that it is difficult to predict dangerous behaviour).[82] Finally, there is the problem of focusing limited mental health resources on one group of patients at the expense of others, for instance, those who could benefit from early treatment. In addition there are the long-standing issues of where to set the boundaries between responsibility and sickness and whether such individuals should be managed in the criminal justice or psychiatric system. Nonetheless, even without legislative change, as psychiatric beds have declined in number, they have increasingly been used for those considered dangerous, including those with psychopathic disorder, a group in which men and those from the lower classes are over-represented.

We can see, therefore that psychopathic disorder has played a very different role from shell-shock in relation to class and gender. Whereas both were initially distinctively male mental disorders, shell-shock, unlike the plebeian psychophathic disorder, was at least as much if not more a disorder of the middle and upper classes as of the lower classes, albeit with its own neurasthenic form for those belonging to the higher classes. Moreover, shell-shock in emerging as a disorder focused on the emotions, and one which called masculinity into question, helped to lay the foundations for the neuroses where women were to feature so strongly. In contrast the focus of psychopathic disorder on conduct and behaviour did not call masculinity into question and the disorder, even in its newer psychiatric formulations, has in practice retained its marked affinities with men.

Conclusion

What this examination of the histories of the use of the categories of shell-shock and psychopathic disorder shows is the myriad ways in which class and gender permeate psychiatric ideas and practice. Categories of mental disorder constitute the changing intellectual framework psychiatrists construct in order to try to make sense of, and deal with, the range of problems that are brought to their attention. When formally delineated these categories follow scientific canons and largely eschew reference to class and gender, or to age and ethnicity. Nonetheless the categories are developed in specific social contexts to deal with specific problems and are applied to individuals who have clear social locations – in the case of shell-shock a military context and in the case of psychopathic disorder a context of dealing with difficult, recalcitrant individuals who have often engaged in criminal behaviour. Psychiatric practice cannot thus avoid reflecting, incorporating, reproducing and sustaining class and gender divisions. Psychiatrists and other mental health professionals need therefore to be very aware of the social contexts in which they operate and the social role they play, making this part of their professional consciousness. Only in this way can they begin to challenge and to change some of the social discrimination their practice reflects.

Notes

1. Feminist scholarship, which did so much to put issues of gender on the map, has tended to concentrate on female mental disorders such as anorexia nervosa, depression and pre-menstrual tension.

2. Data from the subsequent Board of Control, disbanded in 1959, are not so detailed.

3. A.B. Hollingshead and F.C. Redlich, *Social Class and Mental Illness* (New York: John Wiley, 1958).

4. On gender see, for instance, W. Gove, 'The Relationship Between Sex Roles, Marital Status and Mental Illness', *Social Forces*, 51 (1972), 34–44; and P. Chesler, *Women and Madness* (New York: Doubleday, 1972). On ethnicity see, J. Nazroo, *Ethnicity and Mental Health* (London: Policy Studies Institute, 1997).

5. For example, the contrast between the 1960s US model of Community Mental Health Centres providing a range of services for diverse groups of patients under the same roof, and the more differentiated, more traditional British model in the same period of acute psychiatric units in general hospitals, outpatient clinics, and GP care.

6. See, for example, I. Illich, *The Limits to Medicine,* (Harmondsworth: Penguin, 1977); R. Castel, *The Regulation of Madness* (Oxford: Blackwell, 1988).

7. See, Castel, *ibid.*

8. E. Hobsbawm, *The Age of Extremes* (London: Michael Joseph, 1994) starts the century in 1914 and sees it as the short twentieth century.

9. J. Busfield, 'Restructuring Mental Health Services in Twentieth Century Britain', in M. Gijswit-Hofstra and R. Porter (eds), *Cultures of Psychiatry* (Amsterdam: Rodopi, 1998), 9–28. I have made some minor modifications to the periodisation outlined there.

10. G. Esping-Andersen, *The Three Worlds of Welfare Capitalism* (Cambridge: Polity, 1990).

11. *Ibid.,* 26–7.

12. J. Busfield, *Managing Madness* (London: Hutchinson, 1986), Chapter 9.

13. The link between class and mental disorder has been established in a range of twentieth-century epidemiological studies. See, for instance, Hollingshead and Redlich, *op. cit.* (note 3); H. Meltzer. B. Gill, M. Pettigrew and K. Hinds *The Prevalence of Psychiatric Morbidity among Adults Living in the Community* (London: HMSO, 1995).

14. See, for instance, R. Hunter and I. MacAlpine, *Psychiatry for the Poor* (London: Dawsons, 1974).

15. Virginia Woolf provides an interesting example. She was treated by a range of doctors mostly at home and was prescribed rest cures, the avoidance of exhaustion, fresh air and a variety of sedatives (see H. Lee, *Virginia Woolf* (London: Chatto & Windus, 1996), 183.

16. Esping-Andersen, *op. cit.* (note 10), 27.

17. Royal Commission on Lunacy and Mental Disorder, *Report* (London: HMSO, 1926), 15.

18. The one significant therapeutic development prior to this was the introduction of arsenical preparations for the treatment of general paralysis of the insane (GPI).

19. The development of child guidance clinics is documented in N. Rose, *The Psychological Complex: Psychology, Politics and Society in England, 1869-1939* (London: Routledge and Keegan Paul, 1985).

20. Board of Control, *Annual Report, 1936* (London: HMSO, 1937).

21. Data for this period is somewhat limited. The records of Severalls Hospital, Colchester show that more women than men received ECT. From 1948-56, when there was a ratio of roughly three female to two male resident patients, the numbers of women receiving ECT was initially double that of men and treble by the end of the period, see D. Gittins, *Madness in its Place: Narratives of Severalls Hospital, 1913-1997* (London: Routledge, 1998), 199. A recent national survey of the use of ECT showed twice as many women receiving ECT as men (Department of Health, *Statistical Bulletin* 22a, 1999).

22. There had been earlier discussions of boarding-out or fostering long-stay patients and in Scotland this policy had been introduced in the nineteenth century, see H. Sturdy and W. Parry-Jones, 'Boarding-out Insane Patients: The Significance of the Scottish System 1857-1913', in P. Bartlett and D. Wright (eds), *Outside the Walls of the Asylum* (London: Athlone, 1999), 86–114.

23. Whilst many have argued that drugs did not cure mental illness, their role in easing the introduction of the policy of community care is more widely accepted.

24. The eclecticism of British psychiatry was emphasised by Anthony Clare in his popular text *Psychiatry in Dissent* (London: Tavistock, 1976).

25. Esping-Andersen, *op. cit.* (note 10), 27.

26. G. Brown and T. Harris, *Social Origins of Depression* (London: Tavistock, 1978); Meltzer *et al., op .cit.* (note 13).

27. Hollingshead and Redlich's study (*op. cit.* note 3) showed marked class differences in types of treatment and the more limited studies

carried out in the UK suggest a similar picture.

28. Studies indicate that women are prescribed tranquillisers twice as frequently as men (see E. Ettoré and E. Riska, *Gendered Moods* (London: Routledge, 1995), 6.

29. It was paralleled by developments in co-education and can be seen as a way of trying to achieve gender equality. Feminists have argued that such practices have particularly disadvantaged women.

30. In 1964 there were 0.08 clinical psychologists per 100 psychiatric beds; by 1976 there were 0.67 per 100 psychiatric beds (Department of Health and Social Services, *Facilities and Services in Mental Illness and Mental Handicap Hospitals in England, 1974*, and *1976* (London: HMSO 1976; 1980)

31. A survey of community psychiatric nurses shows most adopting bio-medical accounts of mental disorder, see P.M. Godin, 'Doing the Frontline Work: A Sociological History of Community Psychiatric Nursing in Britain', unpublished PhD. thesis (University of Essex, 2002).

32. In the late 1980s seven out of ten recruits into clinical psychology were women, D. Pilgrim and A. Treacher, *Clinical Psychology Observed* (London: Routledge, 1992), 186.

33. J. O'Connor, *The Fiscal Crisis of the State* (London: St Martin's Press, 1973).

34. I. Gough, *The Political Economy of the Welfare State* (London: Macmillan, 1979).

35. For instance, Department of Health and Social Security, *Better Services for the Mentally Ill* (London: HMSO, 1975).

36. J. Higgins, *The Business of Medicine* (London: Macmillan, 1988), 86–8, suggests this change made a major difference to consultants' ability to engage in private work without losing the security and status of NHS contracts.

37. Higgins, *ibid.*, 88.

38. The change was recommended in the 1989 Government review of the NHS. However, as the cost of private medical insurance increases markedly with age this is a disincentive; it is also usually only available to those already insured.

39. Higgins *op. cit.* (note 36), 72–83, argues that the Labour Government's decision to phase out pay beds from NHS hospitals generated this entrepreneurialism, but groups such as BUPA had already become more active.

40. *Ibid.*, 93.

41. In 1984 the Government introduced a limited list restricting GPs' right to prescribe drugs regardless of cost or efficacy, see R. Klein,

The New Politics of the NHS (London Longman, 1995), 164–5.

42. For example, when the National Institute for Clinical Excellence (NICE) made a preliminary decision that Relenza, a treatment for influenza, would not be available for NHS patients on the grounds that it was only of limited value and called for further studies, there were hints from the Chairman of Glaxo Wellcome, the company that produced Relenza, that they would consider moving their factories out of Britain.

43. When NICE reviewed this decision following the further studies it decided that the drug could be prescribed on the NHS but only in limited circumstances.

44. It became increasingly difficult to secure admission for other than sectioned patients.

45. Department of Health, *In-Patients Formally Detained in Hospitals Under the Mental Health Act 1983 and Other Legislation, England 1989-90 to 1999-2000* (Bulletin 2000/19).

46. C.S. Myers 'A Contribution to the Study of Shell-Shock', *Lancet* (Feb 13, 1915), 316–20.

47. Research showed that shell-shock could not result from the physical effects of exploding shells since those physically wounded by shells did not experience the same symptoms. See H. Wiltshire, 'A contribution to the aetiology of shell-shock', *Lancet* (1916) i, 1207-12.

48. J. MacCurdy, *War Neuroses* (Cambridge: Cambridge University Press, 1918), 87.

49. G.M. Beard, *American Nervousness: Its Causes and Consequences* (New York, Arno Press, 1972 [1881]).

50. Hysterical and neurasthenic types of shell-shock involve a contrast between the bodily expression of emotional conflict often held to be more common amongst the working class and its psychological expression more commonly identified amongst the more educated.

51. G.E. Smith and T.H. Pear, *Shell-Shock and Its Lessons*, 2nd edn (Manchester: University of Manchester, 1917), 88–9.

52. See B. Shephard, *A War of Nerves: Soldiers and Psychiatrists, 1914-1994* (London: Jonathan Cape, 2000).

53. Smith and Pear, *op. cit.* (note 51), 89.

54. The term neuropathic referred to disorders with neurological origins.

55. J. Oppenheim, *'Shattered Nerves': Doctors, Patients and Depression in Victorian England* (New York: Oxford University Press, 1991).

56. Estimates vary but around 80,000 British soldiers suffered from shell-shock (see M. Stone, 'Shellshock and the Psychologists', in W.F Bynum and R. Porter, *The Anatomy of Madness* (London: Tavistock,

1995), ii, 242–71.

57. The figures for those suffering from shell-shock after the war were quite high.

58. Oppenheim, *op. cit.* (note 54), 152.

59. See e.g. R.A. Schurman, P.D. Kramer and J.B. Mitchell, 'The Hidden Mental Health Network: Treatment of Mental Illness by Nonpsychiatric Physicians', *Archives of General Psychiatry*, 42 (1985), 89–94.

60. Arguably the construction of femininity became less extreme but, for instance, a belief in the impact of reproductive processes on women's mental states did not entirely disappear, see J. Busfield, *Men, Women and Madness* (London: Macmillan, 1996), ch. 8.

61. Ettorré and Riska, *op. cit.* (note 28), ch. 6.

62. J. Masson, *Freud: The Assault on Truth* (London Faber & Faber, 1984).

63. *The ICD-10 Classification of Mental and Behavioural Disorders* (Geneva: WHO, 1974).

64. B. Wootton, *Social Science and Social Pathology* (London: Allen & Unwin, 1979), ch. 8.

65. The US Epidemiologic Catchment Area study found rates of antisocial personality for men were four times as high as those for women (see D. Regier *et al.*, 'One-month Prevalence of Mental Disorders in the United States', *Archives of General Psychiatry*, 45 (1988), 977–86).

66. For a critical discussion of the overrepresentation of working-class individuals in official statistics of crime, see S. Box, *Deviance, Reality and Society* (London: Holt, Rinehart & Winston, 1971), ch. 3.

67. This was first demonstrated very clearly by Hollingshead and Redlich, *op. cit.* (note 3).

68. J.C. Prichard, *A Treatise on Insanity* (London: Sherwood, Gilbert and Piper, 1835).

69. *Ibid.* This indicates the standard justification usually invoked for viewing behavioural problems as a mental disorder, for whilst the symptoms were behavioural, underlying these behaviours was a judgement of mind.

70. M. Donnelly, *Managing the Mind* (London: Tavistock, 1983), 137–8.

71. *Ibid.*, 133.

72. The term psychopath was used in different ways. In some contexts (as in the term psychopathic hospital) it meant all disorders considered psychological rather than neurological in origin. In others it meant a specific disorder relating to antisocial conduct.

73. Royal Commission on the Law Relating to Mental Illness and Mental Deficiency, *Report* (HMSO 1957).

74. John Bowlby's earliest study, 'Forty-four Juvenile Thieves, their Character and Home Life', *International Journal of Psychoanalysis*, 25, 19 (1944), 19–52, 107–27, was of the affectionless child and the links to subsequent criminality.

75. The Henderson Hospital was the best known of these therapeutic communities.

76. Mental Health Act, 1959, para 4 (4).

77. *Ibid.* para 4(5).

78. Royal Commission on the Law Relating to Mental Illness and Mental Deficiency *op. cit.* (note 72), para 353 (ii).

79. *Ibid.*, para 352. Ramon sees the compulsory powers vis à vis psychopathic patients as particularly coercive because there is no reference to the degree of the disorder. She argues that it was a relatively small group of psychiatrists particularly involved with therapeutic communities who made the case for the inclusion of the disorder in the Act and viewed this as progressive: see S. Ramon, 'The Category of Psychopathy: Its Professional and Social Context in Britain', in P. Miller and N. Rose (eds), *The Power of Psychiatry* (Cambridge: Polity, 1986).

80. Home Office, *Report of the Committee on Mentally Abnormal Offenders* (London: HMSO, 1975).

81. Mental Health Act 1983, para 3(2).

82. Mental Health Act 1983, para 1(3).

83. A. Buchanan, 'Risk and Dangerousness', *Psychological Medicine*, 29 (1999), 465–73.

Index of People and Places

Index of Subjects

A

able-bodied 128
admissions
    Brookwood asylum 227–30,
        232, 233, 235
    Buckinghamshire Asylum 157,
        161
    compulsory 306, 314–15
    and gender 24
    governesses 193-4
    Holloway 232, 233, 235
    Ireland 70–6
    legislation 27, 71, 169, 287–8
    readmissions 228-9, 231
    voluntary 28, 231, 301
    West Riding 125–6
    workhouse 227, 233
aetiology 50, 282, 286, 307–8,
    313
age
    factors 49, 57–8
    profiles 187–8, 194, 196, 201,
        230
alcohol 5–-2, 76, 236, 262, 264
Alleged Lunatic Friends' Society
    190
anorexia nervosa 239
anti-depressants 302
anti-psychiatry movement 45
anti-social conduct disorder 311
anxiety disorders 303, 306
aristocrats 204, 205
Association of Medical Officers of
    Hospitals and Asylums for the
    Insane 154
Asylums Act 1808 154
Asylums Act 1845 154, 253

B

behaviour
    conformity 23, 149–50, 257
    control 149–50
    criminal 273, 311–12
    norms and expectations 11–15,
        113–14
    violent 77–9, 136, 162
bereavement 49–50
bio-medical approach 302
birth rates, feeble-minded 280–2
British Psychiatry, 20th century
    295–322
BUPA (British United Providential
    Association) 305
business failure 137
Butler report *see Report of the
    Committee on Mentally
    Abnormal Offenders*

C

cannabis 241, 242
capacity to work 48–9, 54–8
capitalism 95–6, 104
care
    at home 98, 100–1, 202–3,
        207
    community 28, 296, 301–3,
        304
    private sector 304
case notes as empirical evidence
    125–6
casual poor 278–9
causes
    employment-related 129–31,
        132–3
    feeble-mindedness 277
    of insanity 24

E

F

G